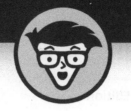

Living Vegan

2nd Edition

by Cadry Nelson

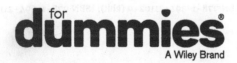

A Wiley Brand

Living Vegan For Dummies®, 2nd Edition

Published by: **John Wiley & Sons, Inc.**, 111 River Street, Hoboken, NJ 07030-5774, www.wiley.com

Copyright © 2024 by John Wiley & Sons, Inc., Hoboken, New Jersey

Published simultaneously in Canada

For general information on our other products and services, please contact our Customer Care Department within the U.S. at 877-762-2974, outside the U.S. at 317-572-3993, or fax 317-572-4002. For technical support, please visit https://hub.wiley.com/community/support/dummies.

Wiley publishes in a variety of print and electronic formats and by print-on-demand. Some material included with standard print versions of this book may not be included in e-books or in print-on-demand. If this book refers to media such as a CD or DVD that is not included in the version you purchased, you may download this material at http://booksupport.wiley.com. For more information about Wiley products, visit www.wiley.com.

Library of Congress Control Number: 2023948611

ISBN 978-1-394-21101-2 (pbk); ISBN 978-1-394-21102-9 (ebk); ISBN 978-1-394-21103-6 (ebk)

SKY10059418_110723

Contents at a Glance

Recipes at a Glance

Desserts

Table of Contents

Introduction

On the surface, going vegan is pretty straightforward. It means not eating meat, dairy, and eggs, or using any animal products. But in practice, it's much more than that. Being vegan is an opportunity. Every time you sit down to dinner, you get to make a decision.

>> Do you want to create a life that's healthy, and full of energy and vitality?

>> Do you want to tread lightly on our planet?

>> Do you want to be mindful of all those who live on it?

If you answered *yes* to these questions, then living vegan is a chance to make choices that are in alignment with your values. It's a way to put your compassion and beliefs into action.

Admittedly, the idea of going vegan can feel a little daunting to most folks. Changing what you eat at every meal, avoiding goods made with animal products, and creating new habits can be intimidating. *Living Vegan For Dummies* is here to help.

About This Book

This book is a comprehensive guide to vegan living at your fingertips. It covers everything you need to successfully navigate the move to a vegan lifestyle. It starts with the basics of what it means to be vegan, and why people choose this way of life. It guides you through how to get started, and what to prepare and eat when everything is new and unfamiliar. It covers the many health benefits associated with veganism, plus which foods you want to reach for to meet all your nutritional needs.

I include pantry guides and grocery lists, as well as tips for reading labels and menu planning. There's advice for dining out at local restaurants and while you're on the road. Many people who consider going vegan worry about saying goodbye to their favorite meat- and dairy-based favorites. So I share how you can eat colorful, varied, and delicious vegan foods that leave you totally satisfied. Are you concerned about the reaction from your friends, family, and coworkers? There's a whole chapter dedicated to navigating any awkward social situations.

Plus, this book includes 38 mouthwatering recipes for breakfasts, entrees, side dishes, and desserts to get you started in your new vegan life. You even find some recipes that kids can help prepare!

This book is for:

- Anyone considering the switch to a plant-based diet
- People who want to live more compassionately, improve their health, and be more environmentally conscious
- New vegans who want to maneuver unfamiliar pitfalls
- Longtime vegans who want to make sure they're ticking all the nutrition boxes
- Non-vegans who want to understand what veganism is all about

Living Vegan For Dummies is divided into seven parts, each covering a different aspect of the vegan way of life.

- Part 1: Getting Started with a Vegan Lifestyle
- Part 2: For the Health of It
- Part 3: Vegan at Home
- Part 4: Tasting Is Believing: Vegan Recipes
- Part 5: Vegan in the Outside World
- Part 6: Veganism in All Walks of Life
- Part 7: The Part of Tens

Finally, as you're reading, be aware that websites listed in this book appear in monofont. If you're reading the book in print, just type the address into your web browser exactly as it's written. If you're reading the digital version and you're connected to the internet, you've got it easy. Simply click the highlighted link to be taken directly to the website.

Foolish Assumptions

In writing this book, I made a few assumptions about you, the reader.

- You're interested in going vegan, and you want to eat delicious and satisfying meals.

>> You're a compassionate person who wants to align your actions with your beliefs.

>> You have a general grasp of how to cook day-to-day meals, but you'd like to expand your repertoire to include plant-based dishes.

>> You're curious about how to thrive on a vegan diet.

>> You're cool with making lifestyle changes, and want tips on dining out with friends and family, traveling, and celebrating holidays.

>> You aren't afraid to take a risk or do something different if it means living a life that's in line with your values.

Icons Used in This Book

As you go through the chapters of this book, you'll find icons in the margins that are designed to draw your attention to valuable bits of information. Here are the icons you can expect to see and what each of them means:

The Tip icon draws attention to handy bits of guidance that inspire, help, and ease your way along the vegan path.

Remember icons are used for the information that's especially important to know. Pay attention to this advice, and file it away for future use.

The Technical Stuff icon points out where I've gone into the science of things. You don't have to read this information to understand the topic at hand, but it can be interesting background information.

The Warning icon directs you to pay close attention. It helps you avoid common pitfalls, and may save you some headaches.

Beyond the Book

In addition to the wealth of information and guidance related to going vegan that's provided in this book, you get access to even more help and information online at Dummies.com. To check out the book's online Cheat Sheet, visit www. dummies.com and search for "Living Vegan For Dummies Cheat Sheet."

Where to Go from Here

With this book, you can make up your own journey of discovery as you go along. You can start at the beginning and keep reading until you reach the back cover. Or you can head to the Table of Contents and seek out the topics that interest you the most.

Of course, Chapter 1 is always a good place to start, but if you're most interested in the health benefits of a vegan diet, you won't want to miss Chapter 3. If you want to get cracking on setting up a vegan kitchen, Chapter 7 is the place to go. If you're worried about missing meat, dairy, or eggs on a vegan diet, Chapter 9 alleviates your concerns. If you'd like to start with your stomach, jump ahead to the recipes in Chapters 11 through 15.

Whether you read this book from cover to cover or bounce from one topic to the next, this information-packed guide contains everything you need to know about living vegan.

1

Getting Started with a Vegan Lifestyle

Get familiar with what it means to be vegan, and find out why folks are drawn to this lifestyle.

Discover how simple modifications to your routine can lead you toward a satisfying vegan life.

Chapter **1**

The Nuts and Bolts of Veganism

There has never been a better time to go vegan.

It wasn't that long ago that vegan specialty products were hard to find outside large cities like New York City or Los Angeles. Even then, you may have needed to visit a health food store to purchase nondairy cheese or find a package of veggie burgers.

Here's where we stand now:

» Big-box stores have whole freezer and refrigerator cases full of vegan products.

» Vegan cheese is available at several mainstream pizza chains.

» Many ice cream shops offer nondairy ice cream.

» Most coffee shops offer nondairy milk.

» Plant-based burgers are sold at certain nationwide fast-food chains.

And every year brings more innovation. Foods or products that were once a stumbling block now have a vegan alternative. You can find vegan eggs that sizzle, cashew cheeses worthy of a showstopping grazing board, high-quality vegan leather purses, and plant-based meats that may make you do a double take.

In 2021, Google identified the search term "vegan food near me" as a breakthrough search in its "Year in Search" report. Because people wanted to find plant-based food in their area, the term grew by more than 5,000 percent that year! In January 2023, a record number of 700,000 people pledged to eat plant-based meals for Veganuary, a monthlong vegan challenge.

Thanks to the internet and various social media sites, it's easier than ever to get informed about where your food comes from, find vegan recipes and products, and locate other like-minded people. The picture of who goes vegan is changing from a hypothetical cartoon to a living, breathing person on the screen of your phone or computer. As people glean more information, they're becoming more open to finding alternatives to the status quo.

With this growing enthusiasm, there's more awareness than ever before of what veganism means. Even my 83-year-old aunt asked me at Thanksgiving, "If two vegans have a fight, is it still called a beef?" (I had to let her down gently . . . "No, that's Beyond Beef.")

In this chapter, you discover what being vegan entails, examine the reasons people choose this lifestyle, and find out that vegan food is all around you. Plus, I reveal that you'll be in very good company if you make this dietary switch!

Knowing What It Means to Be Vegan

Some people are confused about the difference between being vegan and being vegetarian. That's understandable, because they do have some similarities and overlap.

REMEMBER

If you're vegetarian, you don't eat cows, pigs, chickens, turkeys, fish, or any other animals. Vegans don't eat any animals either. Plus, vegans expand that list to include anything that comes from an animal or uses one as a commodity.

>> Vegans don't eat meat, dairy, eggs, or honey.

>> Vegans avoid animal products in clothes, cosmetics, and household goods. They don't buy products that include wool, fur, leather, or animal by-products.

>> Vegans don't support businesses and activities where animals are used as entertainment, like zoos, aquariums, rodeos, horse races, or circuses with animal acts.

Similar to the difference between the words *vegan* and *vegetarian*, when you're vegan, you cut out a few more things than vegetarians do. For example, a vegetarian might eat dairy, eggs, or honey, wear wool, or visit a zoo. But a vegan would not. To put it another way, all vegans are vegetarian, but not all vegetarians are vegan.

Understanding Why People Choose to Go Vegan

People have a wide variety of motivations for going vegan. The most popular reasons are animal welfare concerns, health goals, or to reduce environmental impact. Some people choose a vegan lifestyle for a combination of any or all of those factors. The following sections explain each of these motivations on their own.

For the animals

For many people, choosing to go vegan is an extension of their own care and compassion for animals. Perhaps you love cats and dogs, and it occurs to you that cows, pigs, and chickens also have personalities and feelings. Those animals desire to raise their young, and live out their natural lives without needless suffering.

Or perhaps you saw a video of what happens to animals on farms and in slaughterhouses. When you saw the pain that animals endure, you knew you didn't want to be a part of what's generating demand for meat, dairy, and eggs. For you, going vegan is a way of living your own values of compassion.

TIP

I explore the compassion side of the equation in Chapters 16 and 17, where I share what happens to animals in modern agriculture. Plus, I offer tips on how to avoid animal by-products in clothing, cosmetics, and body products.

For their health

Some people go vegan for their health. Perhaps your doctor suggested it, or maybe you saw a health documentary that piqued your interest.

It may be that you'd like to lower your risk of certain types of cancer, type 2 diabetes, or heart disease. Maybe you want to lower your cholesterol, lower your blood pressure, improve your kidney function, or reap the benefits of a diet filled with antioxidants, fiber, and phytonutrients.

TIP

Whatever the specific reason, if health concerns are your main impetus for considering veganism, be sure to read Chapter 3. That's where I cover the many potential health benefits of a plant-based diet.

For the environment

Others decide to go vegan for the environment. Maybe you realize that while cars and planes get a lot of press, animal agriculture shoulders more of the blame for greenhouse gas emissions and climate change.

According to the United Nations (UN), animal-based foods — most notably red meat, dairy, and farmed shrimp — are responsible for the highest greenhouse gas emissions. Plus, cattle ranching is the biggest driver of deforestation in the Amazon — by as much as 80 percent.

In a report titled *Climate Change 2022: Mitigation of Climate Change,* the UN noted that shifting to a plant-based diet has the potential to greatly reduce greenhouse gas emissions. According to the report, plant-based eating "could reduce pressure on forests and land used for feed, support the preservation of biodiversity and planetary health, and contribute to preventing forms of malnutrition . . . in developing countries."

TIP

If environmental concerns are important to you, check out the section "Addressing Environmental Concerns" in Chapter 16. It lays out what there is to gain by choosing plant foods over animal foods.

KNOWING HOW VEGANISM STARTED

The word *vegan* was coined back in 1944 by Donald Watson, who was part of the Vegan Society of the United Kingdom. They defined veganism as "a way of living that seeks to exclude, as far as possible and practicable, all forms of exploitation of and cruelty to animals for food, clothing, and any other purpose."

However, vegans and vegetarians existed long before the 1940s. They just didn't call themselves that.

There are long histories of cultures which go back thousands of years that abstained from meat in India, where Jainism and Buddhism began, and where the majority of the population practices Hinduism. (Although most of these religious groups are vegetarian, modern India is home to roughly 5 million vegans, according to a 2020 report by the United Nations Food and Agriculture Organization. The report notes that India has the lowest rate of meat consumption globally, largely because 44 percent of India's 1.3 billion population are Hindus.)

Over in Greece, you may remember Pythagoras and his theorem from high school geometry class. But did you know he's also considered to be one of the first ethical vegetarians? Born in 580 BCE, he believed that all animals, not just humans, have souls. In fact, until the term *vegetarian* was popularized in 1847, people would say they were Pythagorean if they didn't eat meat.

Discovering that Vegan Food Is Just Food

Vegan food is anything that doesn't come from an animal. It's fruits, vegetables, mushrooms, nuts, seeds, beans, and grains. Pretty simple, right?

Many people have negative preconceptions about vegan food. I've even heard people say that they don't like vegan food. I have to wonder exactly which food they're talking about, because "vegan food" covers a lot of stuff!

REMEMBER

The truth is, all of us eat vegan food — regardless of whether or not we're vegan. If you've had any of these foods, you've had vegan food:

>> A banana

>> An apple

>> Grapes

>> Peanuts

>> Popcorn or pretzels

>> Vegetable dumplings

>> French fries and ketchup

>> Falafel and hummus

>> A peanut butter and jelly sandwich

>> Potato chips

- » Pasta with spaghetti sauce
- » A bean burrito
- » Tomato soup with crackers
- » Sourdough bread
- » Green salad with balsamic vinaigrette
- » Tortilla chips, salsa, and guacamole

That's all everyday, normal stuff that happens to be free from animal products.

REMEMBER

It's important to remember that food is vegan because of what's absent, not what's present. If it doesn't include meat, dairy, eggs, or honey, it's vegan.

People sometimes assume that to be vegan, you have to eat tofu, tempeh, seitan, veggie burgers, sprouts, or lentil loaves. They think you have to grind flaxseed, sprinkle chia seeds, or juice wheatgrass. But a person can be vegan for decades and never eat any of those things if they don't care to eat them.

I went vegetarian in 2005 and vegan a couple years after that. In many ways, my day-to-day meals aren't so different from what I ate before I stopped consuming meat, dairy, and eggs. Here are some of my typical dinners:

- » Black bean tacos and Spanish rice
- » Big green salad with roasted chickpeas and garlic bread on the side
- » Vegetable stir-fry with cashews and browned tofu
- » Falafel pita stuffed with hummus and cucumber salad
- » Refried bean tostadas with green leaf lettuce, tomatoes, and avocado
- » Chana masala with rice and samosas
- » Baguette pizza (either cheeseless or with nondairy cheese)
- » Ramen with tofu, mushrooms, and bok choy
- » Split pea soup with barley and crusty bread on the side
- » Three bean chili
- » Potato pierogi with sautéed kale

These dishes don't take any longer to make than their non-vegan counterparts. In fact, they often take less time, because most vegetables cook quicker than meat. Plus, they tend to be less expensive than non-vegan food, because they leave out pricey ingredients like meat, dairy, and eggs.

TIP

I cover more about grocery shopping, cooking, menu planning, and saving money on a vegan diet in Chapters 7 and 8.

Realizing Who Goes Vegan

It's estimated that 88 million people in the world are vegan, according to *The VOU* magazine. However, when you imagine someone who is vegan, a specific image often comes to mind. You may picture a woman who's in her 20s, blonde, and living on the coast.

While women do make up the majority of vegans, anyone can choose this lifestyle — regardless of age, gender, race, or where they live. As folks discover the benefits of a vegan lifestyle, more and more of them are choosing to ditch meat, dairy, and eggs, and embrace a plant-based way of life.

According to a 2021 survey from Statista, the largest group of people in the United States eating a vegan diet are college-age adults. When young people venture out on their own, they often feel empowered to explore a vegan lifestyle for the first time. Luckily, an increasing number of college campuses are pivoting to meet students' dietary demands. You can find out more about being vegan as a college student in Chapter 24.

Even though young people are the largest adopters of the plant-based movement, people with a little more age under their belts are gaining on them. The second largest adherents of a vegan diet are people in their 30s.

Older adults in their 40s and beyond have much to gain from adopting a plant-based diet. A 2021 study published in the *American Journal of Lifestyle Medicine* suggests that older adults who are vegan take 58 percent fewer prescription drugs than their non-vegan peers. You can read more about being vegan in middle age and beyond in Chapter 26.

Additionally, many professional and amateur athletes are gravitating toward plant-based diets to fuel their workouts and improve their performance. From professional football players to basketball stars and tennis greats, athletes are turning to the power of plants. You can read more about thriving as a vegan athlete in Chapter 25.

Interestingly, in the United States, Black people are going vegan at a higher rate than the rest of the population. According to a 2016 survey from Pew Research Center, 8 percent of Black Americans define themselves as strict vegetarians or vegans, compared to 3 percent of Americans overall.

Tracye McQuirter, author of *By Any Greens Necessary*, noted in an *Essence* magazine article, "There has been a mighty river of African American leaders and innovators in the plant-based food movement." In the article, McQuirter points to the following examples:

>> Vegetarian Black Seventh-day Adventists in the 1890s

>> Nonviolent civil rights activist Dick Gregory

>> African Hebrew Israelites

>> The Rastafari religion, which started in Jamaica and has plant-based foods as a central tenet

More recently, Coretta Scott King was vegan for the last decade of her life. This author, activist, civil rights leader, and wife to Martin Luther King Jr. was inspired to go vegan by her son Dexter Scott King. Finally, the first vegan cooking show on Food Network was hosted by Black vegan Tabitha Brown, alongside celebrity chef Maneet Chauhan.

There are loads of outstanding Black-owned vegan restaurants and businesses. Here's just a small sampling:

>> Bunna Café in Brooklyn, New York

>> Detroit Vegan Soul in Detroit, Michigan

>> Plum Bistro in Seattle, Washington

>> Rahel Vegan Cuisine in Los Angeles, California (My favorite restaurant of all time!)

>> Souley Vegan in Oakland, California (Chef-owner Tamearra Dyson competed against Bobby Flay in the first vegan episode of Food Network's *Beat Bobby Flay*. She won!)

>> The Southern V in Nashville, Tennessee

>> Stuff I Eat in Inglewood, California

>> Twisted Plants in Cudahy and Milwaukee, Wisconsin

>> V Marks the Shop in Philadelphia, Pennsylvania

IN THIS CHAPTER

» Recognizing your dietary habits

» Figuring out your meals

» Planning your timeline for changing your diet

» Adjusting to the vegan lifestyle

» Reinforcing your motivations for going vegan

Chapter **2**

Making the Move to a Vegan Diet

There are many ways to transition to a vegan diet. Some people do it overnight. For others, it's more of a process. If you've already been vegetarian for a while, you may find it easy to check a few more items off the list in one fell swoop. If you currently eat animals at every meal, you may prefer to change your diet a little more gradually while you get your bearings.

TIP

Whether you decide to go vegan overnight or over a few months' time, just keep moving in that direction. Any movement toward a plant-based diet is a positive step.

In this chapter, I share one of the most common struggles in going vegan. I give you some pointers on how to get started with a vegan lifestyle, and remind you that even though change can feel uncomfortable at first, it will become more natural with time.

Changing Your Habits

Going vegan is about one simple thing: changing your habits. That's both good and bad. It's good, because habits are just habits. They're not necessarily based on what's optimum. They're just what we've gotten used to doing.

Most of us eat the foods we eat, wear the clothes we wear, and buy the products we buy because that's what feels familiar. It's not necessarily because those are the only things we might like or the best way for us to thrive.

But it's difficult too because we like our habits — a lot.

>> We park in the same parking spots day after day.

>> We sleep on the same side of the bed night after night.

>> We sit in the same places in movie theaters, classes, or restaurants.

>> We stay in relationships or jobs that don't serve us because it feels so much easier to do what we've always done.

Doing something different can be hard — even when it's ultimately what you want. That's why every year by the end of January, many folks toss their resolutions in the trash bin along with the year-shaped glasses they wore on New Year's Eve. It takes stamina to commit to real, lasting change.

Therefore, it's no wonder that when someone considers going vegan, one of the biggest hurdles is creating new habits. You're used to running on automatic: tacos on Tuesday, pizza on Friday, ice cream when you're stressed, steak on your birthday, milk chocolate when you need a pick-me-up . . .

When you go vegan, all of a sudden those mundane habits have to be reconsidered — again and again. Going vegan may mean changing what you eat for breakfast, lunch, and dinner. But it can also mean changing what you buy, what you wear, how you honor your holiday traditions, and sometimes even where you go (or don't go) on vacation.

REMEMBER

Don't get overwhelmed. You don't have to figure it all out in one day. Take it one step at a time and have faith that you'll find your way as you go along. Over time, you'll create new habits that reflect your vegan lifestyle. They'll become just as cozy and familiar as your old ways.

Choosing Your Approach

Vegans don't eat animals, their milk, their eggs, or animal by-products. That's the baseline. But beyond that, there are as many types of vegan diets as there are vegans. Some people are more health-minded, and others aren't. Some people eat only whole and unprocessed plant foods, and for others, anything goes (as long as it's vegan).

Within that spectrum, some folks do a mixture of both. They eat a lot of healthy, whole plant foods, but they also pepper their meals with some indulgence items. (That's how I would describe my own eating habits. Whole plant foods make up the bulk of my diet. But I also make room for vegan sausages, nachos with cashew queso, and fries every now and again.)

TIP

Depending on your motivations and goals, see what works for you, and allow that to unfold as time goes on. It may be easier in the beginning to include foods that feel familiar, like vegan chick'n strips, seitan ribs, and veggie burgers that you can really sink your teeth into. Eating those foods may help with the transition period.

On the other hand, you may be vegan for decades and *still* eat and love vegan specialty foods. If having a few vegan chick'n strips on the side makes a huge green salad more inviting, you're still coming out ahead nutrient-wise. (Plus, those chick'n strips have a lot of satiating protein.)

REMEMBER

Dietary habits are always evolving. The way you eat in week 1 of your vegan diet may be totally different by week 52. You may discover new favorites, and other foods may eventually get pushed to the wayside.

Also, keep in mind that people can go vegan for one reason, and then, over time, become more convinced by other motivations as well. For example, maybe you'll go vegan primarily for environmental reasons, and then the more you discover, the more strongly you feel about animal welfare or the many health benefits of a plant-based diet. There are many good reasons for adopting a vegan lifestyle. You don't have to pick just one.

Plus, if you're vegan for ethical reasons, you still reap the benefits of eating phytonutrient-rich plant foods. And if you're vegan for health reasons, you're still reducing the demand for animal products, which means fewer animals being bred onto factory farms.

Anything goes (as long as it's vegan)

If your main reason for going vegan is your concern about animal welfare, you may not particularly care about the health aspects of specific foods, or that may be secondary for you. The main objective for many ethical vegans is reducing harm, and the health component takes a back seat.

For those vegans, their day-to-day diet may look something like this:

>> For breakfast, they might eat cereal with cashew milk.

>> For lunch, they could have a big bowl of vegan ramen with tofu and lots of vegetable toppings.

>> At dinner, they could tuck into a vegan meatball sub with a green salad on the side.

REMEMBER

For ethical vegans, veganism is a way to live their values of compassion and non-violence. It doesn't have anything to do with losing weight, avoiding refined or processed foods, or being on a "diet" in the way many people think of the word.

I've had a vegan food blog since 2009. Some people who come to my site are vegan, and some aren't. Some are super health-minded, and others aren't. Anyway, I had a dessert recipe on my site, and a non-vegan commenter admonished me for having sugar in it. She thought it wasn't healthy enough, and I should just eat dates or something. I told her that I didn't go vegan because I wanted to avoid cupcakes. I have no qualms about them. My cupcakes don't have dairy or eggs in them, but I still eat sweets.

Some folks assume that a vegan diet has to be all kale, all the time. But when your reasons for going vegan are based on ethics, the amount of time/energy/concern you give to the health aspects of veganism varies by person.

Whole-foods, plant-based eating

If your primary reason for adopting a vegan diet is your health, you may feel guided to make decisions based on which foods you think are optimum as fuel or that could provide the most potential health benefits.

REMEMBER

People who choose a plant-based diet for health reasons often gravitate toward a more whole-foods approach.

Their diets include:

» Vegetables

» Fruits

» Whole grains

» Legumes

» Nuts and seeds

They tend to stay away from super-processed foods, processed sugar, refined grains, and oil, and may prefer a minimal amount of salt.

For people who follow a whole-foods, plant-based diet, one day of eating might look like this:

» For breakfast, they might eat oatmeal with blueberries and bananas.

» For lunch, they could have a grain bowl with roasted vegetables and chickpeas.

» For dinner, they could enjoy polenta with sautéed kale and great northern beans.

Transitioning to a Vegan Diet

I've always considered myself an animal lover, but I spent the first 30 years of my life eating meat, dairy, and eggs. Many times I felt uneasy about it. I often felt grossed out while preparing and cooking meat — cutting out tendons, forming ground meat into patties or loaves with my hands, or seeing bright red liquid pooling around steaks on a plate.

It didn't sit right with me that I cherished some animals and ate others for dinner. But instead of changing my habits, I pushed that thought to the back of my mind and tried to compartmentalize it.

To diminish my uneasiness, for a period of time I chose animal products that were marked up with buzzwords like *humanely raised, cage-free, free-range,* or *responsibly sourced*. But then I found out that these taglines were unregulated marketing terms. Similar to *greenwashing* (making products or activities seem more environmentally friendly than they really are), it was *humane washing* (giving the illusion of animal protection while obscuring how much those animals suffer). It made consumers like me feel better, but it didn't offer any guarantees about the ways animals were treated. Plus, the animals' lives ended in the same slaughterhouses — while they were still young and wanting to live.

Then in 2005, I saw a 12-minute video online called *Meet Your Meat*. It showed what happens to animals who are raised for food and the standard farming procedures used. (You can read more about the specifics in Chapter 16.) I saw the fear and terror in the animals' eyes, and how powerless they were against what was happening to them. While I was watching it, something clicked. I knew I could no longer continue paying for that kind of suffering.

So I went vegetarian. From there, I kept studying:

>> I read T. Colin Campbell's book *The China Study,* and *The Food Revolution* by John Robbins.

>> I listened to vegan podcasts and watched documentaries.

>> I thought about the kind of life I wanted to live.

In some ways it was hard to imagine never again eating the foods I'd grown accustomed to in the first 30 years of my life. However, I also knew that at that very moment, I didn't want to consume them.

The more I researched, the more I discovered that the egg and dairy industries involve tremendous suffering too. It became clear to me that the most consistent way of living my values of compassion was to go vegan. So after being vegetarian for about a year and a half, I stopped eating dairy, eggs, and honey, and went fully vegan.

Deciding how you'll go vegan

TIP

As you think about the path that's right for you, here are some timeline options:

>> **You can go "cold Tofurky" today and give up eating animals and animal products all in one go.** Or you can decide to gather more information and then go all in on a specific date like January 1. (Many people celebrate Veganuary for the whole month of January.)

>> **You can start by cutting meat out of your diet first.** Then keep reducing your consumption of any remaining animal products like dairy and eggs until you've gradually removed all of them from your diet.

>> **You can start by being vegan for a month.** Go all in for a month and continue to research veganism and discover more reasons for switching to a plant-based diet. Many people find that when they aren't eating animals, they feel more open to bearing witness to what happens to animals in modern farming. After 30 days, see how you feel. Don't be surprised if you feel amazing and want to keep going.

>> **You can start by reducing your animal consumption footprint.** Because of their size, it takes a lot more small animals like chickens or fish to equal the same amount of meat as larger animals like cows. So you can quit eating small animals first, and then work your way toward giving up the bigger ones.

REMEMBER

An estimated 1 to 2.8 trillion fish are killed for food every year. More than 70 billion chickens are killed annually worldwide. Compare that to the 293 million cows who are slaughtered every year across the globe.

>> **You can start with eating vegan meals once a week, having one vegan meal a day, or eating vegan meals every day until 6 p.m.** Make a variety of plant-based dishes and widen your repertoire. Grow the portions of your plate that are plant-based and crowd out the non-vegan foods. Then, as you gain more knowledge and experience, continue building out the number of plant-based meals you consume until you're fully vegan.

>> **You can start by being vegan at home.** If you have only vegan foods in your home, it's a lot easier to maintain your plant-based diet there. Then, when you're at someone else's home or a restaurant, you can be a little more lax until you have a better handle on how to be vegan in the outside world.

Some people say, "I could go vegan, except for _____." That blank is often cheese, but it can also be ribs, steak, fried chicken, hamburgers, or whatever animal-based food is your favorite. If that's you, don't give up on the idea of going vegan simply because of your attachment to one specific thing.

Instead, start by cutting out all the other animal-based foods you're not as attached to. Cross off the ones that are easy to give up first, gain some confidence, keep reading up on veganism, and trying new recipes and foods. Once you have some momentum, you may realize that _____ doesn't matter that much after all.

Figuring out what to make first

Once you're ready to start preparing vegan meals, the best place to begin is by considering the meals you already make. While cookbooks and online recipes are wonderful and useful resources, you don't necessarily want to page through a cookbook every time you need breakfast, lunch, dinner, or a snack.

TIP

Write down the meals you make consistently. Most of us turn to the same dishes again and again — tacos, pizza, sandwiches, salads, rice bowls, stir-fries. . . . Often with one or two simple substitutions you can "veganize" your go-to standards. Consider what easy plant-based swaps you can make to turn those meals into vegan dishes.

Starting with your regular meals and making a couple of vegan-friendly replacements can feel a lot more manageable than always relying on an outside source for instructions.

Read more about using your go-to meals as a guide in Chapter 8 in the section titled "Starting with the Dishes You Know and Love." I also explain how to veganize dishes in Chapter 9.

Discovering new foods

In addition to tweaking your current favorites, it's good to discover new foods and expand your dietary repertoire. Many people assume veganism is limiting. However, I eat a much more varied diet now than I did before I went vegan. And I know I'm not alone! Many other vegans say the same thing.

That sounds counterintuitive, because when people think about going vegan, they often imagine a lot of *no*.

>> No beef

>> No poultry

>> No fish

>> No pork

>> No dairy

>> No eggs

>> No honey

But what they don't realize is, there's a lot of *yes* too!

When you're hyper-focused on what you're giving up, you don't always notice what you're gaining. A huge world of produce, grains, and legumes suddenly comes into view when you make room for plant-based foods you'd been ignoring.

Before I went vegan, I'd never eaten vegetables like:

>> Celeriac

>> Collard greens

>> Daikon radishes

>> Delicata squash

>> Fennel

>> Jicama

>> Kale

>> Leeks

>> Parsnips

>> Romanesco

>> Swiss chard

>> Turnips

>> Watercress

I'd never prepared tofu. I'd never eaten other plant-based foods like:

>> Adzuki beans

>> Farro

>> Fava beans

>> Great northern beans

>> Jackfruit

>> Mung beans

>> Oyster mushrooms

>> Red lentils

>> Seitan

>> Tempeh

The only split pea soup I'd ever made came out of a can.

Yes, I'm not eating the five or six animals I used to eat, or consuming their milk or their eggs. But breaking out of my old habits and routine gave me license to explore more. The real estate on my plate where animal products used to be was suddenly opened up for business. Every farmers market, every season, and every cookbook offered a new discovery.

REMEMBER

There are more than 20,000 species of edible plants and only a handful of animals that most folks eat in their day-to-day lives. Once you start eating a much wider variety of plant foods, it's easy to see how a vegan diet can feel quite expansive.

Knowing How Long It Takes for Veganism to Feel Natural

The well-worn saying is that it takes 21 days to create a new habit. However, according to a 2021 study published in the *British Journal of Health Psychology*, it takes an average of 59 to 70 days to create new habits. That study reaffirmed older research from 2010 published in the *European Journal of Social Psychology*, which showed that the average time it takes to create a new habit is 66 days.

In the case of the 2010 study, researchers noted that harder habits took more time to cement. For example, developing a habit of drinking water at lunch is a whole lot easier than building a daily running habit. Therefore, it doesn't take as much time for simple habit changes like water drinking to sink in.

The thing to remember about becoming vegan is that it's not just one habit you're changing.

>> You're no longer eating meat, dairy, or eggs. You're opting for plant-based foods for breakfast, lunch, and dinner.

>> You're choosing cleaning products that don't include animal ingredients and weren't tested on animals.

>> You're buying clothes that don't include animal products like wool, fur, or leather.

>> You're seeking out restaurants that are vegan-friendly.

>> You're avoiding attractions that use animals for entertainment.

>> At the holidays, you're making new traditions and bringing new dishes to share.

It's okay if it feels challenging at first. That's to be expected.

The first year, veganism can feel a little like puberty. You may experience some growing pains, awkwardness, and growth spurts. That's part of the process. Then, with time, it becomes natural and seamless.

>> You figure out how to spot non-vegan ingredients on product labels with a glance.

>> You get the hang of making vegan recipes by heart.

>> You discover new favorite restaurants, products, and dishes.

>> You settle in to a full vegan lifestyle.

At some point you'll look back at your old ways and be surprised that it took you so long to make a change.

Remembering Your "Why"

For me, it's easy to stick to a vegan diet, because it's not about me. It's about the animals who I don't want to suffer just so I can have a sandwich. That makes it very simple.

TIP

As you're leaning into a vegan diet, keep your "why" in the forefront of your mind, and focus on what first motivated you to consider veganism. Remember that the actions you're taking are furthering your aim to live more healthfully, be more compassionate, or adopt a more sustainable lifestyle. That awareness makes it easier to go the distance.

It can be helpful to keep reading books, watching documentaries, attending veg fests, and visiting animal sanctuaries. Keeping your "why" at the top of your mind helps prevent you from slipping back into old habits and forgetting the reasons you felt driven to make changes in the first place.

REMEMBER

For many folks, what's easiest wins out. It can be hard to swim upstream, and veganism isn't the default in most homes, restaurants, cities, or offices. It can feel easier to go back to sleep. But fight the urge. Stay awake, continue exploring and discovering, and keep focused on your "why." You'll be rewarded for it with the peace that comes when you live a life that reflects your values.

2
For the Health of It

Chapter **3**

The Health Benefits of a Plant-Based Diet

t's very empowering when you realize that with every meal, you have a choice. You can pick foods that are full of antioxidants, vitamins, and minerals. You can choose foods that are not only delicious but can also make you feel amazing. You can vote for dark leafy greens, whole grains, vibrant fruits, and plant proteins, and reject foods that have been shown to be damaging to your health.

Eating well is its own kind of self-care. It has the power to impact how you feel not only today, but also for the rest of your life. A vegan diet that's loaded with healthy plant foods and low in saturated fat is highly nutritious. It has the potential to improve your heart health, as well as reduce your risk of cancer, type 2 diabetes, and Alzheimer's disease.

According to Harvard Health Publishing, the media and publishing division of Harvard Medical School, "Traditionally, research into vegetarianism focused mainly on potential nutritional deficiencies, but in recent years, the pendulum has swung the other way, and studies are confirming the health benefits of meat-free eating. Nowadays, plant-based eating is recognized as not only nutritionally sufficient but also as a way to reduce the risk for many chronic illnesses."

In this chapter, I share the many ways that choosing a diet rich in nutrient-dense fruits and vegetables can pay serious health dividends.

REMEMBER

As I share the current research, keep in mind that I'm not a doctor. And even though I went to acting school, I don't even play one on TV. Before you make any major changes or embark on a new dietary plan, talk to your primary care physician.

Looking at Longevity

For a window into the benefits of a plant-based lifestyle, we can look at Loma Linda, California, which is considered the U.S.'s only *blue zone,* a community where people live longer and are healthier compared to the rest of the world.

Blue zones are an idea conceived by Dan Buettner, a *National Geographic* explorer and author. Buettner, along with a team of demographers, anthropologists, and scientists, compiled a list of five areas across the globe where people consistently reach age 100. By contrast, the average life expectancy in the U.S. is 76 years, according to a 2022 report from the Centers for Disease Control and Prevention (CDC).

REMEMBER

The reason for Loma Linda residents' long lifespan is generally credited to the vegetarian diet of the many Seventh-day Adventists who live there. Roughly 50 percent of Adventists maintain a vegetarian or fully plant-based diet.

Adventists eat what's called a Garden of Eden Diet. It's a reference to what Adam and Eve ate in the book of Genesis in the Hebrew Bible, as well as the Christian Old Testament. (In the Bible, eating animals was only allowed after "the fall of man.")

Genesis 1:29 states, "Then God said, 'Behold, I have given you every seed-bearing plant on the face of all the earth, and every tree whose fruit contains seed. They will be yours for food.'"

Other beneficial habits of Seventh-day Adventists include getting regular exercise, managing stress, and maintaining community connections, as well as abstaining from alcohol and smoking.

Because of their healthy diet and notable longevity, Adventists are often included in health studies, such as a study of 96,000 Adventists called *The Adventist Health Study.* This study found that Adventists who followed a vegetarian diet had significantly lower risks of high blood sugar, high blood pressure, and obesity than the general population. Other studies have shown vegetarian Adventists have lower rates of heart disease, diabetes, and all forms of cancer.

Even in comparison to other Seventh-day Adventists, vegetarian Adventists come out ahead. Researchers note that Adventists who follow a vegetarian diet have fewer incidences of diabetes, hypertension, high cholesterol, coronary heart disease, and certain types of cancer than non-vegetarian Adventists.

Reducing the Risk of Type 2 Diabetes

In the U.S., 37 million people have diabetes, and 90 to 95 percent of them have type 2, according to the CDC. Diabetes carries an elevated risk of amputation, blindness, and heart disease. While type 2 diabetes usually develops in people over age 45, an increasing number of children and younger people are developing it.

REMEMBER

Research has shown that plant-based diets can lower the risk of type 2 diabetes. Plant-based diets are rich in fiber, magnesium, and antioxidants, which can help with insulin sensitivity and weight management.

>> According to Harvard Health Publishing, "In studies of Seventh-day Adventists, vegetarians' risk of developing diabetes was half that of non-vegetarians, even after taking [body mass index (BMI)] into account." This led researchers to conclude that "a predominantly plant-based diet can reduce the risk for type 2 diabetes."

>> A 2019 meta-analysis published in *JAMA Internal Medicine* looked at nine observational studies with more than 300,000 participants. The researchers wanted to assess how plant-based diets relate to type 2 diabetes risk. The study found that plant-based eaters had a 23 percent lower risk of developing the disease.

The study authors noted, "Greater adherence to plant-based dietary patterns, especially those rich in healthful plant-based foods, is associated with lower risk of type 2 diabetes."

Slashing Cancer Risk

According to the World Cancer Research Fund, 30 to 50 percent of all cancer cases could be prevented with a healthy diet and lifestyle. Since cancer can take 10 or more years to develop, your nutritional choices now have the potential to make a significant difference down the road.

A 2022 article published on the Mayo Clinic's website states, "In research studies, vegans, people who don't eat any animal products, including fish, dairy or eggs, appeared to have the lowest rates of cancer of any diet. The next lowest rate was for vegetarians."

A 2017 review titled *Vegetarian, Vegan Diets and Multiple Health Outcomes* showed that a vegan diet may reduce overall cancer risk by 15 percent.

A 2022 study with more than 470,000 participants revealed that vegetarians (including vegans) had the lowest risk for cancer overall compared to those who ate typical amounts of meat, small amounts of meat, or who chose fish as their primary meat for consumption.

Benefiting from antioxidants and fiber

These benefits could be attributed to the many vitamins, antioxidants, phytochemicals, and abundant fiber in a plant-based diet, which have been shown to be protective against cancer.

REMEMBER

Antioxidants reduce inflammation in the body and help prevent disease. Phytochemicals ward off cell damage, decrease inflammation, and interrupt the mechanisms that lead to cancer production.

Plus, vegan diets are loaded with fiber, and high fiber diets have been shown to lower the risks of breast, prostate, and colorectal cancers.

One large-scale study from 2016, *Dietary Fiber Intake in Young Adults and Breast Cancer Risk,* found that women who ate high amounts of fiber-rich foods during adolescence and young adulthood were 24 percent less likely to get breast cancer later in life, compared to those who ate smaller amounts. For each additional 10 grams of fiber consumed per day, breast cancer risk was reduced by 13 percent. (All plant foods have varying amounts of fiber, but the biggest benefit seemed to be from fiber derived from fruits and vegetables.)

Avoiding the negatives of animal products

Lower cancer risks for vegans could also be attributed to their avoidance of the damaging nature of animal products.

>> In a 2015 press release, the International Agency for Research on Cancer (IARC) stated that red meat is "probably carcinogenic to humans." Red meat like beef, veal, pork, and lamb is linked with prostate, colorectal, and pancreatic cancers.

>> The IARC also noted that processed meat is "classified as carcinogenic to humans, based on sufficient evidence in humans that the consumption of processed meat causes colorectal cancer." Processed meats include hot dogs, ham, sausages, corned beef, and beef jerky. The IARC concluded that eating a 50-gram portion (less than 2 ounces) of processed meat every day increases colorectal cancer risk by 18 percent.

>> The 2022 *Fish Intake and Risk of Melanoma in the NIH-AARP Diet and Health Study* found that higher total fish intake was associated with increased risk for melanoma. The study looked at dietary questionnaires of almost 500,000 people. Melanoma risks were 22 percent higher in the people who ate the most fish, compared to those who ate the least.

WARNING

The researchers noted that more study is needed to confirm their findings. Study commentary pointed out that it's possible mercury or arsenic in fish may bear some of the blame, because previous studies have linked mercury exposure with an increased risk of skin cancer.

>> Men who eat and drink more dairy products, especially milk, have higher risk of prostate cancer than those who consume less or none, according to the 2022 *Dairy Foods, Calcium Intakes, and Risk of Incident Prostate Cancer in Adventist Health Study-2*.

The study showed that men who drank about 1¾ cup of dairy milk a day had a 25 percent increased risk of prostate cancer in comparison to those who consumed ½ cup a week. When you add in vegan men who don't drink dairy milk at all, the group consuming 1¾ cup fared even worse. Heads up: There was no link between nondairy milk and an increased risk of prostate cancer.

Clearing up confusion about soy

Soy has been the focus of a lot of fearmongering in years past, because of the *phytoestrogens* (plant estrogens) it contains. But plant estrogen isn't the same as mammal estrogen. Plant estrogen is much weaker.

It's ironic that consumption of plant estrogen from a bean has created so many myths, but ingesting actual estrogen from other mammals hasn't. All animal products contain varying amounts of estrogen. Eggs are actually a product of an animal's ovary, and dairy milk comes from an animal who's lactating. According to a 2015 study from the National Institutes of Health (NIH), "The main source of animal-derived estrogens (60–70 percent) in the human diet is milk and dairy products."

Plant-based diets have been shown again and again to promote healthy estrogen levels. Plus, research has shown repeatedly that because of their high isoflavone and antioxidant content, soy foods are actually protective against cancer, including breast and ovarian cancers. In fact, studies suggest that breast cancer survivors who eat soy have a lower risk of cancer recurrence compared to those who avoid it.

>> **According to Dana-Farber Cancer Institute:** "Eating soy foods like tofu, edamame, and soy milk has been linked to reduced risk of certain cancers including breast cancer, prostate cancer, and gastric cancer."

>> **According to Mayo Clinic:** "Studies show that a lifelong diet rich in soy foods reduces the risk of breast cancer in women."

>> **According to the American Cancer Society:** "There is growing evidence that eating traditional soy foods such as tofu, tempeh, edamame, miso, and soy milk may lower the risk of breast cancer, especially among Asian women. Soy foods are excellent sources of protein, especially when they replace other, less healthy foods such as animal fats and red or processed meats. Soy foods have been linked to lower rates of heart disease and may even help cholesterol."

>> **According to MD Anderson Cancer Center:** "Research suggests eating soy foods may reduce risk of cancer recurrence — even in patients with estrogen receptor-positive cancer."

Protecting the Brain

Alzheimer's disease (AD) is known for its devastating effects on memory, communication, mood, and a variety of brain functions. Sadly, AD is on the rise, according to the Alzheimer's Association. They estimate that more than 6 million Americans are living with AD in 2023. By 2050, they project that number could grow to as much as 12.7 million.

While some risk factors for developing AD are genetic, others can be modified by lifestyle changes. A growing body of research suggests that plant-based foods may support cognition, and could help in the prevention of AD and other types of dementia.

The 2022 study *Effect of a Vegan Diet on Alzheimer's Disease* considered whether a vegan diet had the potential to prevent neurodegenerative disorders, including AD. The study authors said that, "One of the key lifestyle factors that can be modified to prevent AD is diet."

Researchers noted that vegan diets contain low levels of saturated fats and cholesterol, and are rich in vitamins, antioxidants, and fiber, which may help prevent cognitive decline. According to the study authors, "Several meta-analyses found that the increased consumption of fruits and vegetables can reduce dementia risk and slow down cognitive decline in older adults. Conversely, a low vegetable intake is associated with poorer cognition in AD dementia."

The researchers went on to affirm that the anti-inflammatory and antioxidant properties in fruits and vegetables may be protective against dementia. They noted that, while initial results are promising, long-term research is still needed to draw definitive conclusions.

A 2021 study published in *Molecular Nutrition and Food Research* analyzed the relationship between diet and *cognitive impairment* (an intellectual disability that causes difficulties with memory, decision making, learning new things, and concentrating). The study was carried out over 12 years, and showed that a diet rich in plant-based foods lowered the risk of cognitive impairment in the elderly.

"A higher intake of fruits, vegetables and plant-based foods provides polyphenols and other bioactive compounds that could help reduce the risk of cognitive decline due to aging," said Cristina Andrés-Lacueva, who led the study.

A 2023 study in the *Journal of Alzheimer's Disease* compared the amount of antioxidants in the brains of AD patients versus those without AD. Researchers found that AD patients had half the amount of dietary lutein, zeaxanthin, lycopene, and vitamin E. (Lutein, zeaxanthin, beta-carotene, and lycopene are common *carotenoids*, bright pigments in plants, which lower inflammation and act as antioxidants in the human body.)

"This study, for the first time, demonstrates deficits in important dietary antioxidants in Alzheimer's brains. These results are consistent with large population studies that found risk for Alzheimer's disease was significantly lower in those who ate diets rich in carotenoids, or had high levels of lutein and zeaxanthin in their blood, or accumulated in their retina as macular pigment," said C. Kathleen Dorey, one of the study authors.

"Not only that, but we believe eating carotenoid-rich diets will help keep brains in top condition at all ages," Dorey said.

TIP

You can add more carotenoids to your diet by eating kale and spinach for lutein, corn and orange bell peppers for zeaxanthin, carrots and sweet potatoes for beta-carotene, plus tomatoes and watermelon for lycopene. Keep in mind that eating carotenoids along with heart-healthy fat helps absorption. All the more reason to add avocado, nuts, seeds, or vinaigrette to your salad.

Promoting Heart Health

Every year more than 800,000 people die of cardiovascular disease in the U.S. That comes out to one out of every three deaths. Seventy million Americans struggle with high blood pressure.

WARNING

A high intake of saturated fat can lead to raised cholesterol levels, which increases the risk of heart disease and stroke. Animal products like meat and dairy are the main sources of saturated fats for most folks.

While cholesterol and blood pressure medications are widely doled out, there is another way. Instead of turning to pills, perhaps we should turn to our plates. Studies have shown that eating a healthy, plant-based diet may lower your risk for cardiovascular disease and heart attacks.

>> A 2017 study titled *Vegetarian, Vegan Diets and Multiple Health Outcomes: A Systematic Review with Meta-Analysis of Observational Studies* examined the association between diet and various diseases or ailments. It showed that plant-based eaters have lower BMI (high BMI is a risk factor for heart disease), lower cholesterol (including harmful low-density lipoprotein, or LDL), and lower glucose levels.

Their results found that a vegetarian diet reduced heart disease by 25 percent, and a vegan diet reduced the incidence of cancer overall by 15 percent.

>> A 2019 study published in the *Journal of the American Heart Association* showed that diets higher in plant foods and lower in animal foods were associated with lower risks of developing or dying from cardiovascular disease.

>> A 2018 study in *Clinical Cardiology* found that plant-based diets effectively treat high cholesterol and high blood pressure, and reduce the need for medications. Study participants noticed improvements in just 4 weeks. The study authors noted, "Patients may find this therapeutic approach preferable to conventional and costly drug therapy."

Eating a fiber-rich diet has been shown to be protective against heart disease, according to the American Heart Association as well as the CDC. Eating fiber-filled foods like fruits, vegetables, beans, and whole grains can help lower cholesterol, decrease blood pressure, and reduce inflammation.

TIP

The CDC recommends preventing high cholesterol by:

>> Limiting foods that are high in saturated fats, which largely come from animal products

>> Eating foods that are high in fiber (Only plant foods have fiber.)

REMEMBER

It's worth noting that while eating white meat like chicken or turkey is often given a pass when it comes to cholesterol and saturated fat, research has shown that white meat raises cholesterol levels just as much as red meat.

A study from 2019 in the *American Journal of Clinical Nutrition* revealed that white meat was no better than red in terms of heart disease risk. In their randomized controlled trial, both red and white meat raised LDL cholesterol levels to roughly the same extent, compared to meatless protein options, which didn't.

Improving Gut Health

Gut health doesn't get a lot of fanfare, but it's essential for optimum well-being. Keeping your digestive system in good working order helps with proper digestion, absorption of nutrients, and maintaining a robust immune system. It can even affect mood and mental wellness. Conversely, poor gut health is linked to bloating, constipation, diarrhea, and a variety of health conditions like inflammatory bowel disease and irritable bowel syndrome.

Many studies have shown that plant-based diets rich in phytonutrients, antioxidants, and fiber are great for gut health, because they increase the diversity of your gut microbiota. *Gut microbiota* is the system of microorganisms or bacteria in your digestive tract that helps support digestion and immunity.

REMEMBER

A balanced digestive tract leads to a better immune system, metabolism, and appetite regulation. Gut bacteria depend on fiber, which is only available in plant foods.

Researchers noted in the 2019 study *The Effects of Vegetarian and Vegan Diets on Gut Microbiota,* "A plant-based diet appears to be beneficial for human health by promoting the development of a more diverse gut microbial system, or even distribution of different species."

Researchers concluded that "up-to-date knowledge suggests that a plant-based diet may be an effective way to promote a diverse ecosystem of beneficial microbes that support overall health."

REMEMBER

One way that plant-based eaters promote their gut flora is by eating prebiotics. You've likely heard of *probiotics,* which are the good bacteria that can be found in foods like sauerkraut, miso, and nondairy yogurt. (You can read more about probiotics in Chapter 4.) *Prebiotics* are food for your healthy gut bacteria that help it grow and flourish. They can also help you absorb calcium and ferment the foods you eat.

The following prebiotic foods are especially advantageous to gut health:

» Almonds

» Apples

» Asparagus

» Bananas

» Berries

» Cabbage

» Garlic

» Jerusalem artichokes

» Legumes like chickpeas and lentils

» Onions

» Peas

» Soy like tofu, tempeh, miso, and soy milk

» Whole grains like wheat, barley, and corn

This is a short list of prebiotic-rich foods, but there are many more! The key to creating diversity in your gut and keeping it healthy is to eat a wide variety of plant-based foods.

TIP

Be aware that if you're not used to a lot of fiber, it may take a little time for your body to adjust. However, the health benefits of a fiber-rich diet are worth it. The NIH recommends increasing fiber intake slowly to avoid temporary digestive issues like bloating. Also, make sure to drink plenty of water to keep the fiber moving through your digestive system.

IN THIS CHAPTER

» Knowing what constitutes a serving of fruits and vegetables

» Choosing healthy, nutrient-dense ingredients from the key food groups

» Enhancing flavors with herbs and spices

» Understanding the benefits of fermented foods, nuts and seeds, and healthy fats

» Finding new ways to incorporate an array of whole plant foods into your diet

» Rediscovering foods you think you don't like

Chapter **4**

Eat the Rainbow

For many folks, lunch or dinner is a sea of beige. They have a deli sandwich and potato chips, or perhaps a piece of meat with potatoes and gravy. However, if you want a diet that's packed with *antioxidants* (substances that may help your body fight off harmful free radicals), vitamins, and minerals, fill your plate with color.

When you add splashes of color to your diet, you get a variety of nutrients and *phytochemicals* (chemical compounds found in plants that offer a variety of health benefits), as well as a meal that makes you want to dig in. Colorful fruits and veggies have been shown to protect against heart disease, cancer, hypertension, and other chronic diseases.

As a new vegan, instead of thinking about what you *don't* eat, focus on all the colorful foods you may have ignored in the past. At every mealtime, challenge yourself to try a greater variety of fruits, vegetables, grains, and beans. Make it a game where you literally see how many different colorful foods you can consume in a day. (Dishes like salads, soups, and stir-fries can really help you get a leg up, because you can throw in a little of this and a little of that.)

Turn your plate into a rainbow of red tomatoes, orange carrots, yellow squash, green broccoli, blueberries, blackberries, and purple cabbage. Every fruit and veggie has its own flavor and texture, and brings its own nutrients to the game. Plus, only plant-based foods have fiber!

In this chapter, I offer suggestions for selecting and preparing delicious, nutrient-dense foods. Consider this your sign to try a greater variety of produce, plant proteins, whole grains, and spices at mealtime.

Identifying Serving Sizes

If you haven't been eating much in the way of fruits and vegetables, you aren't alone. According to the CDC, only 1 in 10 American adults eat the daily recommended amounts. Depending on your gender and age, you should be aiming for at least 1½ to 2 cups of fruit every day, and 2 to 3 cups of vegetables. However, most people are getting far less than that.

REMEMBER

Don't know what a serving entails? The serving size for fruits and veggies is roughly four to six ounces.

Here are a few serving sizes according to the American Heart Association:

>> Apple: 1 medium

>> Avocado: Half of a medium

>> Banana: 1 small

>> Grapefruit: Half of a medium

>> Grapes: 16

>> Kiwifruit: 1 medium

>> Mango: Half of a medium

- » Orange: 1 medium
- » Peach: 1 medium
- » Pear: 1 medium
- » Strawberry: 4 large
- » Bell pepper: Half of a large
- » Broccoli: 5 to 8 florets
- » Carrot: 6 baby or 1 medium
- » Cauliflower: 5 to 8 florets
- » Corn: 1 small ear or half of a large ear
- » Leafy vegetable: 1 cup raw or ½ cup cooked (lettuce, kale, spinach, greens)
- » Potato: Half of a medium
- » Squash, yellow: Half of a small
- » Sweet potato: Half of a large
- » Zucchini: Half of a large

Eating Your Veggies

Don't let your produce linger in the crisper. Find ways to incorporate more vegetables into your diet at breakfast, lunch, and dinner. Remember that a mix of both raw and cooked vegetables is healthy and has something to offer.

- » **Breakfast:** Make a tofu scramble with broccoli, garlic, peppers, kale, and/or spinach. Some leafy greens contain omega-3 fatty acids and lutein, which can help fight the inflammation that's at the root of heart disease, coronary artery disease, and macular degeneration. For a quick breakfast on-the-go, add pickled red onions or thinly sliced radishes to avocado toast.

- » **Lunch:** Pile sliced veggies onto a sandwich with romaine, tomato, onion, and pickles. Make a vegetable-packed soup with sweet potatoes, carrots, spinach, butternut squash, or pumpkin, which all boost immunity with beta-carotene. Or put together a colorful rice bowl with roasted veggies, crispy chickpeas, and a creamy tahini sauce to tie it all together.

>> **Snack time:** Whip up a green smoothie with berries, bananas, nondairy milk, and big handfuls of kale or spinach. Or dip sliced bell peppers, radishes, jicama, cauliflower, and/or broccoli into hummus. Broccoli is packed with vitamins A and B6, manganese, potassium, and folate. It's known for lowering the incidence of cataracts, building bones, and supporting cardiovascular health.

>> **Dinner:** Make a vegetable stir-fry: Add sliced mushrooms, bell pepper, broccoli, asparagus, and whatever other vegetables entice you. Asparagus offers folate, phosphorus, potassium, iron, and zinc, as well as vitamins A, C, and E. Or assemble a huge chopped salad with a baked sweet potato on the side.

Enjoying Fabulous Fruits

Continue the colorful noshing with an array of tempting fruits. It's easy to snack on an apple, orange, or banana. Here are a few ways to squeeze even more fruits into your diet:

>> **Breakfast:** Add sliced strawberries to your cereal. Layer cashew yogurt with fresh berries or cherries, like a parfait. Make blueberry pancakes, or mix frozen blueberries and sliced bananas into hot oatmeal. Blueberries contain folate, vitamins C and E, potassium, manganese, magnesium, and *polyphenols* (plant compounds that work as antioxidants).

>> **Late afternoon snack:** Have a handful of peanuts alongside a banana for a tasty mix of salty and sweet.

>> **Dinner:** Add pineapple to pizza or vegetable fried rice. Add orange segments to a spinach salad. Oranges are temptingly juicy and delicious. Plus, they're packed with vitamin C, folate, potassium, and polyphenols. A single orange provides 3 grams of fiber, which is great for your gut, of course. Fiber can also lower cholesterol, help control blood sugar levels, and keep you feeling full longer.

>> **Dessert:** Eat some fruit for dessert! A bowl of cherries, blueberries, strawberries, diced mango, or a slice of watermelon is a sweet finish to a meal. Watermelon is teeming with vitamins A and C, which are good for supporting immunity, skin and eye health, plus nerve function. The lycopene in watermelon also supports eye, heart, and brain health, and fights *free radicals* (unstable molecules that can damage cells).

COLOR ME HEALTHY: THE RAINBOW COLOR CODE

Eating a rainbow of colorful fruits and vegetables offers a variety of benefits.

- **Red:** Strawberries, tomatoes, red bell peppers, radishes, beets, pomegranates, apples, cayenne pepper, cherries, and watermelon. Many red foods contain vitamins A and C, potassium, and lycopene. Lycopene is an antioxidant, which the body uses to fight cancer and cardiovascular disease.

- **Orange/yellow:** Oranges, carrots, winter squash, orange bell peppers, peaches, mangoes, pineapple, cantaloupe, corn, papayas, grapefruit, nectarines, sweet potatoes, and lemons. Orange foods often contain carotenes. Our bodies turn some of the carotenes into vitamin A, which helps eye health. Yellow foods are packed with vitamin C, which fights disease and helps immunity. Citrus fruits provide folate, which helps reduce the risk of birth defects. Oranges, grapefruit, and tangerines are also unexpected sources of calcium.

- **Green:** Edamame, romaine, herbs, collards, Brussels sprouts, cabbage, green beans, cucumber, zucchini, kale, peas, spinach, asparagus, avocados, artichokes, and broccoli. Green foods often contain lutein, potassium, and vitamin K. Vitamin K helps build strong teeth and bones. Many greens are also rich sources of calcium, especially kale.

- **Blue/purple:** Eggplant, figs, purple cabbage, blueberries, blackberries, mulberries, plums, prunes, purple potatoes, purple onions, and grapes. Blue and purple foods often contain *resveratrol* (an antioxidant that promotes heart and brain health) and *anthocyanins* (antioxidants with anti-inflammatory properties that benefit brain and heart health).

- **White/brown:** Cauliflower, garlic, ginger, jicama, mushrooms, onions, parsnips, potatoes, pears, leeks, and turnips. White and brown foods are often high in potassium, fiber, and phytochemicals that benefit heart health and support the immune system.

Discovering Plant Protein: Beans, Lentils, and Soy

Beans, lentils, and soy are rich sources of nutrients and natural energy. They're also some of the least expensive protein options in the grocery store!

>> **Beans:** Whether you make dried beans from scratch or simply pick up a can, beans contain antioxidants, calcium, magnesium, iron, potassium, phosphorus, vitamin E, thiamin, and B vitamins. They also have fiber, which helps them

to be digested slowly. Slower digestion means stable blood sugar levels and sustained energy.

Endless varieties of beans are available. Black beans, pinto beans, and chickpeas are a good place to start.

- Add them to tacos, salads, and soups.

- Turn pinto or black beans into creamy refried beans. Great for dipping or adding to burritos!

- Make a simple black bean salsa with avocado, corn, bell pepper, garlic, cilantro, a squeeze of lime, and a drizzle of extra-virgin olive oil.

>> **Lentils:** Inexpensive and widely available, lentils are a good source of protein, carbohydrates, and fiber. They also have folate, zinc, and iron.

- Add brown lentils to spaghetti sauce for your next pasta night, and enjoy their satisfying texture and terrific bite.

- Use French lentils (or *lentilles du Puy*) for cold marinated salads.

- Include any type of lentils in curries and soups.

>> **Soy:** Just 3 ounces of super-firm tofu offers 14 grams of protein. Tofu also provides calcium, magnesium, and iron.

- Add marinated and browned tofu to a stir-fry.

- Include a dollop of miso paste in homemade pesto.

- Have an appetizer of steamed edamame. (Lightly sprinkle the steamed pods with salt. Then use your teeth to scrape the pods, allowing the beans inside to pop into your mouth.)

Finding Wholly Nutritious Grains

Whole grains provide an excellent source of energy in the form of complex carbohydrates as well as minerals, fiber, protein, and healthy fats. Eating grains in whole, stone-ground, sprouted, split, or cracked varieties ensures that you're getting great nutrition.

Find complex carbohydrates in brown rice, millet, quinoa, barley, wheat berries, and buckwheat. You can also look to whole grain flour products like crackers, bread, pasta, and cereal.

Whole grains and whole grain products bring balanced energy and fantastic nutrition to your everyday diet. Plus, using them couldn't be easier!

>> Make whole grains like brown rice (short grain, long grain, jasmine, and basmati), barley, or quinoa the base of your meal. (Fun fact: Quinoa is technically a seed. Since it isn't a grain, but resembles one, it's known as a *pseudograin*.)

>> Choose whole grain pastas in various shapes and flavors when you're craving noodles.

>> Enjoy cornmeal polenta (or grits) for breakfast, lunch, or dinner. Choose premade polenta in tubes or ground polenta.

>> Pack your freezer with frozen whole grain pancakes, waffles, or pizza crusts for convenient meals.

>> Have whole wheat bread, pitas, and tortillas on hand for easy breakfasts, lunches, and dinners.

>> Start your day with satiating whole grain breakfast cereal or comforting hot porridge. Oats are high in fiber and low in calories. Plus, they come preloaded with protein, magnesium, potassium, and zinc.

Making "Thyme" for Herbs and Spices

Herbs and spices make meals more delicious and add to their signature flavors. After all, what's a taco platter without cumin, paprika, or chili powder? Who wants curry without turmeric, coriander, or ginger? Where would pasta night be without oregano or basil?

But herbs and spices don't just add flavor to recipes. Many of them are also rich in antioxidants and phytochemicals that help fight inflammation and protect against cell damage.

TECHNICAL STUFF

Don't know the difference between an herb and a spice? Herbs come from the leaves of a plant — think cilantro, oregano, basil, thyme, rosemary, mint, or parsley. Spices come from any other part of a plant, like the roots, stem, seeds, flower, fruit, bark, or berries. Examples of spices include cumin, coriander, paprika, chili powder, and cinnamon.

Here's a small sampling of what herbs and spices provide:

>> **Cinnamon** has been credited with reducing inflammation, as well as balancing blood sugar and lowering cholesterol and triglycerides. Sprinkle it on toast, or add a smidge to your morning oatmeal. When you make coffee, try adding a couple dashes to the coffee grounds for subtle but delicious undertones.

>> **Turmeric** is well known for its anti-inflammatory properties. It contains *curcumin,* a powerful antioxidant that fights oxidative damage, which can be a precursor to early aging and disease. Incorporate turmeric in curries, stews, and soups. Consider adding a pinch of turmeric to your post-workout smoothie or afternoon cup of green tea.

>> **Rosemary** is a good source of vitamins A, B6, and C, as well as iron and calcium. It's also rich in antioxidants and anti-inflammatory compounds, which have been shown to prevent cell damage, improve blood circulation, and support the immune system. Add rosemary to roasted potatoes. It's also terrific in stews, soups, and vegetable potpies.

>> **Chili powder** may boost your metabolism, thanks to *capsaicin.* That's the spicy compound in peppers that gives them their heat. Chili powder has also been shown to help alleviate muscle and joint inflammation by way of its anti-inflammatory properties. Use it to season chili, beans, or fajitas.

>> **Cumin** has anti-inflammatory properties and antioxidants that ward off free radicals, which may help with disease prevention. It has been shown to help control blood sugar and may help lower cholesterol. Add it to hummus, tacos, and curries.

Supporting Your Gut with Fermented Foods

Improve your digestion, increase the good bacteria in your gut, and build immunity with fermented foods like sauerkraut, kimchi, miso, kombucha, and nondairy yogurt. These foods contain *probiotics*, which are microorganisms that have been shown to help with digestion, as well as balance your gut after a round of antibiotics.

Sauerkraut and kimchi are briny, cabbage-based foods that add loads of flavor to dishes. Choose the unpasteurized kind to reap the benefits of its probiotics. (*Note:* In heated or canned kraut, all the good bacteria has been lost.) In addition to its probiotic power, sauerkraut is high in vitamin C.

WARNING

Kimchi is a spicy Korean fermented cabbage that's wonderfully flavorful in rice bowls. However, not all brands are vegan. Be sure to read the ingredients label to check for shrimp paste or fish sauce.

Kombucha is a fizzy fermented tea with beneficial bacteria that supports gut health. Miso is an umami-rich paste made from fermented soybeans.

WARNING

To keep the good bacteria in miso, be careful not to boil it. Temperatures above 115 degrees Fahrenheit can harm the probiotics. If you're making miso soup, stir in the paste after the soup has been taken off the heat. You can also use miso paste in uncooked applications like dressings to keep the probiotics intact.

Here's how to incorporate these fermented foods into your diet:

>> Add sauerkraut to a vegan reuben or veggie bratwurst.

>> Throw a dollop of sauerkraut or vegan kimchi onto rice and noodle bowls.

>> Spread sauerkraut over pizza.

>> Gulp down a refreshing glass of kombucha.

>> Make miso soup for lunch or as a starter to a larger meal.

>> Use sauerkraut and miso paste in homemade vegan cheeses for wonderful depth, richness, and salt.

>> Start the day with nondairy yogurt topped with fresh fruit or granola for crunch.

Eating Nuts and Seeds "Walnut" Fail You

Nuts are often lauded as a satiating snack. Here's another good reason to grab a handful of almonds, walnuts, cashews, peanuts, or hazelnuts: They contain healthy fats, vitamin E, B vitamins, and magnesium, which are a boon for cognition and memory.

Nuts and seeds are easy to carry with you. So grab a container or baggie of these filling snacks:

>> **Almonds:** Almonds are a good source of protein, vitamin E, manganese, magnesium, copper, vitamin B2 (riboflavin), and phosphorus. These nutrients may help lower bad cholesterol, reduce the risk of heart disease, and provide protection against cardiovascular disease.

>> **Cashews:** Cashews are lower in fats and higher in antioxidants than most nuts. A good source of monounsaturated fats, copper, and magnesium, cashews promote cardiovascular health.

>> **Chia seeds:** Chia seeds are loaded with fiber, which helps with intestinal health and cholesterol levels. They also contain protein, antioxidants, omega-3 fatty acids, and calcium. Just 2 tablespoons offer 14 percent of your daily value of calcium, 12 percent of iron, and 23 percent of magnesium.

>> **Flaxseeds:** Flaxseeds are a great source of omega-3 fatty acids. They also offer anti-inflammatory benefits and protect against heart disease, breast cancer, high cholesterol, and diabetes. Flaxseeds are rich in fiber and manganese and are a good source of folate, vitamin B6, magnesium, phosphorus, copper, and *lignan* (a compound in plants known for its antioxidants).

TIP

To get the most nutrition and benefit from flaxseeds, grind them fresh with a spice grinder. You also can buy ground flax meal. Just be sure to store it in the refrigerator or freezer between uses to protect the delicate fats from breaking down in heat and light. Ground flaxseed adds a wonderful whippy texture to smoothies.

>> **Peanuts:** Officially a legume, heart-healthy peanuts are a good source of monounsaturated fat, antioxidants, phytosterols, phytic acid, and folic acid. Peanuts also are a good source of vitamin B3 (niacin), folate, copper, manganese, and protein, and they're a significant source of resveratrol, which has been widely studied for its anti-aging effects. Peanuts and peanut butter may help prevent gallstones and protect against Alzheimer's disease.

>> **Pepitas/pumpkin seeds:** Pumpkin seeds are a good source of essential fatty acids, copper, iron, potassium, phosphorus, magnesium, manganese, zinc, protein, and vitamin K. These little green seeds may promote prostate and bone health and offer anti-inflammatory benefits.

>> **Pistachios:** Pistachios are loaded with fiber, potassium, thiamine, and vitamin B6. They're also rich in phytonutrients, which have been shown to protect against a variety of cancers, as well as help in reducing cholesterol.

>> **Sesame seeds:** Sesame seeds and *tahini,* or sesame butter, are rich in beneficial minerals. Tahini is a good source of manganese, copper, and calcium. Good for lowering cholesterol, sesame seeds also are recommended for rheumatoid arthritis.

TIP

To really gain access to sesame seeds' benefits, it's best to grind or smash them before eating. Tahini is already ground into a paste, so it's an easy way to make the most of sesame's goodness.

>> **Sunflower seeds:** Offering anti-inflammatory and cardiovascular benefits, sunflower seeds may lower cholesterol and help prevent cancer. A good source of vitamin E, sunflower seeds also provide *linoleic acid* (an essential fatty acid), fiber, protein, and minerals such as magnesium and selenium.

>> **Walnuts:** Walnuts are an excellent source of omega-3 fatty acids, manganese, and copper. Good for cardiovascular health and lowering cholesterol, walnuts may also help brain function.

WARNING

If you plan to consume your nuts and seeds within a month, feel free to store them at room temperature. However, if you plan to have them on hand for longer, consider storing them in the fridge since they can go rancid with their considerable fat content.

Embracing Healthy Fats

A diet that includes the monounsaturated fats from nuts and seeds, olives, avocados, and extra-virgin olive oil may lower the risk of heart disease, which is still the leading cause of death in the United States.

Fat is a source of energy for the body, supplying 9 calories per gram, which is more than carbohydrates and protein supply. Fat is necessary for many bodily functions, like protecting and cushioning internal organs and helping the body absorb vitamins A, E, D, and K.

Flax, chia, and hemp seeds have ample amounts of omega-3 fatty acids, which are important for treating conditions such as allergies, arthritis, eczema, inflammatory diseases, and depression. Most cooking oils (olive, safflower, soybean, and sesame) are good sources of omega-6 fats. Nuts and seeds also contain omega-6 fatty acids.

WARNING

Cooking oils are highly refined. Therefore, the healthiest option to get omega-6 fatty acids is through whole foods like nuts and seeds. Most of us are getting too many omega-6 fatty acids and not enough omega-3's. A high ratio of omega-6 to omega-3 may be pro-inflammatory. Using minimally processed cold pressed avocado oil or extra-virgin olive oil are healthier options when cooking with oil.

Many health experts believe that the balanced consumption of omega-6 to omega-3 fatty acids should ideally be three to one. Because vegetable oils are common for cooking, it's important to eat omega-3–rich foods often to ensure the proper balance.

Finally, when it comes to good fat, who can forget avocados? I know you didn't need another reason to start the day with avocado toast, but here are some compelling ones: Avocados contain B vitamins, fiber, and heart-healthy fats, which can help with the absorption of nutrients, as well as contributing to your energy reserves. Add avocado to sandwiches, salads, and grain bowls. Of course, it's always welcome on tacos and burritos, especially in the form of guacamole.

Recognizing That Variety Is the Spice of Life

To really enjoy the wealth of flavor, color, and nutrients in a plant-based diet, go for variety. Instead of turning to the same foods again and again, branch out into unexplored produce, grains, and beans. Try new recipes, and visit different grocery stores from your usual standbys. Grabbing a new produce item at the grocery store or sampling a new-to-you cuisine can liven up your meals and add a variety of nutrients to your diet.

Come to new foods with curiosity. When you're thinking about trying something unfamiliar, let go of preconceptions. A lot of foods have bad PR, but that doesn't mean they aren't delicious and worthy of eating.

For example, I didn't grow up eating tofu. Before I'd even tried it, I'd heard countless jokes about it over the years. It took me a while to come around to it, but now it's one of my favorite foods. I eat it multiple times a week. The key was figuring out how to prepare it properly and realizing that tofu is its own thing. It's not chicken. It's not eggs. It needs to be appreciated on its own merits.

Go to the produce section, refrigerated case, or bulk bins, and pick up something that's new to you. Then do a quick Google search to find out how to prepare it. Seeking out information about new foods can be eye-opening and can help you gain a new appreciation.

TIP

To make it easy on yourself, try adding the new ingredient to a dish you already enjoy. Include it in bowls, stir-fries, tacos, burritos, soups, or pizza. If that still feels too complicated, order a dish that includes the unfamiliar ingredient at a restaurant! After being prepared by a pro, you may come to appreciate the food's finer points.

Figuring Out How to Like the Foods You Hate

If you'd asked me when I was a kid about my least favorite vegetable, I would've said spinach. That pile of mushy, waterlogged goop was the absolute worst. I stuck by that sentiment until sometime in my early 20s when I tried fresh spinach for the first time.

You see, up until that point, I'd only had spinach from a can. Canned spinach does that light, leafy green zero favors. Fresh spinach is wonderful in salads or lightly sautéed. It needs hardly any heat at all to wilt in the pan. It's easy to overcook, which canned spinach does times 1,000.

(I don't want to yuck someone else's yum, but Popeye was severely wrong in his affection for canned spinach.)

Prepare it differently

When people tell me they hate a specific fruit, vegetable, grain, or bean, I encourage them to try it prepared a different way.

An alternative preparation can make a huge difference in terms of enjoying a new food. If there's a vegetable you don't like, try it:

>> Raw

>> Roasted

>> Grilled

>> Steamed

>> Sautéed with minced garlic

>> Pickled

>> Shredded or shaved

Just because you didn't like it as a kid, that doesn't mean you won't appreciate it as an adult. Maybe your parents didn't prepare it in a way you enjoyed, or perhaps your palate has changed over time.

Try a different variety

Next, try different varieties of the same type of food.

>> If you hate acorn squash, give delicata a whirl instead.

>> Don't like lacinato kale? Try curly.

>> Not a fan of black olives? See if you like Castelvetrano. (They're incredibly buttery and delicious!)

>> Dislike shiitake mushrooms? Well, remember, there are more than 10,000 different types of mushrooms! Try meaty portobellos or toothsome oyster mushrooms instead.

TIP

They say that kids have to try something 8 to 15 times before they will accept it. I don't think adults are that far off! Give your palate a chance to adjust. It can take time for expectations to adapt.

Start small

When you're acclimating to a food you haven't liked in the past, start small. For example, if kale tastes too bitter, don't start with a big kale salad. Instead, add a handful to a smoothie or stir-fry. Fold sautéed greens into mashed potatoes, or add a handful of finely chopped kale to your favorite soup just before serving. (It will wilt almost immediately in the hot liquid.)

If you're usually put off by Brussels sprouts, mushrooms, or zucchini, don't sit down to a whole plate of them. Instead, slice them thin and have them as part of a stir-fry with other vegetables you enjoy. Mushrooms and zucchini are also delicious in pasta. Finish the dish with a full-bodied sauce that may mask some of the things you don't like about those veggies.

TIP

Some parents have been known to sneak healthy foods into their kids' favorite dishes. Try that on yourself! Sneak in a handful of broccoli or a smattering of cilantro. Over time, you may be surprised by how once-hated foods can become new favorites.

Chapter **5**

Pinpointing Your Protein Needs

"**B**ut where do you get your protein?"

It's the question that vegans are asked over, and over, and over again.

The question may get repetitive, but the answer is easy: You get protein from the same place that "scrawny" mammals like rhinos, hippos, giraffes, horses, and elephants do — plants!

Many people associate protein with meat, dairy, and eggs. However, there are all kinds of plant-based protein sources available. In this chapter, you find out how protein works in the body, as well as how much humans need on a daily basis. You also get detailed lists to help you plan a protein-rich diet.

Examining What You Need to Know

Protein is an essential *macronutrient* (a nutrient the body needs in large quantities to provide energy and function optimally). Every cell in the body contains protein, and it's a large part of the muscles, bones, organs, and skin.

Protein does the following:

» Builds and repairs cells and tissues

» Supports immune function

» Transports oxygen

» Produces enzymes and hormones

TECHNICAL
STUFF

Proteins are typically composed of 50 to 2,000 smaller units called *amino acids*. To form a complete protein, all 20 different amino acids are needed. Your body creates some of these amino acids by itself, but it must receive nine essential amino acids from food.

Luckily, these essential amino acids can all be found in plant foods. As long as your diet is varied, includes a wide array of whole plant-based foods, and provides enough calories, you don't need to worry about getting enough of these building blocks.

Your body creates the specific forms of protein it needs from the dietary protein you eat. When you eat a bunch of nuts, beans, seeds, whole grains or pseudograins (such as buckwheat), seitan, vegan meats, or tofu, your body breaks down that food. It gets digested by the stomach, absorbed, and formed into new proteins. From there, it can use them to perform various bodily functions.

Knowing How Much Protein You Need

There's no doubt about it — Americans are obsessed with protein. At your local supermarket, you can find protein powders, protein supplements, and even protein water! It's enough to make you think everyone is fighting off protein deficiency, but that's not accurate. According to a 2023 article on the GoodRX Health website, "Americans on average get about double the protein they actually need."

People gulp down protein shakes as if they're bodybuilders, and then take a casual walk around the neighborhood or sit down on the couch to catch up on their favorite TV show. There's just no need for all that extra protein!

When people tell me they're supplementing their diet with protein, I ask if they've actually checked to see if they're low in protein. Inevitably, they haven't. There's no reason to ingest more protein than you need since your body can't store it for later. Once your body's needs are met, extra protein is used as energy or stored as fat.

REMEMBER

The current Recommended Daily Allowance (RDA) for protein is 0.8 grams per kilogram of body weight. For a 150-pound person, that would be 55 grams of protein a day (see the formula in the next section). Most Americans are getting closer to 100 to 120 grams a day, which can lead to a whole host of health problems.

Excess animal protein in your diet can lead to heart disease because of the high saturated fat in many protein-dense animal foods. Plus, excess protein taxes many organs, including the liver, kidneys, colon, and heart.

Protein needs for all ages and stages

REMEMBER

The RDA for protein intake is based on a simple calculation used by the National Institutes of Health. The basic formula is this:

1. **Divide your weight by 2.2 to convert pounds to kilograms.**

2. **Multiply your weight in kilograms by 0.8 to determine your RDA for protein.**

TIP

To make it even easier, you can use a handy online protein calculator. This one from the USDA National Agriculture Library includes a field for your current activity level: www.nal.usda.gov/human-nutrition-and-food-safety/dri-calculator.

Using the calculations above, the RDA for a 125-pound woman who gets moderate to light exercise would be about 45 grams of protein. If you're an athlete, pregnant, lactating, or a senior, you may need to increase your daily protein intake.

Your dietary protein requirements change over the course of your lifetime. Protein is especially important for growth in childhood and the teen years, and in advanced years to combat muscle loss as you age. People who are pregnant or lactating also require more protein during this time of life.

Athletes and bodybuilders have different protein needs than the average healthy, moderately active person, but even these fitness enthusiasts don't need excessive amounts. According to a 2023 article on the Mayo Clinic Health System website, "Even athletes often get more protein than they need without supplements because their calorie requirements are higher. With more food comes more protein." (Check out Part 6 for info on vegan dietary needs for all walks of life.)

The problem with too much protein

REMEMBER

The diseases people suffer from in the U.S. and other developed countries are diseases of excess, not deficiencies. The health issues we hear about on a daily basis are things like heart disease, cancer, strokes, obesity, and diabetes. What we don't hear about is *kwashiorkor,* which is what true protein deficiency is called. (Kwashiorkor is seen in people who are starving. Their limbs are emaciated, while their bellies are distended.)

Instead, people in developed countries are eating excessive amounts of animal protein. Recent studies have shown that the damaging effects of excess animal protein may include high cholesterol, kidney stones and renal failure, overstressed liver and kidneys, and a risk of gout.

Understanding the Benefits of Plant-Based Protein

The standard American diet relies heavily on animal-based foods as the main source of protein. At the same time, health experts and doctors have warned that the current onslaught of diseases is a direct result of our diet. These same experts plead with us to eat more fiber and fresh fruits and vegetables as a way to avoid and heal these illnesses.

Plant sources of protein are a wise choice, especially because so many Americans aren't getting enough fiber in their diet. Beans, lentils, split peas, nuts, whole grains, and seeds are rich in fiber and plant-based phytochemicals. (Phytochemicals have protective properties that may help lower the risk of certain types of cancer, type 2 diabetes, and heart disease.)

In his book *The China Study* (published by BenBella Books), T. Colin Campbell draws out the link between cancer growth and protein. Several studies cited in the book show that a diet including animal proteins can lead to cancer cell proliferation. Plant-based sources of protein haven't shown the same link with cancer growth, so a vegan diet can be considered much safer to reduce the risk of certain types of cancer.

The protein sources you choose may even affect fertility. The Nurses' Health Study, a long-term study involving 18,000 women, showed that infertility in women can be greatly affected by the type of protein they consume.

Women who ate more plant sources of protein were much less likely to have infertility issues than women with few plant protein sources in their diet. Infertility was 39 percent more likely in women who ate the most animal protein.

A 2023 study published in the medical journal *Reproductive Toxicology* reviewed the relationship between nutrition, fertility, and in vitro fertilization outcomes. The study found that women who chose animal proteins were more likely to have ovulatory disorders than those who opted for plant proteins. Research showed that eating more veggies improved embryo quality, and more whole grains were associated with higher pregnancy and live birth rates.

Protein in plant foods

Vegans can meet their protein needs with foods like tofu, tempeh, beans, lentils, peas, seitan, vegan meats, nuts, seeds, quinoa (*keen*-wah), and other pseudograins and whole grains.

At one time it was thought that vegans had to combine different types of protein sources within one meal to get a complete protein. But now we know that as long as a person is eating a varied diet, combining foods in meals isn't necessary. Your body will naturally get all the required amino acids throughout the day.

TIP

While people tend to have protein at dinner, it's sometimes pushed to the wayside at breakfast. Consider starting your day with something protein-dense to decrease hunger and cravings. Examples of protein-rich breakfasts include a tofu scramble, nut or seed butter on sprouted whole grain toast, nondairy yogurt, or oatmeal with a sprinkling of nuts or seeds.

TIP

Folks are sometimes wary of "processed" vegan foods like plant meats. However, they can be a really convenient way to get a lot of protein in one go. Exact protein amounts vary by brand, but here are some general examples:

» A ⅓ cup serving of soy chorizo has 8 grams of protein.

» Three vegan chicken strips have 13 grams of protein.

» A meaty veggie burger has 19 grams of protein.

» A seitan bratwurst has 26 grams of protein.

Enjoy these protein-packed foods alongside whole foods like vegetables and whole grains for a meal that offers the best of both worlds.

REMEMBER

Protein heavy hitters like tofu and seitan are just as digestible as the protein in animal products. Other plant proteins like beans, whole grains, and vegetables are a little less digestible. In addition to protein, when you choose a variety of these sources, you get the added benefits of fiber, phyotchemicals, minerals, and vitamins.

Protein-rich vegan favorites

Once you look at the list of vegan foods in Table 5-1 and their protein content, you'll feel much more comfortable creating healthy menus.

Grab a pen and paper, and figure out how much protein you need according to the formula listed earlier in this chapter. Put together a few days' worth of menus that include the listed foods to reach your daily needs for protein.

TABLE 5-1   **Protein Values of Popular Vegan Foods**

Food	Quantity	Grams of Protein
Almonds, roasted	¼ cup	7
Beans, black	1 cup	15
Beans, chickpeas	1 cup	15
Bread, whole grain	2 slices	10
Broccoli, cooked	1 cup	4
Cashews, raw	¼ cup	5
Hempseed	1 ounce	9
Lentils	1 cup	18
Nutritional yeast	1½ tablespoons	8
Pasta, whole grain, cooked	1 cup	8–10
Peanut butter	2 tablespoons	7
Quinoa	1 cup	9
Rice, brown	1 cup	5
Seitan	3½ ounces	24
Sesame seeds	1 ounce	5

Food	Quantity	Grams of Protein
Soy milk (enriched)	1 cup	8–11
Spinach, cooked	1 cup	5
Sunflower seeds	¼ cup	6
Tahini	2 tablespoons	5.8
Tempeh	1 cup	31
Tofu (super-firm)	3 ounces	14
Veggie burger	1 patty	8–22

Source: U.S. Department of Agriculture's FoodData Central

Meeting Protein Requirements with Ease

It can be very eye-opening when you realize how easily you can meet your protein needs without going to any great lengths.

Consider the earlier example of a 125-pound woman who gets moderate to light exercise (see the section "Protein needs for all ages and stages"). She could meet her RDA of 45 grams of protein with this menu:

Breakfast: Avocado toast on sprouted whole grain bread with seasoned tofu slices (13.5 grams of protein)

Lunch: 2 black bean tacos with chips and salsa (15 grams of protein)

Snack: A handful of peanuts and a banana (7 grams of protein)

Dinner: Brown rice bowl with falafel, hummus, salad, and tahini dressing (17 grams of protein)

Total protein for the day: 52.5 grams

As you can see, it doesn't take a lot of work to meet your RDA of protein. If you have higher protein needs, you could meet them by adding a soy latte at breakfast, including seitan or soy chorizo in your tacos, or having a side of refried beans or quinoa with lunch. For a snack, you could have steamed edamame or protein-rich nondairy yogurt.

Chapter **6**

Getting Essential Nutrients on a Vegan Diet

As you embark on a vegan lifestyle, you may have a number of questions like:

» How will I get calcium without cow's milk?

» Where will I get iron without burgers?

» Can I get omega-3s without eating fish?

Fear not. While many vitamins, minerals, and nutrients are associated with animal foods, that doesn't mean animal products are the only or even the optimum way to get them. You can meet your nutritional needs on a plant-based diet with ease.

In this chapter, I illuminate how you can comfortably get a sufficient amount of calcium, iron, vitamins D and B12, omega-3s, and iodine on a vegan diet.

REMEMBER

Building Strong Bones with Calcium

Calcium is the most abundant mineral in the body. It's the main building block for bones. It's also needed for clotting blood, as well as many muscle and nerve functions. Almost all of it is stored in the bones and teeth, which is what gives them hardness and structure.

Most people associate calcium with milk, particularly cow's milk. It's no secret why. From a young age, we've been told that milk makes strong bones. We're led to believe it's essential.

However, calcium is a mineral, and minerals come from the earth. After all, where do you think cows get calcium? Once cows are past the age of weaning, you don't see them nursing on their mothers. Instead, when they're old enough for solid food, cows get calcium from grass.

TIP

You can also go to the earth for your calcium in the form of plant foods. Plants pull minerals up from the ground with their roots and into their leaves. Choose foods like collard greens, kale, mustard greens, broccoli, beans, okra, peas, Brussels sprouts, seeds, and almonds for your calcium needs.

TECHNICAL STUFF

Plus, plant sources of calcium offer better *bioavailability* than dairy products. That means our bodies have an easier time absorbing and using the calcium in greens than from dairy products. Also, with greens you get the added benefit of magnesium, which helps with bone building.

Yes, we've been told for years that cow's milk is a miracle food in terms of calcium. However, these days, most dairy cows aren't grazing on green grass. They're in feedlots. (When you see cows in grassy fields nowadays, they're generally cows used for beef.) Since they're not in the fields eating calcium-rich grass, their feed is supplemented with calcium. Calcium supplements for cows come from things like limestone, oyster shells, and bone meal. (They know cows are herbivores, right?)

In terms of resources, it doesn't make a lot of sense to supplement cows' diets so that they can produce calcium-rich milk for humans to drink. Instead, we can just supplement our own diets with calcium from plant sources and leave the cows out of it.

Meeting your body's calcium requirements

According to the National Institutes of Health (NIH), recommended amounts of dietary calcium vary by age and life stage.

>> Birth to 6 months — 200 milligrams (mg)

>> 7 to 12 months — 260 mg

>> 1 to 3 years — 700 mg

>> 4 to 8 years — 1,000 mg

>> 9 to 18 years — 1,300 mg

>> 19 to 50 years — 1,000 mg

>> Adult women 51 to 70 years — 1,200 mg

>> Adult men 51 to 70 years — 1,000 mg

>> Adults 71 years and older — 1,200 mg

>> Pregnant and breastfeeding teens — 1,300 mg

>> Pregnant and breastfeeding adults — 1,000 mg

Note that calcium recommendations vary by health organization or what part of the world you're in. According to a 2022 article from *Harvard Health Publishing*, the World Health Organization recommends 500 mg daily for adults (about half the U.S. Recommended Dietary Allowance [RDA]), and the UK sets the goal at 700 mg.

To meet your dietary calcium requirements, eat a variety of the foods in Table 6-1 on a regular basis.

TABLE 6-1 ## Vegan Sources of Calcium

Food	Amount	Calcium (mg)
Vegetables		
Collard greens, boiled	1 cup	268
Turnip greens, cooked, boiled	1 cup	197
Kale, cooked, boiled	1 cup	177
Okra, frozen, cooked, boiled	1 cup	170
Bok choy, cooked, boiled	1 cup (shredded)	158
Broccoli, frozen, cooked, boiled	1 cup	93.8

(continued)

TABLE 6-1 *(continued)*

Food	Amount	Calcium (mg)
Fruits		
Prunes, uncooked	1 cup (pitted)	74.8
Oranges	1 fruit (151 grams)	64.9
Apricots, dried	1 cup (halves)	71.5
Blackberries	1 cup	41.8
Figs, fresh	4 figs (large)	89.6
Beans and Grains		
Cornmeal, yellow, self-rising	1 cup	483
Soybeans, cooked, boiled	1 cup	175
Kidney beans, canned, drained solids	1 cup	152
Oats, regular and quick, unfortified	1 cup	42.1
Chickpeas, canned, drained solids	1 cup	114
Nuts and Seeds		
Almonds, whole	½ cup	192.5
Sesame seeds, whole	1 tablespoon	87.8
Walnuts, black	½ cup (chopped)	38.1
Pecans, halves	½ cup	34.65
Tahini, from roasted kernels	2 tablespoons	128
Brazil nuts, whole	½ cup	106.5
Hazelnuts, whole	½ cup	77
Almond butter	1 tablespoon	56
Flaxseed, whole	1 tablespoon	26
Sunflower seeds, dried	½ cup	54.5
Soy Foods		
Tofu	½ cup	434
Edamame (soybeans), cooked	1 cup	98
Soy yogurt, plain	1 cup	309
Soy milk (Silk Organic Unsweetened)	1 cup	299
Other		
Blackstrap molasses	1 tablespoon	191

Source: U.S. Department of Agriculture's FoodData Central

Spinach, amaranth, rhubarb, chard, and beet greens, which may seem like good sources of calcium, all contain *oxalic acid*, which can bind with calcium and reduce its absorption. These foods are healthy, of course, but they shouldn't be considered good sources of calcium. Other greens like kale, broccoli, mustard greens, and bok choy are better calcium choices.

Avoiding foods that leach calcium

Calcium isn't the only player in the bone health game. Watch out for excess acids, sodium, and alcohol, which can cause your body to leach calcium out of your bones. This can impact your bone health over time.

Here are some foods to omit, reduce, or enjoy in moderation:

>> Alcohol

>> Caffeine

>> Salt/sodium

>> Soda

REMEMBER

The maximum RDA for sodium is 2,300 mg. However, most Americans get at least 4,000 mg of sodium per day. Don't blame your salt shaker right away. Instead, look at prepared and packaged foods. That's where Americans get more than 70 percent of their dietary sodium.

When you take in too much sodium, your body gets rid of it in your urine along with calcium. This, in turn, depletes calcium stores in your body.

Pumping Up Your Iron Intake

Iron is vitally important for energy. It's used to make *hemoglobin,* which blood cells use to transport oxygen.

REMEMBER

There are two forms of iron: heme and nonheme. *Heme iron* is found in animal flesh foods like meat and fish. *Nonheme iron* is found in plant foods like vegetables, fruits, nuts, seeds, grains, and beans.

Obviously, as vegans, we're eating only nonheme iron. Foods that are rich in nonheme iron include lentils, black-eyed peas, chickpeas, cashews, leafy greens, quinoa (*keen*-wah), tofu, and tempeh. Plus, when those foods are eaten with vitamin C powerhouses like lemons, oranges, or red bell peppers, iron absorption is increased.

To get you on track with your iron intake, the following sections provide information on how much to consume, which sources are best, and how to optimize absorption.

Knowing how much you need

According to the NIH, daily iron needs vary by age, sex, life stage, and diet. Here are their default amounts:

» Birth to 6 months — 0.27 mg

» 7 to 12 months — 11 mg

» 1 to 3 years — 7 mg

» 4 to 8 years — 10 mg

» 9 to 13 years — 8 mg

» Teen boys 14 to 18 years — 11 mg

» Teen girls 14 to 18 years — 15 mg

» Adult men 19 to 50 years — 8 mg

» Adult women 19 to 50 years — 18 mg

» Adults 51 years and older — 8 mg

» Pregnant teens — 27 mg

» Pregnant adults — 27 mg

» Breastfeeding teens — 10 mg

» Breastfeeding adults — 9 mg

REMEMBER

The iron needs shown above are for people who include meat in their diets. According to the NIH, "The RDAs for vegetarians are 1.8 times higher than for people who eat meat." This is because nonheme iron isn't absorbed as well as the heme iron found in a meat eater's diet.

Luckily, it isn't difficult to get sufficient iron from plant foods. And vegans aren't any more likely than the general population to develop *anemia*, a dangerous blood disorder caused by iron deficiency. Because vegan diets tend to be high in vitamin C, their ability to absorb iron is improved. (Read more about improving iron absorption with vitamin C later in this chapter.)

Most folks in the U.S. get enough iron. However, these groups are more likely to struggle with getting enough iron and should pay special attention to their daily intake:

- » Frequent blood donors

- » People who have cancer, gastrointestinal disorders, or heart failure

- » Infants

- » People with heavy menstrual periods

- » Pregnant people

TIP

If you are pregnant, talk to your midwife or doctor about taking prenatal iron supplements, eating iron-rich foods, and gauging your specific iron needs. (You can read more on vegan pregnancies in Chapter 21.)

WARNING

If you are in one of the above groups that struggles with iron deficiency or if you have concerns about your iron levels, talk to your doctor about doing a blood test. If your physician deems it necessary, they can recommend iron supplements. (Too much iron can be harmful. So don't take iron supplements without talking to your doctor first.)

Finding iron in plant foods

A diet full of various whole foods and vegetables will easily satisfy your daily iron requirements. Take a look at Table 6-2 to start adding up your needs.

TABLE 6-2   **Vegan Sources of Iron**

Food	Amount	Iron (mg)
Beans and Grains		
Soybeans, boiled	1 cup	8.8
Lentils, boiled	1 cup	6.6
Quinoa, cooked	1 cup	2.76
Tempeh	1 cup	4.48
Black beans, canned	1 cup	4.56
Pinto beans, canned, drained solids	1 cup	3.68
Chickpeas, canned, drained solids	1 cup	2.71
Bulgur, cooked	1 cup	1.75

(continued)

TABLE 6-2 *(continued)*

Food	Amount	Iron (mg)
Vegetables		
Spinach, cooked, boiled, drained	1 cup	6.43
Swiss chard, cooked, boiled, drained	1 cup (chopped)	3.96
Potatoes, baked, flesh and skin	1 medium	1.87
Peas, cooked, boiled, drained	1 cup	2.46
Brussels sprouts, cooked, boiled, drained	1 cup	1.872
Broccoli, cooked, boiled, drained	1 cup	1.046
Nuts, Seeds, and Fruits		
Prune juice, canned	1 cup	3.02
Tahini, from roasted and toasted kernels	2 tablespoons	2.68
Dried apricots	1 cup	3.46
Dried figs	1 cup	3.02
Cashews, dry roasted	½ cup	4.11
Raisins	½ cup (packed)	2.135
Almonds	½ cup	2.65
Other		
Blackstrap molasses	1 tablespoon	3.6
Beyond Burger	1 patty	4
Beyond Sausage, hot Italian	1 cooked link	3.8

Source: U.S. Department of Agriculture's FoodData Central

Helping iron absorption with vitamin C

Iron doesn't work alone. It needs the help of another nutrient to do its work efficiently. When vitamin C is present with nonheme iron, the body can absorb it up to six times better. Luckily, a well-rounded vegan diet provides this nutrient in abundant quantities.

It just so happens that many sources of nonheme iron are naturally high in vitamin C as well. Most leafy greens like broccoli and bok choy are full of both iron and vitamin C, making the iron in these foods more easily absorbed.

Think of all the iron-rich foods you already eat. Then consider the foods you eat with them. You'll probably find that you're already eating iron and vitamin C together, which is why vegans can do so well nutritionally.

Here are some easy ways to eat vitamin C and iron-rich foods together:

>> Squeeze lemon juice over leafy greens.

>> Enjoy a brown rice bowl with tofu, broccoli, and avocado.

>> Have a bean burrito with salsa.

>> Make chili with lentils or beans and canned tomatoes.

>> Nosh on a spinach salad with bell peppers and tomatoes.

TIP

Vitamin C isn't the only nutrient that improves iron absorption! Eating iron-rich foods with alliums and foods high in carotenes also helps. (Foods that are rich in carotenes include bell peppers, carrots, sweet potatoes, and pumpkins. Examples of allium vegetables are garlic, onions, and shallots.)

COAXING OUT IRON WITH CAST-IRON COOKING

Cooking food in a cast-iron skillet is a good way to add iron to your diet, according to a 2021 review published in the *Nepal Journal of Epidemiology*. By examining previous studies on cast iron, researchers found that foods increased their iron content when cooked using cast-iron pots or ingots like *Lucky Iron Fish*. (These fish-shaped blocks of cast iron are placed in cooking liquids to leach elemental iron into food.) The increase was especially notable with acidic foods that are high in vitamin C.

Researchers found that 90 percent of foods contained more iron when cooked in cast-iron pans than in glassware. Foods that were most likely to absorb higher amounts of iron were acidic foods (often high in vitamin C), foods with moisture, and foods cooked for longer periods of time.

Note: Acid increases the iron intake, but it can also increase the metallic flavor in your final dish, especially if foods are cooked for a long period of time. That's something to be aware of if you're sensitive to that tinny flavor. Cooking in cast iron can also cause some high oxalate foods like beets, rhubarb, and spinach to turn brown.

Be aware that children who are 1 to 3 years old only need 7 mg of iron per day. So it's not advisable to go overboard. Don't cook all their meals in cast iron.

Staying away from iron blockers

Vitamin C helps your body absorb iron, but some foods and unhealthy habits can lead to poor absorption. One of the main foods to avoid is cow's milk, which isn't a problem for vegans, of course.

TIP

If you take a calcium supplement, do it when you're not having iron-rich foods, because calcium inhibits iron absorption.

The tannins and caffeine found in tea and coffee also can block iron absorption. Try drinking herbal or decaf teas and coffees instead if your iron levels are a concern.

Phytates are compounds naturally found in many plant foods, including soy and other beans, nuts, seeds, and grains. Phytates can bind with minerals like iron, making it more difficult for the body to absorb them. Luckily, cooking, sprouting, soaking, and fermenting can help disable phytates.

Unhealthy behaviors like smoking and excessive alcohol consumption also can block your body's ability to absorb and properly use iron.

Shining a Light on Vitamin D

Proper vitamin D intake is essential for bone health. It can reduce or prevent the onset of the bone-weakening disease *osteoporosis*. Vitamin D promotes bone formation by helping the body use calcium and phosphorus.

Vitamin D is also essential for a healthy immune system and for improved cardiovascular, skin, and prostate health. It's a fat-soluble vitamin that's stored in the liver, and it can be used by the body during the dark winter months.

Soaking in those rays

Vitamin D is created in your body after your skin is exposed to sunlight or UVB and UVA rays. Without these ultraviolet rays, your body can't naturally produce this essential nutrient.

Most people with lighter skin need only about 15 to 30 minutes in the sun to make enough vitamin D. However, people with darker skin or who live far from the equater may need a longer time in the sun to produce enough vitamin D.

TIP

Avoid using sunblock for those times each day that you're restoring your body's vitamin D. The rays that are blocked are necessary for vitamin formation. Keep the sunblock handy for later in the day, or just apply it to your face.

Supplementing with vitamin D

If you live in any northern location where you rarely see the sun all winter, or if you cover every square inch of your body with clothing when you're outside, consider getting vitamin D from food or supplements.

Vitamin D comes in two forms: D2 and D3. The *cholecalciferol* form of vitamin D3 that's derived from lanolin in sheep is not vegan. However, vitamin D3 derived from lichen and vitamin D2, ergocalciferol, derived from a yeast are both vegan.

Many studies suggest that D2 is as effective as D3 in raising blood serum levels of vitamin D, when taken in large enough amounts. Get your blood levels tested to determine how much vitamin D supplementation you need, if any.

REMEMBER

You can get your daily dose of vitamin D with fortified nondairy milks, fortified cereals, and certain mushrooms that have been exposed to sunlight or another source of UV light. (When buying fortified cereal, check that it's made with a vegan form of vitamin D.) Or take a vitamin D supplement.

TIP

Be aware that if you take calcium supplements, you're likely getting vitamin D from them as well. Check the label to make sure.

Getting a Boost with B12

Vitamin B12 is a must for healthy nerves, blood cells, and neurological functioning. The body also uses B12 in the following ways:

>> To protect and regenerate nerve fibers and repair nerve damage

>> To help maintain the nerves' *myelin sheath*, a protective sleeve of fat and protein

>> To synthesize DNA and RNA

>> To metabolize and use carbohydrates, fat, and protein

Vitamin B12 is made by bacteria, not by plants or animals. Nowadays, food is sterilized and the soil, once rich in B12, is exposed to more pesticides. Therefore, plant-based foods are not a reliable source of B12. Produce was a more reliable source of B12 before humans washed their produce well and when the soil was replete with B12.

Bacteria is attracted to flesh. It's produced in a mammal's digestive tract. Animals who graze may also pick up B12 from manure in the field, and their food is often supplemented with B12. For all these reasons, B12 is found in meat.

TIP

In your new vegan life, to ensure that you're getting all the nutrients you need, take a B12 supplement or vegan multivitamin that includes B12.

The human body doesn't need a huge amount of vitamin B12. However, it does need a little bit on a regular basis. The RDA for B12 is 2.4 micrograms (mcg) a day. You may notice that the amounts in supplements are much higher. They can range from 250 mcg up to 1,000 or even 2,500 mcg per tablet because the absorption of B12 from oral supplements is very low. If you're unsure how much to take, check with your healthcare provider. Some nutrition experts suggest 100 to 250 mcg a day or 1,000 to 2,000 mcg a few times a week.

Vitamin B12 is available in two forms: cyanocobalamin and methylcobalamin. Either one will work. You can find B12 supplements in any drugstore or in the supplement aisle of your favorite natural foods store. Choose from the following oral supplement options: capsules, vegan gummies, sprays, chewable tablets, lozenges, or liquid.

Taking a vitamin supplement is the most reliable option. However, you can add to your B12 reserves with certain fortified products like:

>> Fortified cereals

>> Fortified nutritional yeast flakes

>> Fortified nondairy milks and yogurts

>> Fortified vegan meats made from wheat gluten or soy

Note: Some fermented soy foods like miso, natto, and tempeh, as well as some sea vegetables, have been reported to contain vitamin B12. However, the type of vitamin B12 in these foods are inactive B12 analogs, similar in structure to vitamin B12, but not an active form of the vitamin.

WARNING

Vitamin B12 deficiency isn't common, but can be serious, leading to irreversible neurological damage, nerve damage, and anemia. B12 deficiency can take years to develop, so it's best to avoid it with regular supplementation.

Older people, regardless of the way they eat, sometimes have difficulty absorbing vitamin B12. Also, certain medications can interfere with its absorption.

TIP

If you're concerned about your vitamin B12 status, you can ask for a B12 test as part of your blood work panels. Note that there is a test called *methymalonic acid* (MMA) that is thought to be a better predictor of B12 status than a serum B12 test. Ask your healthcare provider about it. If oral supplements aren't enough to keep your levels adequate, talk to your doctor about B12 injections.

Squeezing in Omega-3s

Omega-3 fatty acids are heart-healthy fats. They help promote brain and heart health, reduce inflammation, and are linked with lower rates of heart disease and certain cancers.

Omega-3s are often associated with fish. But do you know why some fish have omega-3 fatty acids in their bodies? It's because those fish eat algae. As I said earlier about calcium, the minerals we need are plant-based. Fish eat algae and phytoplankton. That's why their flesh contains omega-3 fatty acids.

What does this mean for vegans? You can rely on plants for your heart-healthy omega-3s by consuming chia seeds, flaxseed, hemp hearts, and walnuts.

A vegan diet is already very protective in terms of heart health, but adding plant-based omega-3–rich foods is another great step. Plus, it means you don't have to worry about how much mercury in your diet is "safe," which is a concern associated with eating fish.

TECHNICAL STUFF

Plant-based foods are loaded with a type of omega-3 fatty acid called *linolenic acid* (ALA). The other two essential omega-3 fatty acids are *eicosapentaenoic acid* (EPA) and *docosahexaenoic acid* (DHA). A small percentage of ALA can be converted to EPA and DHA in the body. The amount converted depends on the individual.

Here are some ways to incorporate omega-3–rich foods into your diet:

>> Blend ground flaxseed or chia seeds into a fruit smoothie.

>> Top oatmeal with ground flaxseed.

>> Make chia pudding using chia seeds and nondairy milk.

>> Make salad dressing with flax oil.

>> Add walnuts or hemp hearts to salads.

>> Enjoy a handful of walnuts as a snack.

>> Sprinkle hemp hearts on smoothie bowls or nondairy yogurt.

>> Use walnuts as a substitute for ground beef in tacos or chili.

TIP

If you're concerned about your omega-3 levels, ask your healthcare provider about having an omega-3 index test done to see if you're getting enough. If your levels are low or if you're unsure of your omega-3 levels, consider taking an algae-based omega-3 fatty acid supplement.

Adding Iodine for Thyroid Health

Iodine is an essential trace mineral that's found in the ocean and in soil. Because it's not made in the body, you must get your RDA by eating food or supplements that contain it.

Iodine has many functions in the human body. It helps make thyroid hormones, which keep our cells healthy and regulate blood pressure, heart rate, and metabolism.

Not having enough iodine in your diet can lead to swelling of the thyroid gland (a *goiter*), or an under- or overactive thyroid, which can result in *hypothyroidism* or *hyperthyroidism*.

The RDA for iodine is 150 mcg for adults 19 and older. If you're pregnant, you'll need 220 mcg. If you're lactating, you'll need 290 mcg.

Some people look to non-vegan sources of iodine like fish, eggs, and dairy products. Here's how these animal products get iodine:

>> Fish who swim in seawater absorb it from the water. Amounts vary depending on the water source or if they are farmed fish. Some get it through the algae they eat.

>> Egg yolks contain iodine because iodine is added to chicken feed.

>> Dairy products contain iodine because cows are given iodine supplements in their feed. Plus, disinfectants that contain iodine are used to sterilize milking equipment and wash udders to help with infections like mastitis. Because of that, more iodine ends up in cow's milk.

It seems rather silly to give chickens and cows supplements, so that humans can get those nutrients from eating eggs or milk. Instead, you can cut chickens and cows out of the equation, and simply eat iodine-rich foods yourself.

You can reach your RDA with any of the following methods:

>> **Eat seaweed like kombu (also known as kelp), wakame, and nori.** They're all good natural iodine sources, because they soak in seawater. The iodine content in sea vegetables can vary greatly so check the label or with the manufacturer to make sure you're getting enough or not too much. (The upper tolerable limit is 1,100 mcg a day for adults 19 years and older.)

>> **Use iodized sea salt.** You need ½ to ¾ teaspoon of iodized salt a day to reach the RDA. Check your table salt to see if it's iodized.

Iodine started being added to sea salt in the 1920s to fight against iodine deficiency, which was common in some areas. Approximately 120 countries now have mandatory iodization of all food-grade salt. (In the U.S. iodine fortification is voluntary. Be aware that most processed foods use non-iodized salt.)

Vegans can meet their iodine needs through iodized salt, by adding sea vegetables throughout the week or taking a multivitamin. However, if you have higher needs because you're pregnant or lactating, talk to your doctor about taking a prenatal multivitamin that contains sufficient iodine. (It's sometimes listed as potassium iodide or sodium iodide, or the ingredients list contains kelp, an iodine-rich seaweed.)

Taking a Daily Multivitamin

A well-planned vegan diet is loaded with nutrients. However, you may still want extra insurance by way of a daily multivitamin. It's an easy way to cover your bases. Check the label to ensure that your multivitamin is vegan-friendly (including the vegan version of vitamin D).

WARNING

Unless your doctor recommends it, steer clear of multivitamins that include iron. Too much iron can be as detrimental as too little.

Many supplement companies make quality vegan products. Deva Nutrition, Veg-Life, Garden of Life, Hippo7, and Country Life are just a few brands to consider.

REMEMBER

Talk to your doctor about getting some simple blood tests that can pinpoint specific health concerns to address. Then inquire about any supplementation you may need.

3
Vegan at Home

Stock your kitchen with plant-based staples and basic cooking equipment, and make daily meal preparation a cinch.

Get the lowdown on visiting grocery stores, decoding food labels, and planning your weekly vegan meals.

Satisfy your palate with plant-based versions of foods you already love.

Celebrate all year round with vegan alternatives at holidays and festive gatherings.

IN THIS CHAPTER

» **Stocking your vegan pantry**

» **Shopping for weekly groceries**

» **Storing your fresh produce and pantry items properly**

» **Becoming a savvy vegan shopper**

» **Gathering the basic cooking supplies you need to maximize your success**

Chapter **7**

Gearing Up for Grocery Shopping and Cooking

Vegan cooking is a whole lot easier when you've got a fully stocked pantry, refrigerator, and freezer. With all the essentials at hand, you can whip up plant-based meals in a snap.

This chapter offers the lowdown on stocking your pantry with plant-based staples, as well as what to look out for on food labels. It also helps you choose the tools you need and figure out how to get started.

Feeling confident in the kitchen and knowing that you have basic ingredients at the ready will empower you to create satisfying and delicious meals.

Filling Your Pantry

In this section, I cover the many options that can be included in a vegan pantry. While you could buy everything listed, I don't recommend it! You won't use everything all at once, and it's not indicative of your weekly needs. Think of this section as a road map — it will help you navigate your way toward a vegan kitchen.

After you plan the meals you want to make for a week, buy only the ingredients you need. (For a sampling of what I buy regularly, check out "Getting Weekly Vegan Groceries" later in this chapter.)

Grains, breads, and pasta

Grains, breads, and pasta are an excellent start toward a satisfying meal. With them as the base, you're halfway to breakfast, lunch, or dinner.

>> **Barley:** Pearl (or pearled) barley tends to be more widely available and cooks quicker. However, hulled barley has more vitamins and minerals. Choose whichever one suits your needs.

>> **Bread:** Sandwich bread is a must for toast and sandwiches. Look for simple, easily recognizable ingredients. I especially like Silver Hills Bakery and Dave's Killer Bread. Baguette and sourdough are delicious all-purpose breads that are almost always vegan. Pita is handy for filling with *falafel* (fried chickpea or fava bean patties) or dipping in hummus.

>> **Cereal:** For an easy breakfast, keep one or two types of cold cereal on hand. Cascadian Farm or Nature's Path Raisin Bran cereals are popular options. Nature's Path Crispy Rice is good for making Strawberry Crispy Rice Treats. (You can find the recipe in Chapter 15!)

>> **Crackers:** Water crackers, golden crackers, and saltines are my standard choices. They're good for serving with nondairy cheese or crumbling into chili. For a boost of fiber and nutrients, opt for whole-grain crackers or crackers made with nuts and seeds.

TIP

Surprise! Although they have a buttery flavor, most golden crackers (like Ritz Original) are free of animal products. Of course, it's always best to read the ingredients label to double-check before buying. I usually buy golden crackers from Trader Joe's, which don't include high fructose corn syrup or palm oil.

>> **Noodles:** There are a huge variety of shapes and ingredient options. I usually opt for whole-wheat pasta, but sometimes only plain will satisfy. You can also branch out and try pastas made with legumes like chickpeas, lentils, or edamame, which offer a variety of nutrients. For shapes, choose between

elbow, rigatoni, fusilli, spaghetti, lasagna, linguine, fettucine, farfalle, penne, couscous, rice noodles, and more.

TIP

Most dried noodles are vegan, unless they are specifically labeled as egg noodles. Still, it's always best to read through the ingredients to be sure.

>> **Oats:** Choose steel cut or rolled, depending on your preferences.

>> **Polenta or corn grits:** Great for breakfast, as a side dish, or as the base layer of a one-bowl meal.

>> **Popcorn kernels:** Pop on the stove or in an air popper for a tasty snack.

>> **Rice:** Brown, pink, white, or wild are good starting points.

>> **Tortillas:** Choose between flour, corn, or crunchy hard shells for tacos and burritos.

REMEMBER

When buying prepared items (like bread, cereal, crackers, noodles, and tortillas), be sure to read the ingredients label. That's the easiest way to know for sure if a product is vegan-friendly.

Baking ingredients

If you enjoy baking, you may already have a lot of the items on this list. Many of these baking ingredients are staples in any kitchen.

>> **Agave syrup:** This liquid sweetener is a good substitute for honey.

>> **Baking powder:** This leavening agent is used to lighten the texture in baked goods, as well as increase volume. Baking powder includes both sodium bicarbonate and an acid (like cream of tartar). The reaction of the two ingredients helps baked goods to rise. Baking powder typically includes cornstarch as well to prevent the acid and base from activating during storage.

>> **Baking soda:** Unlike baking powder, which is a mixture of ingredients, this leavening agent is simply sodium bicarbonate and nothing else. It's generally used in recipes where there's already an acid to activate it.

>> **Chocolate chips:** Look for dairy-free semisweet or dark varieties.

>> **Cocoa powder:** This unsweetened chocolate powder is made from ground cocoa beans. When you look at the ingredients label, there should be just one item — cocoa powder. Equal Exchange Organic Baking Cocoa is my go-to option.

WARNING

TIP

Be aware that cocoa powder is different from hot cocoa mix, which usually contains cocoa powder, sugar, and dehydrated milk.

Look for cocoa powder and chocolate with *Fairtrade certification*. This ensures that the farmers received fair pay, and that the cocoa was procured with ethical means, which met environmental standards and prohibited slavery and child labor.

» **Dry active yeast:** This is the most common type of active yeast. It's widely available in stores, and used often in recipes. This all-natural form of yeast creates light, airy textures in dough. If you don't plan on baking bread, you can probably skip this one.

» **Flours:** All-purpose flour and whole wheat flour are popular options. However, you may want to consider using the following as well:

  ● **Gluten-free 1-to-1 baking flour or gluten-free all-purpose flour:** If you plan on doing gluten-free baking, you'll want to pick up a gluten-free flour blend, which is a mix of flours, starches, and *xanthan gum* (a thickening agent). Gluten-free all-purpose flour is good for recipes with yeast, and gluten-free baking flour is good for recipes without yeast.

  ● **Specialty flours:** Depending on your needs, you may want specialty flours like rice flour, teff flour, oat flour, almond flour, spelt flour, cake flour, or quinoa flour.

» **Maple syrup:** Made from the sap of maple trees, this syrup is a delicious multi-purpose sweetener that is a terrific vegan replacement for honey. And of course, it's always welcome on pancakes and waffles. Be sure to choose real maple syrup, not pancake syrup, which is often made with corn syrup, artificial flavors, and colors.

» **Molasses:** Add rich sweetness to baked goods with this thick, dark syrup. I especially love it in chocolate chip cookies! It's also surprisingly nutrient-dense for what is essentially a by-product of the sugar making process. It is rich in calcium, potassium, iron, and antioxidants.

WARNING

Some people do not consider molasses to be vegan if the sugarcane being processed was filtered through *bone char*, a material produced by charring animal bones. If this is a concern for you, look for organic molasses, because organic sugar can't be filtered through bone char.

» **Sugars:** Granulated sugar is the default, all-purpose sugar that's expected when a recipe calls for sugar. Brown sugar is that same white sugar but with molasses added into it. (Depending on the color, more or less molasses has been added.) Powdered sugar is also known as icing sugar or confectioner's sugar. It's simply white sugar that's been finely ground until it becomes a powder. It's great for making frosting for Wacky Cake. (Get the recipe in Chapter 15.)

Some sugars are refined through bone char, but the options listed here are vegan-safe: organic cane sugar, beet sugar, coconut sugar, organic brown sugar, or organic powdered sugar. When in doubt, look for unrefined, raw, or organic sugar if you'd prefer to avoid sugar refined through bone char. For more information about bone char, see the sidebar "Is sugar vegan?" in Chapter 10.

>> **Thickeners:** Cornstarch, potato starch, tapioca starch, or arrowroot are good to have on hand for thickening pie fillings and puddings. In addition to being used as thickeners, they're also useful in gluten-free baking to help with binding.

>> **Vanilla extract:** Choose pure vanilla extract in a glass bottle. It can last several years longer than the kind sold in plastic bottles. Pure vanilla extract is made with vanilla, water, and alcohol. Steer clear of "imitation vanilla," which can add a synthetic, bitter flavor to your baked goods.

Beans and lentils

When it comes to beans and lentils, you can choose between dried, canned, or other precooked options.

For beans, I usually choose canned, because they're convenient and ready to go. You just have to drain and rinse. However, dried beans are sometimes cheaper. Plus, you can control the amount of sodium used in the cooking, as well as how soft you would like the beans to be. It's your call.

You can also find *edamame* (soybeans) in the refrigerated and freezer sections. Either are good options.

There are many types of beans, but here are a few of my favorites:

>> **Black beans:** Great for refried beans, burritos, and Black Bean Tacos. (Recipe in Chapter 12.)

>> **Black-eyed peas:** Use these white and black beans for soups, salads, dips, and black-eyed pea fritters. I especially love cooking black-eyed peas with collard greens and seitan bacon, serving them over grits.

>> **Cannellini beans:** These mild-flavored beans are delicious in soups, pot pies, pasta salads, and cold bean salads.

>> **Chickpeas (also called garbanzo beans):** These are a must for homemade hummus, and they're terrific in soups and stews. You can also use them to make Roasted Chickpeas, a delicious snack. (Get the recipe in Chapter 14.)

- » **Great northern beans:** These delicately flavored beans take on the flavor of whatever is cooked with them. That makes them terrific for soups and stews. They're also lovely cooked with garlic, leeks, sun-dried tomatoes, and handfuls of baby spinach.

- » **Kidney beans:** Perfect for soups, side dishes, and hot or cold salads. They're ideal for making baked beans from scratch.

- » **Pinto beans:** Another good choice for chili, refried beans, tacos, and burritos.

- » **Split peas:** There's nothing like a cozy bowl of split pea soup in cold weather months using either green or yellow split peas. (For smoky flavor, add a tiny splash of liquid smoke.) Split peas are also wonderful in Ethiopian *wots* (stews).

With lentils, I usually use dried. However, vacuum-packed steamed lentils are very convenient for quick meals. Here are a few lentil options:

- » **Brown or green lentils:** These all-purpose lentils are good for soups, salads, and tacos or for adding to pasta sauce instead of ground beef.

- » **French lentils (or *lentilles du Puy*):** These tiny lentils keep their shape during cooking. Use them for salads, soups, and side dishes.

- » **Red lentils:** These lentils don't hold their shape once cooked, which makes them really good for soups or curries, but not for anything where firmness is needed.

Nuts and seeds

Nuts and seeds are handy for snacking, adding to salads, and throwing into curries or stir-fries. If you have a high-speed blender, you can make your own nut butters — as well as nut milks, vegan cheeses, and sauces — from scratch.

- » **Almonds:** Roasted almonds are good for snacking. Raw work well for whipping up nut cheeses and almond milk.

- » **Cashews:** I like to get both raw and roasted cashews. You can enjoy roasted cashews by the handful or add them to stir-fried vegetables. Raw cashews are perfect for making creamy sauces, cashew milk, and vegan cheeses.

- » **Chia seeds:** These omega-3–rich seeds make a good egg replacement (along with water) in baked goods. They can also be added to smoothies for a whippy viscosity. Plus, you can use them to make homemade chia pudding.

- » **Flaxseed (ground or whole):** Use ground flaxseed and water as an egg replacer in recipes. Flaxseed is also a healthy addition to smoothies.

For instructions on how to use chia and flaxseed as egg replacers, turn to the section titled "Binding without eggs" in Chapter 9.

>> **Hemp hearts:** Add these to smoothies or sprinkle them on salads.

>> **Peanuts:** Great by the handful or sprinkled on Cold Peanut Noodles in Chapter 12.

>> **Pecans:** A delicious topper for salads, as well as a protein-packed snack.

>> **Pine nuts:** Add toasted pine nuts to salads, pasta, and rice dishes.

>> **Pistachios:** These delicious nuts are wonderful by the handful, or use them in Basil Pesto Pasta in Chapter 12.

>> **Pumpkin seeds or shelled sunflower seeds:** Tasty for snacking!

>> **Sesame seeds:** Sprinkle on stir-fries, rice bowls, and tofu.

>> **Walnuts:** This all-purpose nut is good for snacking, adding to salads, or turning into vegan taco meat.

Additional pantry items

The following shelf-stable items will last for months or even years in sealed packaging, so stock up when they're on sale:

>> **Artichoke hearts:** Get them packed in water, marinated, or oil-packed. I especially like the grilled variety.

>> **Capers:** These pickled unopened flower buds have a briny flavor that's reminiscent of green olives. Add them to olive tapenade or vegan "chicken" piccata. They're also great on pizza or pasta.

>> **Chickpea flour:** This flour is made with dried garbanzo beans. It can be used as a binder in veggie burgers and falafel. It's a component of seitan, and it's wonderful in savory pancakes such as Italian *socca* or Indian *besan chilla*.

>> **Coconut milk:** Add unsweetened canned coconut milk to curries, soups, and sauces for body and rich coconut flavor.

WARNING

Be aware that the fat content and texture of canned coconut milk is different from the kind sold in cartons for drinking or adding to cereal.

>> **Coffee:** Choose whole bean or ground coffee.

TIP

Look for Fair trade and organic labels to ensure that the beans were ethically sourced without child labor, the farmers were paid fairly, and the beans were produced without pesticides.

- » **Cooking oils:** You have lots of options when it comes to cooking oils. And of course, if you prefer oil-free cooking, you can skip this ingredient. I always have these two types on hand:

  - **Avocado oil:** This is my preferred all-purpose oil for cooking, because of its neutral flavor and high smoke point. You can even fry with it.

  - **Extra-virgin olive oil (EVOO):** This antioxidant-rich oil is good for dressings, dips, and general-purpose cooking. It also makes a delicious bread dip with seasonings and balsamic glaze.

- » **Dolmas:** These stuffed grape leaves make a nice snack or addition to a *mezze* (Mediterranean appetizer) platter. Look for leaves stuffed with rice, not meat.

- » **Hearts of palm:** Harvested from the inner core of certain palm trees, this ingredient is usually sold in cans or jars. It has a flaky texture and mild flavor that makes it especially good for vegan versions of seafood dishes like crab cakes, fried shrimp, lobster rolls, or ceviche.

- » **Hot sauce:** Add a kick to your dishes with hot sauce. Arizona Gunslinger Red Jalapeño Pepper Sauce is my favorite all-purpose hot sauce. It's great for adding to chili or sprinkling on tacos. TRUFF Sauce is also amazing if you like the flavor of truffles. If you like buffalo flavors, pick up a bottle of Frank's RedHot Sauce. Simply mix it with melted nondairy butter for vegan buffalo sauce. Then use it on browned tofu, breaded cauliflower, seitan, or vegan chicken.

TIP

  I like to make my own vegan buffalo sauce. But if you'd prefer a store-bought version, Frank's Buffalo Wings Hot Sauce is vegan; the "natural butter type flavor" listed on the ingredients is actually vegan.

- » **Jalapeños:** Pickled jalapeños add heat and briny crunch to nachos, tacos, and sandwiches. Although I prefer homemade pickled jalapeños, having a jar of store-bought peppers in the pantry is convenient.

- » **Jams, jellies, and fruit butters:** Options include strawberry, blackberry, apple butter, and pumpkin butter.

- » **Ketchup:** Naturally sweetened is best!

- » **Liquid smoke:** Add a tiny splash anywhere you'd like a smoky flavor, like in collard greens, barbecue sauce, or split pea soup. A little bit goes a long way!

- » **Mustard:** There are many varieties to choose from, including yellow, stone-ground, or spicy.

- » **Nut and seed butter:** Choose between options like almond, peanut, sunflower seed, or cashew.

- » **Nutritional yeast flakes:** Nutritional yeast can be a supplement or a major component in a cheesy sauce or *seitan* (wheat meat). It can also be used as a seasoning on popcorn. (Read more information about nutritional yeast in the section "Get cheesy with nutritional yeast" in Chapter 9.)

>> **Olives:** Try a variety of types, like Castelvetrano, kalamata, Cerignola, or Niçoise.

>> **Pasta sauce:** Jarred sauce makes a quick pasta dinner so much easier! Use it on spaghetti, vegan ravioli, or vegan lasagna. It's also a delicious dipping sauce for garlic bread or vegan cheesy bread.

WARNING

Be sure to read check the ingredients list for dairy or meat products. Dairy-based cheese has a way of sneaking in!

>> **Pickles:** Choose dill, kosher, gherkins, sweet, bread and butter, or cornichons. Depending on the type, you can use them on vegan charcuterie boards, sandwiches, salads, or for snacking.

>> **Ramen:** Look for vegan varieties from organic brands like Koyo. My preferred flavor is shiitake mushroom. If you want to splash out, try one of Sun Noodle's ramen kits, sold in the refrigerated section of the grocery store. The kits include fresh noodles, which can't be rivaled.

>> **Salsa:** Jarred salsa is super convenient as a snack with chips. You can also spoon it onto vegan quesadillas or nachos.

>> **Soy sauce:** Wheat-free tamari is my go-to soy sauce. Other alternatives include Bragg Liquid Aminos or coconut aminos.

>> **Tomatoes:** Choose between diced, crushed, or whole. They're sold in cans, cartons, and jars. While tomato paste is often sold in jars, toothpaste-style tubes are easier to use and last longer once opened.

>> **Tahini:** This sesame seed butter is a must for making hummus, as well as for adding creamy body to sauces, soups, and dressings. Soom and Seed + Mill are my preferred brands.

>> **Tea:** Caffeinated teas like English breakfast or green tea are nice for an afternoon pick-me-up, while decaffeinated teas like chamomile or rooibos are ideal for winding down at night. (Fun fact: Rooibos and chamomile aren't technically teas. They're officially herbal infusions or tisanes.)

>> **Toasted sesame oil:** This nutty oil is delicious in stir-fries, sauces, and dips. Don't use it for high-heat cooking.

>> **Tortilla chips:** Good for snacking with salsa or guacamole.

>> **Vegan Worcestershire sauce:** Most Worcestershire sauce isn't vegan. Look for brands like Annie's and The Wizard's, which don't include anchovies or fish sauce.

>> **Vegetable bouillon or broths:** Better Than Bouillon, in either No Chicken Base or No Beef Base, is great for soups, stews, and gravies. If you'd prefer, use vegetable broth or other types of vegetable bouillon.

>> **Vinegar:** It's good to have a variety of vinegars for dressings, sauces, and homemade pickles. Consider options like balsamic, red wine, apple cider, rice, or white.

>> **Vital wheat gluten:** This high-protein flour is essential for making homemade seitan. It's made from wheat flour that's been processed to remove everything but the gluten. Bob's Red Mill is my preferred choice.

Spices, seasonings, and herbs

Seasonings help you achieve the flavors you crave — whether it's cheesiness, smokiness, or spiciness. When you add a dash of this or that, suddenly your meal develops new levels of interest.

However, when you're stocking a vegan pantry for the first time, you may want to err on the side of simplicity. Buy a few spices that have a multitude of uses to get the most bang for your buck.

If I was getting only a handful, my short list of dry seasonings would be:

>> **Ancho chili powder:** Typical chili powder is a spice mix that varies by brand. However, ancho chili powder is made from one ingredient: ancho chilies. (When they're fresh, they're called poblano peppers.) Ancho chili powder adds warmth and deep rich flavors without amping up the heat.

>> **Basil:** Dried basil brings a nice balance to dishes like tomato soups and sauces.

>> **Cumin:** This spice-of-all-trades is an essential ingredient in cuisines from India to the Middle East, and Mexico to Portugal. It's used in tacos, curries, hummus, and *baba ghanoush* (roasted eggplant dip).

>> **Granulated garlic:** I always have fresh garlic cloves on hand, but granulated garlic is useful in smooth sauces or when you want a less intense flavor than fresh provides. I prefer granulated over powdered garlic, because the larger, coarsely-ground granules offer bolder notes of garlic.

>> **Granulated onion:** Similar to onion powder, this flavor agent adds deliciousness to savory dishes. I prefer granulated over powdered, because the coarse texture offers a stronger punch of onion flavor.

>> **Kala namak:** Also called black salt, *kala namak* is a sulfurous salt that gives food an eggy taste and smell. (If you didn't like the taste of eggs, obviously you'll want to skip this one.) Even though it's called black salt, the color straight out of the bag is pink (but don't confuse it with Hawaiian pink salt). Look for kala namak in Indian grocery stores or online.

>> **Oregano:** This fragrant herb has a distinctive smell that's strongly associated with pizza and pasta dishes. You see oregano in all kinds of cuisines, including Mediterranean dishes and Latin food.

>> **Paprika:** Bursting with bright red color, paprika is packed with nutrients. It's made from grinding mild peppers, but its flavor doesn't overwhelm. If you crave a bit of smokiness, smoked paprika adds a beautiful edge, reminiscent of a campfire.

>> **Rosemary:** Rosemary adds a wonderful piney scent and flavor to everything it touches.

>> **Salt:** Sea, kosher, smoked, or iodized are all excellent salt options. (Read more about the benefits of iodized salt in the section "Adding Iodine for Thyroid Health" in Chapter 6.)

>> **Thyme:** This herb is well suited to winter holiday dishes and soups.

Other seasoning options include allspice, bay leaves, black pepper, cardamom, cayenne pepper, celery seeds, chili powder, cinnamon, cloves, coriander, curry powder, dill, dried ginger, fennel seeds, garam masala, marjoram, red pepper flakes, saffron, sage, and turmeric.

TIP Feeling overwhelmed by seasoning options? Think about the types of cuisines that you love the most, like Italian, Mexican, Thai, or Indian. Then stock up on the spices most commonly used in that cuisine's dishes. (If you need ideas, look up recipes online or buy a vegan cookbook focused on that specific cuisine.)

TIP You can also buy smaller amounts of spices by using the bulk bins at the grocery store and getting only what you need for a recipe. Or pick up small spice packets at stores like World Market, which can be more cost-effective than committing to a full-sized jar.

In addition to dried herbs, it's also nice to have some of the following fresh herbs on hand for garnishes, sauces, salads, and spreads:

>> Basil

>> Chives

>> Cilantro

>> Dill

>> Oregano

>> Parsley

>> Rosemary

» Sage

» Thyme

Fresh produce

Fresh produce makes up the bulk of most vegans' diets. Challenge yourself to try some new-to-you items, and fill your plate with fruits and veggies. However, because fresh produce has a limited shelf life, don't overbuy.

» Avocados

» Bell peppers (red, yellow, or orange)

» Broccoli

» Brussels sprouts

» Cabbage

» Carrots (orange, purple, red, white, or yellow)

» Cauliflower

» Celery

» Collard greens

» Cucumbers

» Fruit (apples, bananas, blackberries, blueberries, cherries, grapefruit, grapes, kiwi, lemons, limes, melons, oranges, pears, pineapple, strawberries)

» Garlic

» Jalapeños

» Kale (curly, lacinato, or purple)

» Mushrooms (cremini, portobello, oyster, white button, or shiitake)

» Onions (yellow, white, or red)

TIP

One of my favorite ways to enjoy red onions is by quick pickling them. They add amazing tang to salads, sandwiches, bowls, or a vegan charcuterie board. Because quick-pickled veggies aren't canned (and therefore aren't shelf stable), you must store them in the refrigerator. You can find my favorite recipe for easy pickled red onions on my website, https://cadryskitchen.com/easy-pickled-red-onions.

» Potatoes (russet, yellow, red, or fingerling)

» Salad greens (spinach, romaine, or green leaf lettuce)

>> Sweet potatoes

>> Tomatoes (red, pink, orange, yellow, green, or purple)

>> Winter squash (butternut, acorn, delicata, or kabocha)

Tofu, tempeh, and vegan meats

Tofu, tempeh, and vegan meats are mostly found in the refrigerated or frozen sections of the grocery store. They are often protein-rich, and can easily replace meat in recipes.

>> **Jackfruit:** If you're planning on using jackfruit as a meat substitute, look for canned young or green jackfruit that's been packaged in water or brine, and avoid ripe jackfruit packed in syrup. It's much too sweet for savory applications.

>> **Seitan:** This high-protein vegan meat comes in a variety of flavors. Get store-bought seitan or make your own from scratch.

>> **Soy chorizo:** This highly seasoned crumbly sausage is wonderful in tacos, nachos, burritos, and Ultimate Homemade Chili in Chapter 12.

>> **Tempeh:** This traditional Indonesian food is made with fermented soybeans that have been formed into a cake or patty. Some types of tempeh include a grain as well. Use it for tempeh bacon or tacos. It's also tasty cooked with barbecue, teriyaki, or peanut sauce.

>> **Tofu:** Super-firm vacuum-packed tofu is my favorite, because it doesn't need to be pressed. (Depending on your needs or local availability, you may prefer water-packed or silken tofu.) You can also buy flavored tofu (like teriyaki or sriracha) that has already been baked and can be enjoyed right out of the package.

>> **Vegan chicken:** You can find breaded tenders, as well as chunks and filets without breading.

>> **Vegan deli meats:** Deli slices are a handy option for sandwiches or vegan charcuterie boards.

>> **Vegan ground beef:** You can choose between kinds that can be easily formed into patties for burgers, as well as preformed patties and crumbles.

>> **Vegan meatballs:** Serve vegan meatballs with pasta or in a sandwich.

>> **Vegan sausages and vegan hot dogs:** Look for vegan bratwurst, Italian sausages, breakfast sausages (patties or links), frankfurters, and more. They're sold in the refrigerated or frozen sections of the grocery store.

Additional perishable items

Fill your fridge with these plant-based items:

>> **Hummus:** Make your own or get store-bought hummus in a variety of flavors like plain, garlic, roasted red pepper, sun-dried tomato, or kalamata olive. Use it as a dip or spread. Here's my basic hummus recipe: `https://cadryskitchen.com/homemade-hummus/`.

>> **Miso paste:** This fermented soybean paste is a delicious addition to soups, sauces, and vegan cheeses. I use white miso paste most often, but depending on the recipe, you may also want yellow or red.

>> **Nondairy butter:** This can be used 1-to-1 for dairy-based butter. It comes in tubs as well as sticks. Nondairy butter is usually made from a blend of vegetable oils or natural ingredients like nuts or seeds. If you don't want to buy nondairy butter, there are loads of recipes online to make your own.

WARNING

Some vegans avoid nondairy butter made with palm oil, out of concerns for its environmental impact, habitat loss for animals like orangutans (among other animals), and human rights violations. However, some nondairy butter brands that use palm oil promote that they only use sustainably sourced and socially responsible palm oil. These are things you may want to consider when buying nondairy butter.

>> **Nondairy milk:** Loads of nondairy milks are available. Popular options include soy, almond, oat, or cashew milk. Drink it by the glassful, add it to cereal, use it in recipes, or add it to coffee. (If you prefer, grab nondairy creamer for your coffee needs.)

>> **Nondairy sour cream:** It's not an essential, but a dollop is nice on tacos, nachos, or baked potatoes.

>> **Nondairy yogurt:** Choose plain unsweetened or flavored nondairy yogurt for breakfast or a snack. It can be made from a variety of bases like soy, almond, cashew, or coconut milk.

>> **Sauerkraut:** This probiotic-packed condiment is a must for vegan reubens or veggie bratwursts. It's also a tasty addition to rice bowls. Be sure to get the refrigerated kind, not canned, to reap the benefits of the probiotics.

>> **Vegan cream cheese:** Plain and flavored options are made from a variety of bases like almond, cashew, coconut, or soy. Miyoko's Creamery Savory Scallion is my favorite choice for spreading on bagels.

>> **Vegan eggs:** Options like JUST Egg and WunderEggs are ideal when you want the plant-based version of a fried, scrambled, or boiled egg.

>> **Vegan kimchi:** This spicy Korean fermented cabbage is a delicious addition to rice bowls. Not all types are vegan. Be sure to check the ingredients for shrimp paste or fish sauce.

>> **Vegan mayonnaise:** Vegenaise is my favorite among the many options available.

>> **Vegan ravioli:** These stuffed noodles contain delicious fillings like cashew cheese, mushrooms, or butternut squash.

>> **Vegan salad dressings:** Make your own or buy premade dressings for easy salads. You can find three of my favorite salad dressing recipes in Chapter 14.

For the freezer

When time is short and hunger is high, the freezer can be a terrific resource for quick meals. Stock your freezer with any of the following:

>> **Appetizers:** Some of my favorites include vegetable pot stickers, samosas, and spring rolls.

>> **Fruits:** Great for smoothies! Look for blueberries, strawberries, tropical fruits, and pitted cherries.

>> **Nondairy ice cream:** Choose from endless flavors and bases like cashew, almond, sunflower seed, oat, soy, and more. I particularly love a vegan ice cream sandwich on a summer day.

>> **Pizza:** There are many types of vegan frozen pizza available with a variety of topping options — including vegan pepperoni and sausage.

>> **Potatoes:** For easy side dishes, pick up fries, tater tots, or hash browns.

>> **Rice:** While you can easily make rice from scratch, having frozen rice on hand is a convenient shortcut. You'll find options like basmati, Spanish, and rice mixed with vegetables. You can even get cauliflower rice, which isn't technically rice. It's simply cauliflower that's been finely chopped until it's rice-sized.

>> **Vegetables:** When you're in a rush or your favorite veggies are out of season, look for frozen corn, edamame, mixed stir-fry vegetables, peas, and more.

Getting Weekly Vegan Groceries

It's easy to get overwhelmed by the many vegan grocery options listed previously in this chapter, but let's break it down. Most of the time you won't need to pick up staples like seasonings, flours, and condiments. Once you have a fully-stocked pantry, you only have to buy whatever ingredients you need for that week's meals and snacks.

Figure 7-1 is an example of what I buy on my weekly grocery run. Depending on your needs, you may want more, fewer, or different products. You can use my shopping list as starting point.

Produce
- ☐ Apples
- ☐ Avocados
- ☐ Bananas
- ☐ Basil (fresh)
- ☐ Bell peppers
- ☐ Broccoli florets
- ☐ Brussels sprouts
- ☐ Cabbage (shredded)
- ☐ Carrots
- ☐ Cauliflower
- ☐ Celery
- ☐ Cilantro (fresh)
- ☐ Collard greens
- ☐ Cucumbers
- ☐ Garlic
- ☐ Grapefruit
- ☐ Kale
- ☐ Lemons
- ☐ Lettuce (romaine or green leaf)
- ☐ Mushrooms
- ☐ Onions
- ☐ Pineapple
- ☐ Potatoes
- ☐ Tomatoes
- ☐ _____
- ☐ _____
- ☐ _____
- ☐ _____
- ☐ _____
- ☐ _____
- ☐ _____

Refrigerated
- ☐ Nondairy milk
- ☐ Nondairy yogurt
- ☐ Soy chorizo
- ☐ Tofu

- ☐ Vegan deli slices
- ☐ _____
- ☐ _____
- ☐ _____
- ☐ _____
- ☐ _____

Frozen
- ☐ Rice (brown or Spanish-style)
- ☐ Strawberries
- ☐ Vegan chick'n strips
- ☐ Vegetable pot stickers
- ☐ _____
- ☐ _____
- ☐ _____
- ☐ _____
- ☐ _____
- ☐ _____

Pantry
- ☐ Baguette
- ☐ Beans (canned black, pinto, and chickpeas)
- ☐ Cashews (roasted)
- ☐ Lentils (dried brown, red, or French)
- ☐ Pasta
- ☐ Pasta sauce
- ☐ Peanuts
- ☐ Salsa
- ☐ Sandwich bread
- ☐ Tortilla chips
- ☐ Tortillas
- ☐ _____
- ☐ _____
- ☐ _____
- ☐ _____
- ☐ _____
- ☐ _____

FIGURE 7-1: My weekly grocery list.

Following the Storage Guidelines

Proper storage of whole foods, dry seasonings, and fresh herbs is important to ensure that they stay fresh as long as possible. This section provides an overview of how to store your vegan ingredients appropriately. Consider the following guidelines:

>> **Dry grains and legumes:** Keep beans, lentils, and grains in well-sealed containers away from light, moisture, and heat.

>> **Crackers and chips:** Store in a cupboard and seal with a clip to keep them from going stale.

>> **Shelled nuts and seeds:** If you plan to consume your nuts and seeds within a month, store them at room temperature in sealed containers. However, if you plan to have them on hand for longer, consider storing them in the fridge. With their considerable fat content, they can go rancid over time.

>> **Whole grain bread:** Bread without any preservatives is more likely to mold. If you can't finish it in a few days, store it in the freezer to help it last longer.

>> **Fresh fruits and vegetables:** Most produce should be stored in the crisper drawer of your fridge. Exceptions are bananas, stone fruits like peaches, and tomatoes, which lose flavor in the fridge.

TIP

To ripen avocados, leave them on the counter. You'll know they're ready to use when they yield slightly to pressure from your thumb. Once they feel ripe, move them to the refrigerator to slow ripening so they don't go bad before you can use them.

>> **Potatoes, onions, ginger, and garlic:** These ingredients are fickle, but when stored properly, they stay fresh for a long time. Store garlic heads in a cool, dark place to prevent sprouting. (A countertop garlic keeper works beautifully!) Potatoes and onions should be kept separate from each other in a cool, dark place to reduce contact spoiling. Ginger keeps well in the freezer. It can be grated while frozen.

>> **Dry seasonings:** Herbs and spices (or other dry seasonings) should be stored in sealed containers in a dark cabinet or drawer away from moisture and the heat from the stovetop or oven.

TIP

To organize your seasonings, you can either move those you use most often to the front of the pantry, or you can organize them from A to Z in a spice rack so you always know where to find them.

>> **Fresh herbs:** Store fresh herbs in plastic storage bags or other sealable containers in the crisper drawer of your fridge. Don't wash them until you're ready to use them, because moisture promotes spoilage. When it's time to use them, wash the herbs and dry them completely. They're much easier to chop when dry. (I recommend using kitchen shears for easy chopping.)

>> **Oils:** Since heat and light can cause oils to go rancid quickly, store them in a cool dark place, away from heat (not next to the dishwasher or stove). For oils with high omega-3 content, like flax or walnut oil, store in the refrigerator.

Buying Groceries: A Vegan Shopping Guide

In this section, I highlight the best places to seek out plant-based food, and I give you the lowdown on reading food labels. (Chapter 17 deals with shopping for vegan nonfood items.)

These days there are tons of options when looking for vegan groceries. Of course, produce has always been available at any grocery store. But now vegan specialty products are popping up at more mainstream places. Some spots to check out include:

>> **Health food or natural food stores:** You're sure to find loads of organic produce, bulk bins, and vegan specialty products at natural food stores. Many of these stores offer deli counters with vegan options, as well as fresh juice and smoothie bars. These stores also are a good place to buy cruelty-free health and beauty products.

>> **Co-ops:** These natural food stores are cooperatively owned by the people who shop there. Member owners usually get some kind of discount for their membership fee. However, anyone can shop there — with or without a membership. Co-ops are often filled with local produce, making them almost an offshoot of the farmers market. They tend to carry a lot of vegan specialty items as well.

>> **Farmers markets:** Don't miss the farmers market in your community! It overflows with fresh and in-season local produce. Usually held during warm-weather months, farmers markets offer a variety of fruits and vegetables, baked goods, condiments, and sometimes soy products.

TIP

One of the fun things about the farmers market is the sheer variety of produce. Vendors offer much more than what you see at a brick-and-mortar grocery store. Garlic *scapes* (long green shoots that grow from the garlic bulb), squash blossoms, or *purslane* (a trailing plant that's unusually high in omega-3) may not be on your everyday menu. Give something new a whirl!

>> **Community supported agriculture:** Also known as CSA, this is a way to support your local farmers and get a great deal on produce at the same time. You pay for a share of the farmers' crops at the beginning of the season. Then, as food ripens, you pick it up at the farm (or a designated pickup point like a farmers market).

For the most part, you don't get to choose what you're getting with CSA. It just depends on what's ready at the time. It's a good way to diversify your diet and eat a variety of produce.

>> **Mainstream grocery stores:** Options keep getting better at your average grocery store, where you may find vegan-friendly products, as well as organic produce sections, bulk bins, and international aisles. If your grocery store has a health food section, check out their fresh, frozen, and pantry sections.

TIP

Is there a specific item you'd like that's not currently available? Talk to your local grocery store manager and request it.

>> **Big-box stores:** Look for vegan meats, nondairy cheeses, plant milks, and snacks at Target, Walmart, and other big-box stores. Sometimes vegan specialty products are in their own special section. Other times they're commingling with the non-vegan products. Vegan products are peppered throughout the refrigerated, dry goods, and frozen sections.

>> **Indian markets:** These stores offer lentils, herbs, spices, fresh produce, and whole grains. They're a great place to pick up kala namak (black salt) for adding eggy flavor to dishes.

>> **Chinese, Japanese, and Korean markets:** These markets offer huge varieties of leafy green veggies, spices, soy foods and tofu, noodles, teas, grains, and beans. I love going there for frozen udon noodles and shelf-stable rice noodles for stir-fries.

>> **Middle Eastern markets:** Middle Eastern markets offer hummus, beans, stuffed grape leaves, olives, and breads.

>> **Warehouse and membership stores:** These stores may offer great deals on certain bulk purchases, such as grains, beans, soy foods, and even organic produce.

TIP

If you don't already have a membership to one of these stores, find out whether any of them offer special sneak previews for nonmembers. A sneak preview allows you to explore the aisles to look for items you would buy, which in turn helps you decide whether the membership is worth the price.

Shopping smarter, not harder

Make grocery shopping easier and more enjoyable with these tips:

>> **Take a list to stay on track.** It's exasperating to get home and realize you forgot the one thing you went to the store to get. Plus, a list can help prevent you from veering too far off with impulse purchases.

>> **Shop during off-peak hours.** If possible, skip weekdays during the 5 o'clock rush and weekends when everyone else is buying for the week.

>> **Avoid shopping when you're hungry.** Your stomach has a way of convincing you to throw a lot of foods into the cart that you may have skipped otherwise. Eat a snack before you leave the house.

>> **Choose stores that offer the best deals on the foods you always buy.** Take some time to visit different stores and figure out who has the best deals on the groceries you buy week after week. Even small savings add up over time.

>> **Activate digital coupons or member deals on store apps.** If you use apps like Target Circle, see what promotions and discounts are available on vegan products. Activate digital coupons and member deals before heading to the store so that they're ready at checkout time.

>> **Consider using a grocery delivery service.** When you're short on time, grocery delivery services can bring everything you need for a week of meals right to your door. Many grocery stores have their own delivery service, or you can use apps like Instacart.

TIP

Follow along on your app as the shopper gathers your groceries. That's when they'll ask if any substitutions will work for items that aren't available. It's good to keep an eye on the chat to make sure they don't trade out your vegan items with non-vegan ones.

>> **Use grocery store pickup.** Many grocery stores and big-box chains offer grocery pickup outside their stores. It's generally cheaper than delivery, and in some cases, free. Order groceries online or use the store's app. Then drive over when the groceries are ready. Pull into one of the designated pickup spots in the parking lot, and a team member will bring your groceries right to the car.

TIP

If you're particular about your produce, you may want to use grocery delivery or pickup only for shelf-stable or frozen items.

Reading labels

Reading labels is essential for vegans, but really, it should be a habit for everyone — regardless of how you eat! You should know what's in your food, so you can make informed decisions.

REMEMBER

When you're looking at the ingredients on a food label, remember that they're listed in descending order by weight. That means the ingredient listed first is the largest in the package by volume. The second item is the next largest, and so on, down to the smallest component.

In general, healthier products have fewer and more easily identifiable ingredients. Lean toward products that contain whole grain flours or whole grains, and natural sweeteners.

When you first go vegan, reading labels can take a bit of time. But after a while, you know what to watch out for, and the process goes pretty quickly. (These days I can look at a food label and know in seconds if it's vegan or not. Non-vegan ingredients just jump out at me.)

It's very handy when products note on the front of the package that they're vegan or have a "Certified Vegan" logo, but most do not. Get good at reading food labels, and find out for yourself which products are vegan-friendly.

TIP

I like to start by looking at the allergens in bold just underneath the ingredients list. If you see it contains milk, eggs, fish, or shellfish, you know it's an immediate no.

After that, read through the ingredients list.

If there is an ingredient you don't recognize, do a simple Google search to find out if it's vegan-friendly or not.

TIP

Buying online? Many stores include the food label with the product listing. Take a peek at the ingredients before adding the product to your cart.

Knowing what to avoid

When you're reading the ingredients label, you obviously want to avoid foods that include any type of meat, dairy, eggs, or bee products.

Here are some of the less obvious ingredients to watch out for when grocery shopping:

>> **Albumen:** This comes from egg whites and is sometimes found in cakes, candies, cookies, or wine (as a clarifying agent).

>> **Carmine/cochineal:** It's made from grinding cochineal scale insects to make a red dye used in certain foods (such as drinks and candies) and make-up.

>> **Gelatin:** Derived from boiled animal bones, tendons, and ligaments, it's often found in gummy candies and marshmallows.

>> **Honey or beeswax:** These bee-made products are not vegan.

>> **Isinglass:** This filtering (or *fining*) agent made from fish bladders is used to remove impurities in some types of beer and wine (see the nearby sidebar).

>> **L-cysteine:** This is made from bird feathers or human hair, and sometimes pops up in breads as a dough conditioner.

>> **Shellac or confectioner's glaze:** A secretion from the female lac insect, it's often used as a glaze to make foods shiny.

>> **Vitamin D3:** This is common in fortified foods like cereal, but it's usually derived from lanolin, which is a by-product of the wool industry. (A vegan form of vitamin D3 made from lichen exists. However, animal-based D3 is far more prevalent in fortified foods.)

>> **Whey, lactose, milk protein, or casein:** These are all forms of dairy.

ARE BEER AND WINE VEGAN?

Many people assume that beer and wine are automatically vegan, because obviously, there's no steak floating around inside the bottle or can. It's just grapes or grains, right? Unfortunately, that isn't always the case.

The issue is in the way beer and wine are filtered. Sometimes animal products are used during processing. It's usually things like isinglass, gelatin, casein, or egg whites. Sometimes beermakers will add honey to their products as well.

Because alcohol is exempt from labeling requirements, it's not as easy as just reading the ingredients label. Luckily, you have a great resource at https://www.barnivore.com/. Check it out to see if a specific beer or wine is vegan. If you're at a local brewery or winery, ask the brewmaster or winemaker what they use for refining.

Because it's distilled and not filtered, hard liquor is almost always vegan (unless it's a cream-based liqueur). You're generally safe with options like vodka, gin, schnapps, rum, tequila, bourbon, and whiskey.

Understanding cross-contamination

Some prepared foods note on their packaging that they're made on equipment shared with non-vegan products like dairy or eggs. You may see a warning like:

>> "Produced in the same facility as . . ."

>> "May contain traces of . . ."

>> "Manufactured in a facility that processes . . ."

>> "Made on shared equipment with . . ."

If you have an allergy to a listed ingredient, obviously you should steer clear of it. But if you don't, it's generally not a concern.

Manufacturing plants are often shared by different companies that use the production lines for their various products. However, manufacturing equipment is fully cleaned between runs of different types of foods.

Even after sanitizing and cleaning production areas, it's possible that trace amounts of allergens could be left behind. That can be a problem for people who are highly sensitive to those foods (that is, have a food allergy or Celiac disease). To protect their own liability and their customers' health, manufacturers may include a warning about the risk of trace amounts of allergens on food labels. (This is voluntary and not regulated. Manufacturers aren't legally required to do it.) This is a matter of safety. It doesn't affect a product's vegan-ness.

Gearing Up with Basic Cooking Equipment

Now that you have all your groceries in hand, it's time to start cooking! Choosing and using the appropriate kitchen gear will get you on your way to cooking mouthwatering plant-based fare.

If you aren't already comfortable in the kitchen, don't worry about purchasing fancy gadgets. Instead, focus on the basics. If you cook somewhat regularly, you probably own many of these items.

Pots and pans

The following list can help you start your collection of pots and pans. As you build your collection, you can add more as you need them. Here are some of the essentials:

>> **Two 10- to 12-inch ceramic nonstick fry pans or skillets with lids:** Use these skillets for frying, sautéing vegetables, and making sauces, pilafs, and risottos.

>> **3-quart saucepan:** Steam vegetables or cook grains and pastas in this pan.

>> **5-quart saucepan:** Buy a large saucepan for cooking soup, stew, and chili.

>> **13-x-9-inch glass baking dish:** Bake casseroles, lasagna, and other entrees in this dish.

>> **One or two baking sheets:** Use rimmed baking sheets for roasting vegetables, baking biscuits, or making Happy Pigs in a Blanket (recipe in Chapter 13). If you like, flat baking sheets can be used for cookies.

Bakeware

If you like baking, consider buying this bakeware:

>> 9-x-5-inch metal loaf pan

>> 9-inch round cake pan (to bake layer cakes)

>> 8-inch square cake pan (for brownies and other cakes)

>> 9-inch metal pie pan

Cooking implements and utensils

Having the right tool for the job streamlines your cooking. You can accomplish just about any basic vegan cooking task with the following cooking implements:

>> **Colander:** Use your colander for rinsing veggies and fruits, as well as draining pasta.

>> **Dry measuring cups:** Look for a six-piece set with 1 cup, ¾ cup, ⅔ cup, ½ cup, ⅓ cup, and ¼ cup sizes. These cups can be used to measure dry ingredients like whole grains, flour, or chopped nuts.

>> **Fine-mesh bowl-shaped strainer:** This tool can be used for washing grains and lentils.

>> **Kitchen tongs:** Tongs make it easy to flip vegetables or skewers on the grill, toss or scoop noodles, or serve salads.

>> **Liquid measuring cups:** Liquid measuring cups are made of glass or plastic. Depending on what you buy, they can hold 1, 2, 4, or 8 cups of liquid. Use them to measure liquids like water, maple syrup, vinegar, and cooking oil.

>> **Measuring spoons:** Look for sets with 1 tablespoon, ½ tablespoon, 1 teaspoon, ½ teaspoon, ¼ teaspoon, and ⅛ teaspoon.

>> **Mixing bowls:** Stainless steel bowls are lightweight and easy to clean. However, heavier glass or ceramic bowls stay put as you stir.

>> **Rolling pin:** If you plan on rolling out dough for pie crusts, pizza crusts, or other baked goods, a wooden rolling pin gets the job done.

TIP

If you don't have a rolling pin, a wine bottle (empty or corked) will work in a pinch!

>> **Rubber or silicone spatula:** Have at least one or two rubber or silicone spatulas on hand to get every last bit of vegan mayo from a jar or to remove sticky nut butter from a blender. It helps to reduce food waste because nothing gets thrown away that could have been eaten.

>> **Spatula:** This is a must for flipping pancakes and getting underneath veggie burgers. (That burger crust is the best part! You don't want it to get left behind on the pan or grill.) If you're using an outdoor grill, choose a metal spatula. If you're using a ceramic nonstick skillet, choose silicone instead.

>> **Steaming basket or steamer pot:** These baskets are wonderful for steaming veggies. I especially like stainless steel pots that include a steamer insert. That way, you can boil pasta and steam broccoli at the same time, as shown in the recipe for Basil Pesto Pasta with Roasted Chickpeas in Chapter 12.

>> **Vegetable peeler:** A lightweight vegetable peeler with a sharp blade is useful for peeling carrots, potatoes, sweet potatoes, and more. If the peeler has a pointed end, it can be used for removing potato eyes and hulling stems on strawberries.

>> **Whisk:** Whisking allows for the proper combining of liquids such as homemade salad dressings or the adding of wet ingredients into dry.

>> **Wood, bamboo, or composite cutting board:** A board of at least 12 x 14 inches works well for most of your cooking needs. I especially like the kind from Epicurean, because they can go straight into the dishwasher, unlike wood or bamboo cutting boards. Avoid cutting board with feet, so that you can use both sides of it.

TIP

If your cutting board doesn't have rubber corners, place a damp kitchen towel underneath for traction while you chop your veggies.

>> **Wooden spoons:** Wooden spoons are useful for stirring without fear of scratching ceramic non-stick surfaces on pans. Plus, because they don't conduct heat, they won't get too hot to handle when stirring a pot of chili or soup.

TIP

My favorite use for a wooden spoon is to prevent water from boiling over when making noodles. Simply lay the wooden spoon horizontally across the top of an open pot. The wood acts as a water repellant to the bubbles, which causes them to stop rising once they reach the spoon. Since the wood is cooler than the water, it causes the steam to condense and break the bubbles.

>> **Zester or rasp-style grater:** This is perfect for zesting citrus fruits, as well as grating ginger, garlic, or nutmeg. I use my Microplane zester constantly for grating garlic into salad dressings and sauces.

WARNING

After grating sticky ingredients like fresh garlic, be sure to clean your zester right away. Otherwise, the garlic can get dried on and difficult to remove.

Knives

A few good knives are essential for every home cook. I use the following knives most often:

>> 10-inch serrated bread knife

>> 8- to 10-inch chef's knife (for chopping vegetables)

>> Small serrated knife (for cutting thin-skinned produce like tomatoes and bell peppers)

You may also want to get a sharpening steel to sharpen your knives. High-carbon steel knives are easier to sharpen at home.

REMEMBER

Sharp knives are safe knives! Have your knives professionally sharpened one or two times per year, and then use your steel at home regularly. The sharper the knife, the less pressure you need to cut.

TIP

Go to a kitchen store and hold several brands and styles of knives to get a feel for which ones you like best. Consider how heavy the knife feels, how easy the grip feels, and whether you like the balance of the weight as you rock it back and forth across a cutting surface.

Special equipment to consider

The preceding sections cover the basics, but in this section, I introduce you to a few kitchen gadgets that can make your cooking time easier or more fun. These specialized tools include the following:

>> An air fryer for making food crispy in a hurry. It cooks in a lot less time than the oven, doesn't require preheating, and doesn't heat up the whole house during the cooking process.

>> An electric rice cooker for cooking all kinds of grains and saving space on the stove.

>> A garlic press for those times when you don't feel like mincing garlic by hand. (If you already have a garlic grater, you may not need both.)

>> A handheld citrus juicer for juicing lemons, limes, or oranges (depending on the juicer size) with the squeeze of hand.

TIP

When using this style of juicer, remember to insert the citrus cut side down toward the holes.

>> A toaster oven for quick reheats and toasting without using the whole oven or the microwave.

>> A food processor for chopping, grating, and mixing large quantities quickly.

>> Washable kitchen scissors for cutting herbs, pizza, and flatbreads, opening food packaging, and trimming veggies.

>> A silicone funnel set for pouring homemade sauces, purees, and bulk spices into smaller receptacles. (Funnels with wide mouths are especially easy to use because food doesn't get stuck in the spout.)

>> A coffee grinder or spice grinder for grinding whole coffee beans and whole spices.

>> A pressure cooker like an Instant Pot for cooking soups, stews, grains, and beans in a hurry.

>> A slow cooker for making a hands-off meal over several hours. It can also be used as a warmer at holiday functions.

>> An immersion or stick blender for blending soups in the pot. It's very handy if you don't want to transfer hot liquid to a countertop blender.

>> A high-speed blender like a Vitamix for making nut-based sauces, spreads, and cheeses. A high-speed blender can easily break down fibrous leafy greens in fruit smoothies and make completely creamy cashew sauces. Standard blenders sometimes struggle with these tasks.

TIP

High-speed blenders come with a higher price tag (usually several hundred dollars). If you don't have room in your budget for one just yet, here are a couple good workarounds for standard blenders:

- When making green smoothies, blend the dark leafy greens on their own with nondairy milk first. Once that mixture is fully blended, add the other smoothie ingredients.

- To make creamy nut-based sauces, grind nuts like raw cashews in a clean coffee grinder until they have the texture of a powder. Then add the ground nuts to your standard blender along with the remaining ingredients.

Chapter **8**

Deciding What's for Dinner: Meal Planning

I remember standing in my kitchen the morning after I officially went vegan, trying to come up with a plan for breakfast. I didn't know where to even start. It was way too early in the morning to pull out a cookbook. I wasn't awake enough for a big production with homemade seitan sausages, a tofu scramble, and hand-shredded hash browns. I just wanted to make something simple . . . but somehow that concept felt complicated!

Do you know what the problem was? I was figuring out my breakfast at the wrong time! When you're starting a new lifestyle, the best time to make a plan isn't when you're in your pajamas with the coffee still brewing. No, the ideal time to get everything sorted is when you have the energy and faculties to pull it all together. Build the rails, and then in the morning, you just have to step on the train.

Waiting until you're hungry to decide what to eat is a recipe for disaster. (Sorry, recipe. You get one star.)

You see, many of us choose what we eat based on habits. We get used to grabbing the same things again and again without too much consideration. But when you change your diet, those habits get jostled. The stuff you'd just throw together in the past may not work anymore.

At some point in your vegan future, you'll create new habits. But until then, make things easier for yourself by sorting out your meals ahead of time. It's much less stressful and a lot more enjoyable.

In this chapter, I share how to plan well-rounded meals, do some practical food prep, and have a few easy backup meals in your back pocket. Plus, you find out how to do it all while staying on budget!

Considering How Many Meals You Need

Before you plan out your menu for the week, think about how many meals you'll actually need. If you just assume you'll need seven breakfasts, lunches, and dinners, you may end up with more perishables than you can use. Consider these questions first:

>> Will you be dining out some nights?

>> Will you finish leftovers for lunch or dinner?

>> Do you have any lunch meetings at restaurants?

>> If you have kids, will they be eating in the school cafeteria or taking packed lunches?

It can be stressful to spend a lot of money on groceries, only to have them frittering away in the refrigerator because you overbought. By outlining the types and amounts of meals you need, you can save yourself from paying for the same meal twice — once in the grocery store and again in an unplanned night out at a restaurant.

REMEMBER

Before your grocery run, think about how much produce you can use, and make a general plan for the week. Even something as simple as deciding you'll get salad ingredients for four nights, or easy side dishes for three lunches, can help. That way you won't walk away with more perishable stuff than you can finish before it goes bad.

If you have kids, look at their extracurricular obligations. If you know that Wednesday night you have to go straight from swim practice to dance class, think about getting ingredients for a dinner that can be eaten on the go. Cold sandwiches or pasta salads are convenient options. Another option is to plan to have soup waiting in the slow cooker for a hot meal that's ready when you walk in the door.

Once you know how many meals you need for the week, you can move on to the next step.

Starting with Dishes You Know and Love

First, think about the meals you already make regularly. Like I said, we're creatures of habit. So don't fight that. What simple tweaks can you make to your go-to standards to turn them vegan?

Say you have spaghetti for dinner every Monday. Use the same boxed spaghetti as always. If your usual jarred sauce includes any animal products like cheese, pick up a different all-vegetable sauce. Then swap out any meat in your usual recipe with veggies like mushrooms, bell peppers, and onions. Or you can replace the meat with a plant-based alternative like vegan sausage. Serve it with a green salad and garlic bread made with vegan butter.

If you always have ground beef tacos on Tuesday, replace the meat with soy chorizo, chickpeas, pinto beans, or black beans. Then season your filling with the same spices as usual. Spoon it onto tortillas and finish with shredded cabbage, tomatoes, and guacamole on top. Serve your tacos with seasoned rice or chips and salsa.

Love having a burger every Friday night after work? Pick up some plant-based ground beef. Season it the same way you used to season meat and throw it in a grill pan. The buns, lettuce, tomatoes, onions, and mustard all stay the same. Serve with corn on the cob, salad, or french fries.

When you look at your regular meals and then make a couple substitutions, it can feel a lot more manageable than constantly searching for a recipe. (For more tips on veganizing meals, be sure to check out Chapter 9.)

That said, it's fun to try something new too! While you're making your meal plan for the week, find a recipe or two from Part 4 of this book, check out a vegan cookbook from the library, or look online. Seek out recipes that fit your taste preferences and cooking abilities.

TIP

Have something specific in mind? Do a search on Google or Pinterest. If there's a dish that you love, it's almost certain that someone has made a vegan version of it!

TIP

When you're just starting, I recommend selecting simple foods that don't require a lot of time, sophisticated cooking tools, or techniques. A project can be fun, but maybe not for a Monday night.

Finally, write out the ingredients you need for these meal ideas and recipes.

Mulling Over Menu Ideas

As you're thinking about what your weekly meal plan will look like, here are some easy ideas for breakfasts, lunches, dinners, and snacks.

If you're a person who loves cooking, you may be happy picking more time-intensive dishes. However, if you don't cook often, gravitate toward simpler meals that can be thrown together in 15 or 20 minutes. Or challenge yourself with a healthy mix of complicated and simple meals!

Choose simple breakfast options

Growing up, I never cared all that much about breakfast. After going vegan, it's my favorite meal of the day!

What I like about breakfast is that I can eat the same meal day after day and never tire of it. Most days, I eat avocado toast topped with pickled red onions, a sprinkling of nutritional yeast flakes, and salt. For a protein-dense side, I make tofu seasoned with *kala namak* (black salt), nutritional yeast, and black pepper. (See Chapter 11 for my Avocado Toast with Baked Tofu and Eggy Tofu recipes.)

You can choose between many delicious options for a filling breakfast. Here are some ideas:

>> Breakfast burrito with seasoned tofu, potatoes, and black beans

>> Peanut butter toast with fruit

>> Blueberry Banana Oatmeal (Get the recipe in Chapter 11.)

- » Fruit smoothie
- » Nondairy yogurt
- » Breakfast sandwich with vegan sausage, JUST Egg, and nondairy cheese
- » Cold cereal with nondairy milk and banana slices or berries
- » Breakfast quesadilla stuffed with Eggy Tofu, sliced bell pepper, chopped onion, spinach, and nondairy cheese (The Eggy Tofu recipe is in Chapter 11.)
- » Hummus Bagel Sandwich with green leaf lettuce, thinly sliced radish, chopped onion, sliced tomato, and slices of bell pepper. (Recipe in Chapter 13.)
- » Veggie-Packed Tofu Scramble (See the recipe in Chapter 11.)
- » Frozen waffles warmed in the toaster
- » Grits or polenta

For even more breakfast ideas, check out the recipes in Chapter 11.

Pack lunches for work and school

The key to fast, no-fuss lunches is a combination of planning, a well-stocked kitchen, and a few convenience foods.

Some of my favorite lunches include:

- » Sandwiches with vegan deli slices, vegan tuna salad, vegan chicken salad, or vegan egg salad
- » Leftovers from dinner
- » Ramen topped with browned tofu and veggies (Get the Dressed Up Ramen Noodles recipe in Chapter 13.)
- » Burritos or tacos with beans, rice, lettuce, salsa, and avocado
- » Big salad with roasted chickpeas and garlic bread (Kale holds up especially well for packed lunches.)
- » Vegan ravioli or other pasta with mushrooms, vegan sausage, and jarred marinara
- » Brown rice bowl with baked falafel, baby spinach, and tahini dressing (Get the Easy Tahini Dressing recipe in Chapter 14.)
- » Soup (Pack homemade or keep a can at the office for an emergency lunch.)
- » Vegetable stir-fry
- » Pasta salad
- » Veggie wrap with hummus, romaine, pickled veggies, and *bulgur* (cracked wheat)

Figure out quick dinner ideas

Dinnertime is hectic in many households. With late worknights, evening activities, traffic jams, and chores, fixing a healthy meal can seem overwhelming.

Consider these easy dinner menus to keep stress to a minimum:

>> **Soup and crusty bread:** Make a batch of Vegan Chicken Noodle Soup (recipe in Chapter 12), potato soup, lentil barley soup, tortilla soup, tomato soup, gnocchi soup, wild rice soup, split pea soup, chili, or corn chowder.

>> **Dinner-sized salad:** Toss together your favorite veggies, leafy greens, and something protein-dense like baked tofu or vegan chick'n strips.

>> **Burrito bowls:** Pile seasoned beans, guacamole, shredded cabbage, cilantro, and salsa on top of brown rice.

>> **Veggie burger:** Make a Classic Vegan Cheeseburger topped with pickles, lettuce, and onion. (Grab the recipe in Chapter 12.) Serve it with steamed broccoli and baked fries.

>> **Stir-fried veggies and tofu:** Serve over rice along with store-bought vegetable pot stickers.

>> **Baguette pizzas:** Top with marinara, vegan pepperoni, onion, and sautéed mushrooms. (If you like, sprinkle with nondairy mozzarella!)

>> **Mezze platter:** Lay out a spread of hummus or *baba ghanoush* (eggplant dip), pita bread, *tabbouleh* (herb and cracked wheat salad), kalamata olives, falafel, marinated artichokes, and cucumber tomato salad.

>> **Dinner of side dishes:** Fill your plate with roasted potatoes, red wine infused mushrooms, and garlicky broccolini.

>> **Breakfast for dinner:** Whip up a Veggie-Packed Tofu Scramble (see Chapter 11) and top with avocado. Serve it with toast and veggie sausage.

>> **Vegan cheese and crackers:** Arrange vegan cheese(s), crackers, vegan deli slices, olives, pickles, carrot and celery sticks, red bell pepper slices, and berries on a platter.

>> **Chickpea curry:** Heat chickpeas and veggies in your favorite curry sauce and serve over rice along with store-bought vegetable samosas.

>> **Homemade or boxed vegan mac and cheese:** Serve with barbecued tofu and Sautéed Kale with Garlic (recipe in Chapter 14).

TIP

Change the flavor profile of dishes by using a different sauce! Start with the same base of veggies, beans, seitan, and/or tofu. Then add any of these sauces for entirely different taste experiences: barbecue, curry, marinara, vegan pesto, chimichurri, cashew cheese, gravy, teriyaki, sweet and sour, or buffalo sauce.

Having a few convenient sauces (or sauce recipes) on hand can help you completely reimagine the same few ingredients. Serve with your choice of rice, noodles, or potatoes, depending on the dish.

Prepare easy snacks

When hunger strikes, it's nice to have some staple items on hand for convenient and filling snacks. Choose from this handy list:

>> Fresh or dried fruit

>> Banana with nut butter or a handful of peanuts

>> Nondairy yogurt

>> Fruit smoothie

>> Trail mix, nuts, or seeds

>> Bagel with hummus or vegan cream cheese

>> Toast with peanut butter, jelly, or nondairy butter

>> Chips and salsa, bean dip, or guacamole

>> *Dolmas* (stuffed grape leaves)

>> Pita bread or pita chips with hummus or baba ghanoush

>> Vegan cheddar cheese, crackers, pickles, and/or olives

>> Popcorn with melted vegan butter, nutritional yeast, and salt (For a lighter option, top plain popcorn with a squeeze of lime juice and sprinkle of salt.)

>> Carrots, celery, or red bell peppers with Ranch Dressing (Get this vegan dressing recipe in Chapter 14.)

>> Heated frozen pot stickers with tamari dipping sauce

>> Roasted Chickpeas (Grab the recipe in Chapter 14.)

>> Store-bought baked tofu in flavors like teriyaki or sriracha

>> Cold cereal and nondairy milk

Use menu charts

Planning a week of menus can really take the guesswork and stress out of shopping trips. If you already know what you're having for dinner each night, you don't need to worry about running by the crowded grocery store on the way home from work.

Use the menu chart in Figure 8-1 to help guide your shopping trips.

Monday Date:	Notes	Grocery List
Breakfast:		☐ _____
Lunch:		
Dinner:		☐ _____
Snack:		
		☐ _____
Tuesday Date:		
Breakfast:		☐ _____
Lunch:		
Dinner:		☐ _____
Snack:		
		☐ _____
Wednesday Date:		
Breakfast:		☐ _____
Lunch:		
Dinner:		☐ _____
Snack:		
		☐ _____
Thursday Date:		
Breakfast:		☐ _____
Lunch:		
Dinner:		☐ _____
Snack:		
		☐ _____
Friday Date:		
Breakfast:		☐ _____
Lunch:		
Dinner:		☐ _____
Snack:		

Saturday Date:	Sunday Date:	☐ _____
Breakfast:	Breakfast:	
Lunch:	Lunch:	☐ _____
Dinner:	Dinner:	
Snack:	Snack:	☐ _____

FIGURE 8-1:
Sample menu
chart.

Performing Food Prep

After you've picked up all your produce, beans, grains, and other cooking essentials, it's time for food prep. While many people assume food prep has to be an hours-long affair on Sundays, there are endless ways of doing it. Food prep may be a lot easier than you think! Here are a few options that you can store in the refrigerator:

>> Make several full meals and put them into individual containers to grab and go.

>> Prepare individual ingredients for easier meal preparation later.

>> Cook some staples (like a big batch of rice or roasted potatoes) that will make it simpler to put together dinners during the week.

Whichever way you choose to go, doing some food prep makes the rest of the week a whole lot less hectic.

An added bonus? You're more apt to choose healthy foods if they're convenient and quick. When you're hungry, it's tempting to grab the easiest thing. If a frozen pizza is all that's around, that wins out. But if a big salad is prepped and ready to eat, that becomes lunch instead.

Check out these simple meal-prep ideas. Then set yourself up for streamlined lunches and dinners throughout the rest of the week.

Wash and chop vegetables while unpacking groceries

When you get home from the grocery store, instead of putting all your produce into refrigerator bins to be dealt with later, wash and chop the sturdy vegetables you bought. Having them ready to go means you're more likely to use them later in salads, stir-fries, bowls, and snacks.

>> Cut celery, radishes, carrots, and bell peppers into sticks, dices, or slices.

>> Break down heads of cauliflower and broccoli into florets.

>> Peel and dice onions.

>> Peel, seed, and cut hard winter squash like acorn, butternut, or delicata.

>> Trim and slice cabbage and Brussels sprouts.

Store the cut produce in covered containers in the refrigerator. Hardy vegetables like carrots and celery can be stored in water to keep them crisp. Be sure to change out the water every few days.

TIP

Chopped onion should be stored in its own container. It has a way of transferring flavors.

Once your veggies have been sliced, put them to the front and center in the fridge. Carrot and celery sticks, bell pepper slices, and cauliflower florets are perfect for dunking in hummus.

REMEMBER

Keep in mind that some cut vegetables last longer than others. Sturdy vegetables like carrots, broccoli, cauliflower, cabbage, and Brussels sprouts last throughout the week. Once cut, softer vegetables like bell peppers, cucumbers, and tomatoes should be eaten within three days or so.

TIP

No time to chop? Most grocery stores sell vegetables that are sliced and ready. If shortcuts like buying precut vegetables will make you eat more of them, do it! Some people worry that cut vegetables lose nutrients, but you know what loses *more* nutrients? Not eating them at all! If using precut vegetables means you're getting more veggies in your diet, that's a big improvement.

Prep for future meals while cooking dinner

Meal prepping isn't just for weekends! You can easily incorporate it with your daily cooking. When you need only half an onion, cut a whole one instead. Then save the extra half in the fridge for another time. When you need one bell pepper, cut two instead.

When you've already got the cutting board out, it doesn't take that much more time to chop an extra veggie. However, it means you won't have to set aside special time in your schedule for food prep.

Cook batches of grains or lentils

Take half an hour or so and make a big batch of rice, pearl barley, bulgur, farro, *freekeh* (a nutty, chewy grain), or lentils on the stove. They keep well in the refrigerator or freezer. Throughout the week, you can add them to bowls, stir-fries, and salads.

TIP

Want an even easier shortcut? Buy a box of frozen brown rice or precooked lentils! I always have store-bought frozen rice in the freezer and vacuum-sealed lentils in the fridge. They're extremely convenient for lunches and dinners.

Whip up a big salad

Make a huge salad in a large mixing bowl. Have some for dinner, and then keep the rest in an airtight container in the fridge for easy salads throughout the week.

While you're at it, make one or two homemade dressings, like vegan ranch dressing, tahini dressing, or balsamic vinaigrette. (Check out the dressing recipes in Chapter 14.) Store them in sealed salad dressing bottles.

Having a salad at the ready makes it easy to get your recommended amounts of leafy greens every day.

Make staples that can easily be repurposed

Prepare one or two dishes that can be enjoyed in a variety of ways to keep leftovers from getting monotonous. Things like chili, spicy black beans, or seasoned chickpeas can be repurposed and used in burritos, rice bowls, loaded fries, nachos, tacos, taco pizza, or taco salads.

Make a big batch of hummus or refried beans for dipping veggies, tortilla chips, or crackers. Or you can spread them onto sandwiches or wraps.

Double the recipe you're making

Instead of just making enough for one night, cook twice the amount you need. Doubling a recipe makes exponentially more meals, but at a fraction of the labor since you're still just cleaning one cutting board, pan, and knife afterward.

Store the leftovers in the refrigerator to enjoy throughout the week. Or if it's a freezer-friendly meal, freeze it for another time when you need a homemade lunch in a hurry. Think of it as a gift to your future self.

Air fry or bake several potatoes

I never cook just one potato in the air fryer. It's every bit as easy to cook four! Russet potatoes cook in 35 to 40 minutes in the air fryer at 390 degrees. Baby potatoes take even less time — about 12 to 17 minutes at 400 degrees.

Don't have an air fryer? Bake russet potatoes in the oven at 425 degrees for 45 to 60 minutes, until they can be easily pierced with a fork.

Don't forget to puncture medium or large potatoes a couple times with a knife or fork before baking or air frying them!

Baked potatoes aren't just for side dishes! They can be a satisfying and delicious main course. Plus, they can be repurposed throughout the week. Have a baked potato bar one night with nondairy sour cream, chives, browned seitan bacon, and/or vegan chili. Take a potato to work for lunch the next day. Then dice any remaining cooked potatoes for breakfast burritos, or a quick hash with peppers and onions.

Roast seasonal vegetables

Another great way to maximize the vegetables on your dinner table is by roasting them en masse. Think roasted asparagus, zucchini, onions, sweet potatoes, broccoli, cauliflower, winter squash, bell peppers, and Brussels sprouts.

Buy whatever vegetables are in season. Then cut them into roughly equal-sized pieces, and throw them on a parchment paper–covered baking sheet with a drizzle of oil. For best roasting, be careful not to overcrowd the pan. If you like, sprinkle the vegetables with salt, dried herbs, or your favorite seasoning mix. Roast at 400 degrees until tender, giving them a stir halfway through. The cooking time will vary, depending on the density of the vegetables and size of the pieces.

Keep containers of roasted veggies on hand for quick side dishes or additions to bowls and wraps.

When the weather is nice, you can grill veggies on an outdoor grill instead using a grill basket or skewers. (For cooking instructions, check out the recipe for Grilled Vegetable Skewers in Chapter 14.)

Stock the freezer with prepared meals

Lots of staples freeze well. Make a big batch of chili, beans, soup, or stew and ladle it into meal-sized containers for the freezer. (To avoid freezer burn, store beans in their cooking liquid.)

My favorite soups for freezing include split pea, potato, butternut squash, sweet potato, and anything tomato-based. Then just thaw, heat, and eat.

Keeping the Costs Down on Vegan Meals

If you're looking to save money, stick with whole plant foods with lower price tags like beans, grains, veggies, and fruits. Think of high-end vegan cheeses, meatless meats, and other prepared foods as occasional splurges, not daily staples.

TIP

If you want to eat vegan meats and cheeses, try making your own! It's not hard to make seitan from scratch or simple tofu- or nut-based cheeses (such as Cashew Parmesan in Chapter 14).

Gravitate toward foods that you make yourself rather than premade refrigerated and frozen items. Often, making food from scratch comes with a cost savings. When you have someone else make the food for you, you're paying for their labor on top of the food cost.

Use bulk bins

Another way to save money is by buying from bulk bins. Most natural grocery stores (and some mainstream ones) have bins of dried beans, grains, flours, teas, herbs and spices, as well as dispensers for nut butters, coffee beans, and oils. You just take the amount you want, and then pay for it by weight. Since less packaging, plastic, and cardboard is required, stores are able to pass the savings on to you.

Buying just the amount you need is ideal when you're trying a new recipe and don't want to commit to a full jar or package of something. (I especially like this option for spices that I don't use often.) If you end up loving the ingredient, you can buy it in larger amounts the next time you need it.

REMEMBER

If you choose to refill your own clean glass jar at the store, be sure to have the cashier weigh it before you fill it, so they can subtract the weight of the container from the total cost at checkout.

Shop in season

When you buy straight from the farmer, produce often costs less because farmers don't have a grocery store taking a percentage. So farmers can sell to the consumer for less. Visit your local farmers market, and buy in season. Cherries and asparagus are a whole lot more affordable in spring and summer than they are in January. When you buy out of season, you're paying for produce to get shipped around the globe.

Not only does buying local help the farmers in your community, but it's also a great way to ensure optimum freshness of your ingredients. Produce that's shipped from across the country has already spent a lot of its life on trucks or grocery store shelves. Local seasonal produce will last that much longer in your kitchen, giving you time to use it.

Continuing with that line of thought, consider growing your own herbs, fruits, and veggies. Growing your own food is a good way to save money and enjoy the freshest produce. Setting up a little container garden of herbs in your window is easy and inexpensive, and it looks great with any décor.

TIP

If you don't have the space to grow food yourself, see if there's a community garden in your town, where you can rent a garden plot.

Choose stores wisely

Some grocery stores are almost museum-level in terms of their beautiful array of produce, artisanal breads, and high-end ingredients. They have irresistible desserts, flashy juice bars, and wine available by the glass. That's lovely and all, but you're likely going to be paying a premium for that environment.

TIP

Do a little tour of the grocery stores in your area. See who has the best prices for staples and who has the freshest produce. After all, food that spoils quickly wasn't really a bargain if it goes to waste.

Even if you buy most of your groceries at one store, you may find that other markets are good for a few specific products. Some pricey natural food stores have their own generic lines, which tend to be equal in quality but cheaper than name brands.

In the warm-weather months, I buy primarily from the farmers market and a CSA (community supported agriculture). When the farmers market is out of season, I do most of my shopping at Trader Joe's. I fill out the rest of my grocery needs at my local co-op, Target, Walmart, an Indian grocery store, and a Korean grocery store. Spread your purchases among various businesses to find the best value for you. Read more about where to do your vegan grocery shopping in Chapter 7.

Eat your food

According to a 2020 study from the *American Journal of Agricultural Economics*, the average household wastes about a third of the food they buy. It's wild to think about! Food is bought with good intentions, but often fritters away in the refrigerator until it's unusable.

TIP

One simple way to save money is by not overbuying. Cook what you get, and find ways to use all of it from root to stem. If you don't think you'll get to a perishable item in time and it can be frozen, stick it in the freezer to expand its shelf life. When you go to a restaurant, take home any leftovers, and eat them.

It sounds simple, but it really makes a world of difference. When you take home fresh foods only to have them go bad before you can use them, it's a lot of wasted time, energy, and resources — both for you and for the farmers who grew it.

WHY IS VEGAN FOOD EXPENSIVE?

A while back, a fast-food place started offering plant-based burgers. The reaction I heard time and again from non-vegans was that the price was too high. They couldn't understand why the plant-based burger was so much more expensive than the meat-based one. They wondered how a burger that includes the costs of feeding, housing, and raising a cow can be less expensive than the one made only from plants.

The answer is that animal products are artificially cheap. Meat, dairy, and eggs get subsidized by the U.S. government. That makes them seem cheaper, but in actuality, we're paying for these subsidies through taxes. Plant-based foods don't get the same level of treatment, so they seem more expensive.

The U.S. government spends $38 billion in tax money to subsidize the meat and dairy industries, according to a 2015 paper from UC Berkeley's Sutardja Center for Entrepreneurship and Technology. However, the fruit and vegetable industries only see about .04 percent of that sum (or $17 million). Soybeans are subsidized but only for use as animal feed — not for tofu, tempeh, or edamame. That's an enormous difference that makes the playing field anything but level.

Plus, the mass farming of animals lowers production costs by cramming as many animals as possible into very small spaces. Animals are given food that will make them grow as quickly as possible and produce more milk and eggs in less time. It saves money, but at a huge cost — to the animals.

Meanwhile, new vegan products require research and development. Innovation costs money. They're targeting a niche market, and they have to spend more to reach consumers who may be totally unfamiliar with what they're offering.

Finally, many vegans opt for organic foods over conventional ones, and organic products often come at a premium.

(continued)

(continued)

Even considering all that, a lot of the most expensive things on a non-vegan's grocery bill are the animal products. A report from data and consulting company Kantar showed that home-cooked vegan meals cost 40 percent less on average and take a third less time to prepare than non-vegan meals. It also showed that even when people were buying some pricier vegan specialty products, the other cost savings more than made up for them.

The takeaway? If you choose wisely by sticking with simple whole plant foods (beans, grains, fruits, and veggies), eating vegan can be a lot less expensive than buying meat, dairy, and eggs at the grocery store.

Chapter **9**

Anything You Can Make, I Can Make Vegan

One of the cool things about going vegan is figuring out how to turn the dishes you grew up eating into new plant-based favorites. It often doesn't take much more than a swap or two to transform a meaty dish into a vegan one.

These days there are vegan products and recipes for almost any non-vegan food or dish that exists. Veganize it yourself, or do a recipe search and see if someone else has already done the work for you.

Over the years, I've made vegan versions of Philly cheesesteaks, Reubens, BLTs, fried chicken drumsticks, eggnog, eggs Benedict, crab rangoon, crab cakes, and bacon-wrapped dates. I've even made a vegan version of the sandwich my family prepared all grilling season long — a bacon burger dog. That's a hot dog surrounded by hamburger and wrapped up with a strip of bacon. (With vegan ground beef, veggie dogs, and vegan bacon, it's easy to do!)

In this chapter, I show that you can veganize almost anything. If you're worried about giving up a particular dish, don't be. Just reimagine it.

Recognizing Why Vegans Eat Foods That Taste Like Meat

People are often confused about why someone who goes vegan would want to eat something that tastes like meat. After all, if they're rejecting milk, meat, and eggs, isn't it because they hate the flavor of those things? Not necessarily.

Personally, I really enjoyed those flavors. When I was considering going vegan, I had a hard time imagining never eating some of my favorite foods again. If you've been vegan for any length of time, you've definitely heard someone say, "Oh, I couldn't live without cheese!" I probably said it before I went vegan too.

No matter where you grew up, there's a solid chance that meat, dairy, or eggs featured heavily in your regional dishes. People sometimes make the excuse that they can't go vegan because they're from (insert literally anywhere here). Maybe you grew up eating pork chops in Iowa, fish tacos in California, lobster in Maine, brisket in Texas, meat pies in Australia, haggis in Scotland, or schnitzel in Austria. If you wanted, you could point a finger at a place on a map, and that could be your excuse for not choosing a plant-based diet.

The fact is, people usually have attachments to the foods they grew up eating. They like their family favorites and old standards. They associate those dishes with happy memories, cherished loved ones, and fun-filled holidays. For many vegans, the reason they stopped eating meat- and cheese-filled family favorites isn't because they didn't like the taste or texture. It's because they don't want to harm animals when there's another choice.

I grew up eating steaks, bratwurst, and bacon burger dogs, but over time, I became uncomfortable with animals being killed for my dinner. So if I can eat a plant-based version of those foods instead, in which no one gets harmed in the process, why wouldn't I choose that? After all, my issue is with animal suffering, not grilled and smoky flavors, or chewy textures.

REMEMBER

You may think of vegan meats as a fairly new thing, but they've been around for a loooooong time. The origins of wheat meat, also known as *seitan*, date back to the year 535 BCE. Then tofu came along between 206 and 220 BCE.

All that said, some vegans don't like foods that mimic meat, dairy, and eggs. Maybe they never enjoyed those things in the first place, and that was part of their reason for going vegan. Or perhaps they associate those flavors, tastes, or textures with cruelty, and that's a turnoff to them.

If you're not a fan of vegan substitutes, don't eat them! You can still find plenty of other plant-based foods to enjoy.

Giving meaty names to vegan dishes

Similarly, people are sometimes confused about why vegans give their food meaty, cheesy, or eggy names like vegan steak, vegan cheddar, or vegan deviled eggs. These naysayers assert that vegans should come up with new names for their plant-based versions.

Here's the thing: Associations and comparisons are common in language. They're helpful. They let people know what a food tastes like or how it should be used.

That's why there are turkey burgers, bison burgers, and veggie burgers. It's a point of reference. People may expect a burger made from a cow, but instead it's made with turkey, bison, or veggies.

Consider these common names with food descriptors in them:

>> Peanut *butter* is a creamy spread.

>> Coconut *milk* is a smooth liquid.

>> The *flesh* inside a coconut is called *meat*.

>> *Egg*plant was so named because it looks like a goose's egg.

>> *Grape*fruits grow in clusters like grapes.

>> *Spaghetti* squash comes apart in strands like noodles when it's cooked.

>> Candy *corn* is shaped like kernels.

>> Jelly*beans* are shaped like pintos.

>> *Spaghetti* strap dresses have skinny noodle-like straps.

By drawing comparisons, people understand something about the object's size, shape, texture, flavor, or use.

Because most of us weren't born vegan, we know what specific animal products taste like and the kinds of dishes in which they'd be used.

>> If I call something vegan mozzarella, people will sprinkle it on pizza or add it to baked pasta.

>> If I say it's vegan chicken, they know they can batter and fry it for vegan fried chicken, or chop it and mix it with eggless mayo for vegan chicken salad.

>> If I call a dish vegan meatballs, people know to serve them with pasta, or throw them on a sandwich with marinara sauce.

Also, when people are new to veganism, they often look online for recipes or products that fulfill a particular craving. They use familiar terms and then put the word "vegan" in front of them. For example, if someone wants an alternative to pork sausage, they google "vegan sausage." If they want an alternative to ribs, they google "vegan ribs."

Naysayers sometimes suggest that vegans come up with their own unique names for plant-based foods, but that's not how people perform Google searches. Instead, people search with terms they already use and understand. When someone wants vegan pepperoni, they don't google "vegan spicy wheat log." And when they want vegan cheese, they don't google "creamy cashew block."

According to keyword research site KeySearch.co, every month 74,000 people search for "vegan cheese" on Google. That number goes even higher if you include searches for "vegan ricotta," "vegan mozzarella," or "vegan parmesan cheese." But do you know how many people search for "creamy cashew block"? If you guessed zero, you're right. There's no point in creating a recipe or product and then calling it something that people would never search for.

Considering the shapes of vegan food

Folks also wonder why vegans form their food into the same shapes that meat eaters do. They think we should just be eating rice, beans, and veggies — not forming those same ingredients into circular burgers.

But the fact is, there isn't a *nugget* part of a chicken. There's no *burger* part of a cow. People form ground meat into round shapes for meatballs, disc shapes for burgers, and box shapes for meatloaves. Meat eaters don't own the concept of circles or rectangles.

Round patties fit nicely on buns. Small nuggets are good for dipping. (By the way, chicken nuggets got their name because of their resemblance in shape and color to nuggets of gold.)

While people criticize vegans for making plant-based food in the shape of hot dogs or burgers, meat eaters shape their food too. They sometimes prefer that it show no resemblance to its original form. I've known many meat eaters who are uneasy when their dinner looks too much like the living animal it used to be.

Some people feel uncomfortable being served a whole lobster or whole fish. They don't want their dinner staring back at them. Other meat eaters feel ill at ease seeing plastic-wrapped cow tongues, pig ears, or chicken feet in the meat department at the grocery store. They're uneasy when roasted ducks are hanging by their necks in restaurant windows or when brains are on the menu.

I know people who eat animals but don't like eating any meat off the bone, or who don't like meat that's called the same name as the animal (like turkey or chicken). Forming meat into a circle or rectangle or slicing it into a "chop" makes it easier to forget who's on the dinner table.

Pinpointing your cravings

Over the course of your life, you've surely had times when you craved a specific food. You couldn't get it out of your head until you ate it. Cravings can be especially strong when you're stressed, tired, or crabby. Sometimes you want a food to mask something you're feeling, or you see a commercial that makes you want to put down the remote and drive to a restaurant STAT.

Just because you go vegan doesn't mean those cravings and impulses will vanish in a day. While some of your cravings may be for things that are already vegan like potato chips, other cravings may not be.

TIP

When a craving pops up, the first thing to do is identify it. Is it for something salty, smoky, or chewy? If so, is there a plant-based food that would satisfy it? If you want to sink your teeth into something, have breaded or fried seitan, vegan barbecued ribs, or a smoky vegan BLT.

TIP

Once you examine the craving, you may discover that a lot of what you desire has more to do with the toppings and sauces that go on a dish than the meat itself. Ask yourself if you're craving the shrimp or the fried breading around it and the cocktail sauce for dipping. Are you craving the bratwurst, or are you craving the sauerkraut and grainy mustard? Many times, it's not the meat you're really desiring. It's what goes along with the meat. Maybe you're craving:

>> Breading

>> Horseradish

>> Sauerkraut

>> Mustard

>> Ketchup

>> Pickles, onions, or hot peppers

>> Barbecue sauce

>> Cocktail sauce

If the part of the experience you're craving is a plant-based sauce, topping, or breading, you can simply replace the animal-portion of the meal with vegan meat, tofu, or tempeh.

TIP

Another thing to try is using the same spices from the dish you're craving on plant-based ingredients. Think about tacos. What really stands out in the flavor of tacos is cumin, chili powder, and paprika. When it comes down to it, while the meat gives it a particular texture, the dominant flavors are of the plant-based spices, onions, and garlic.

So, cook vegan ground beef, vegan chorizo, or beans with the aforementioned spices, onions, and garlic. Spoon the filling into warmed tortillas or taco shells. Finish with toppings like lettuce, tomatoes, pickled onions, cilantro, and guacamole. You won't be able to tell the difference!

Acknowledging the power of umami

Sometimes when people have cravings for meat, what they're really missing is umami. You know how foods are salty, sweet, sour, or bitter? Well, there's a fifth taste called *umami*. It's the deep, savory flavor that's often associated with meat. However, plant-based foods also have umami.

When the craving for umami hits, try one of these:

>> **Fermented foods:** Reach for sauerkraut, vegan kimchi, tamari, vegan Worcestershire sauce, vinegar, miso paste, tempeh, wine, or beer. (Remember that wine and beer aren't just for drinking. They add robust flavor to dishes.)

>> **Garlic and onions:** Sauté garlic and onions, roast garlic until it's spreadable, or make caramelized onions. Add granulated onion and/or granulated garlic to a dish.

>> **Mushrooms:** Shiitake, portobello, cremini, and white button are particularly high in umami, but all mushrooms have it. Grilling mushrooms amps up their umami quality. You can also use dried mushroom powder in soups and sauces.

>> **Nuts and seeds:** Toasting nuts and seeds brings out their umami flavor.

>> **Sea vegetables:** Check out *nori* (dried seaweed) and *kombu* (dried kelp).

>> **Tomatoes:** Tomato paste, sun-dried tomatoes, and ketchup are especially rich in umami.

>> **Yeast foods:** Cook with *nutritional yeast,* an inactive yeast that adds cheesy richness to sauces, dips, and spreads. When making soup, add one of the vegan varieties of Better Than Bouillon, which contains yeast extract. If you're a fan of Marmite or Vegemite, add it to stews or smear a thin layer on toast.

Checking Out Vegan Meat Alternatives

For many people, the centerpiece of the meal is meat. So when they consider going vegan, they don't know what they're going to put in that focal point of the dinner plate. Will dinner just consist of two little side dishes and that's it?

Many vegan meat alternatives are available for quick and easy veganizing. Longtime staples like seitan and tofu have been eaten for centuries, and newer meat-free darlings are winning over fans day after day.

Make tofu the "meat" of the meal

Often when folks think of vegetarian or vegan food, *tofu* (also known as bean curd) is the first thing that comes to mind. Tofu is made in a way that's similar to the way dairy cheese is produced. Where dairy cheese is made by curdling an animal's milk, tofu is made by curdling soy milk.

Tofu is a blank canvas that can change its flavor and texture depending on how it's prepared. In vegan cooking, tofu can replace meat or eggs, because of its high protein and iron content. (Read more about how to replace eggs with tofu later in this chapter.)

Like cheese, tofu is a fully cooked product. You can eat it right out of the package without doing anything to it. But because it has a neutral flavor, some seasoning, marinating, saucing, or cooking usually improves it.

Tofu varies by softness and uses.

>> **Silken tofu:** Very soft and used in desserts and sauces, this type is usually sold in *aseptic* (sterile) packaging in the center aisles of the grocery store or in the refrigerated section with other varieties of tofu.

>> **Super-firm, extra-firm,** and **firm tofu:** Used in savory dishes, this type is sold in the refrigerated section of the grocery store. It can be shredded, crumbled into chunks, or cubed. It's then fried, grilled, browned, baked, or eaten cold in sauces.

TIP

Vacuum-packed super-firm tofu is my favorite. Unlike other types of tofu, it isn't packed in water. If your plan for tofu is to brown, bread, fry, bake, or scramble it, vacuum-packed super-firm tofu is a good default option. You can just remove it from the package and use it right away.

Knowing how to use water-packed tofu

If you can't find vacuum-packed tofu, use water-packed tofu instead. It's the most common variety of tofu. The only thing to remember with water-packed tofu is that you often need to press it to remove the water before cooking with it.

If you've never worked with tofu, you may wonder why pressing is necessary. See, tofu is like a sponge. It can take on the flavors of any marinade you soak it in. Tofu that's stored in water is like a water-soaked sponge. You want to squeeze the water out, so it has room for picking up other flavors.

Pressing water-packed tofu also gives it a denser texture. When you squeeze out the water, you get a more toothsome bite. Finally, pressing it helps with browning. If you've ever fried anything, you know that wet things are difficult to brown, and water causes splatter.

Taking steps to press water-packed tofu

Plan an extra half hour into your prep time for pressing the water out of your tofu.

PRESS TOFU BETWEEN KITCHEN TOWELS

While you can find store-bought tofu presses on the market, start with the old-school method that uses stuff you already have on hand in your house. No extra purchases required!

1. **Cut open the tofu package and drain it.**

2. **Cut the block into half-inch slices and lay them on a clean towel-covered plate.**

3. **Top the tofu slices with another clean kitchen towel.**

4. **Lay something firm and flat on top of it.** A thick hardcover book, plate, or cutting board works well.

5. **For a final layer, add extra weight, like a hand weight or cans of soup.**

I recommend pressing for at least a half hour. An hour is better if you have the time. If you're really short on time, 20 minutes will do. (If you're going to press it for a while, move it to the refrigerator.)

After the tofu slices have been pressed, you can marinate, bake, grill, or bread and fry them.

USE A STORE-BOUGHT TOFU PRESS

If you'd prefer to splash out on something slicker, buy a tofu press. Some of them are just a box with a lid and spring.

You put a whole block of water-packed tofu into the box. When you place the lid on the box, it provides gentle pressure, pushing out the liquid. The liquid stays contained in the box, so it's easy to drain it off afterward.

Freezing tofu

One more option for tofu prep is freezing it. It's really simple: You just put a whole block of firm, extra-firm, or super-firm tofu into the freezer — either in its package or in a freezer-safe container. Then let it freeze.

When you're ready to use it, move it to the refrigerator to thaw for at least 8 hours. Once it has thawed, you can use your hands to squeeze the water out. (You'll be surprised at the amount of water that's released!)

Freezing tofu changes the texture completely. It becomes dry and kind of rough inside. The places where the water froze inside it leave holes. This dense tofu has a meaty texture that works particularly well crumbled in chili or used in a vegan chicken–style sandwich.

TIP

Freezing tofu is also a good way to extend its shelf life. You can freeze it for up to 5 months.

Try protein-packed tempeh

Tempeh (*tem*-pay) is made with whole fermented soybeans that are pressed into firm cakes. In addition to soybeans, this traditional Indonesian food is often fermented with some type of grain, nut, or seed.

TIP

Look for tempeh in the refrigerated section at the grocery store. It's often near the tofu.

Tempeh has a nutty, earthy flavor that's sometimes compared to mushrooms. Because it's fermented, it smells vaguely like yeast when you open the package. The fermentation creates enzymes that make it more digestible and give it a good amount of B vitamins.

Tempeh is lauded for its protein, fiber, and *prebiotics* (plant fibers that promote the growth of healthy bacteria in your gut). It's also enjoyed for its satisfying chewy texture and versatility. It can be sautéed, baked, grilled, or fried in crumbles, strips, triangles, or squares. Depending on how it's seasoned, it can take on an endless array of flavors. I like to use tempeh to make tacos, as shown on the cover of this book!

REMEMBER

For the most part, tempeh is beige in color, but you'll occasionally see dark gray or black spots. That's a natural part of the fermenting process and nothing to worry about.

TIP

Some people find tempeh to have a bitter aftertaste. To soften that, you can either briefly steam it before using it, boil it in water, or cook it in a flavorful liquid until it has absorbed the liquid's flavor and cooked off any bitter edge.

Discover seitan and store-bought vegan meats

Seitan (pronounced *say*-tan) is also known as wheat meat, because it emulates the flavors and textures of meat. It's a great source of protein and is very low in fat.

People are sometimes wary of seitan because it's unfamiliar to them. But the ingredients and process of making it aren't a world away from bread. It's basically a dense, savory bread that has been cooked by baking, steaming, or boiling. Where bread is light and fluffy, seitan is toothsome. It has bite. It's also the "meat" of a meal.

When it was invented, seitan was produced by rinsing dough made from regular flour until you were left with the protein-dense remnants. But nowadays, you can make it much easier on yourself by using *vital wheat gluten*, a flour that's made with the main protein in wheat.

REMEMBER

Since seitan is pretty much straight gluten, you'll want to stay away from it if you or someone you are feeding has a gluten sensitivity.

If you don't feel like making your own, premade seitan can be found in the refrigerated section at natural grocery stores, as well as in big-box stores. Depending on how it's seasoned and formed, seitan can be made into jerky, sausage, hamburger, bacon, chorizo, chicken, deli meats, holiday roasts, meatballs, pepperoni, hot dogs, and more.

Because it's so dense, it's great for grilling, as well as cooking in soups, stews, and sauces.

In addition to seitan, there are lots of other types of vegan meats made with pea protein or soy protein.

Many options are available and new ones are popping up all the time. Here are a few delicious options for plant-based meats:

>> **Holiday roasts:** Field Roast, Gardein, or Trader Joe's

>> **Plant-based beef and burgers:** Beyond Meat, Impossible Foods, Field Roast, Gardein, or Trader Joe's Korean Beefless Bulgogi

>> **Plant-based hot dogs and sausages:** Beyond Meat, Field Roast, Impossible Foods, Herbivorous Butcher, or Tofurky

>> **Seitan bacon:** Herbivorous Butcher or Upton's Naturals

>> **Seitan pepperoni:** Herbivorous Butcher or BE-Hive

>> **Seitan ribs:** Herbivorous Butcher

>> **Vegan chicken:** Beyond Meat, Impossible Foods, Tofurky, Gardein, May Wah, Butler Soy Curls, or Trader Joe's Chickenless Crispy Tenders

>> **Vegan deli slices:** Tofurky, Field Roast, or Unreal Deli

>> **Vegan jerky:** Beyond Meat, Herbivorous Butcher, or Louisville Vegan Jerky Company

>> **Vegan seafood:** Gardein

Note that some vegan meats are high in sodium. If that's a concern for you, choose tofu, tempeh, or beans instead. (Or at least more often!)

WARNING

DRAWING THE LINE: ANIMAL TESTING OF PLANT-BASED FOODS

Over the past decade, we've seen amazing innovation in the world of plant-based specialty products. With innovation comes the development of new ingredients. Unfortunately, the U.S. Food and Drug Administration (FDA) essentially requires that novel ingredients be tested on animals before they're given the Generally Recognized As Safe (GRAS) designation.

Although some people claim that the GRAS all clear is optional, when the FDA signs off on a new ingredient, it assures consumers that the ingredient is safe to eat, and it satisfies requirements of large-scale retailers, fast-food chains, and governmental bodies.

Even if a brand isn't creating new ingredients, they're often relying on animal testing that's been done in the past to give their products' ingredients a pass. Ingredients that

(continued)

(continued)

have been tested on animals include pea protein isolate, oat protein, and rice protein. (It's a similar situation to prescription and nonprescription medications, like common painkillers, which have all been tested on animals.)

When a new plant-based product comes on the scene, some vegans raise a red flag if it has been tested on animals, like the Impossible Burger and JUST Egg. In the case of JUST Egg, mung bean protein was fed to rats to test its digestibility. While Impossible Foods used rats to test their plant-based heme (soy leghemoglobin), which is part of what gives the Impossible Burger its meaty flavor. (Now that mung bean protein and soy leghemoglobin have been tested on animals, other food companies that want to use those ingredients in the future won't have to do animal testing to ensure their safety.)

There are disagreements amongst vegans about the ethics of purchasing plant-based foods that were tested on animals. Some say the FDA's requirements should be getting the brunt of vegans' ire, and vegans should implore the FDA to change rules around animal testing. Others argue that ground-breaking plant-based products convince people to give up eating animal products, even if only for occasional meals, which reduces demand for them. Finally, there are those who say that if a product is tested on animals, it can't possibly be called vegan. They may go even further to assert that if a vegan product is sold by a non-vegan company (like a maker of meat, dairy, or eggs), vegans should avoid it too. Ultimately, you'll have to decide for yourself where you draw the line.

Amp up your recipes with beans

While beans aren't really a meat substitute in terms of their taste or texture, they do add protein and bite to a meal. Another benefit of using beans as an alternative to meat is that most people are already very familiar with them, so the learning curve is small. Plus, beans are inexpensive, especially in comparison to some high-end vegan meats.

Keep dried or canned beans on hand for soups, stews, salads, salsas, and tacos.

Use beans to make:

- » Falafel and hummus
- » Black or pinto bean tacos
- » Bean burgers
- » Refried bean burritos
- » Three bean chili
- » Roasted Chickpeas (recipe in Chapter 14)

- » Black-eyed peas with collard greens

- » *Chana masala* (chickpea curry)

- » White bean soup with pasta

- » Vegan tuna salad sandwiches

- » Red beans and rice

- » Beans on toast

Get the scoop on jackfruit

A vegan meat alternative that's become surprisingly popular in recent years is *jackfruit*, which comes from Southeast Asia. Jackfruit is the largest tree-borne fruit. It can weigh up to 80 pounds and looks like a huge spiky watermelon.

Usually when people think of fruit, they imagine something sweet. However, when jackfruit is used in vegan cooking, it isn't ripe yet. Green jackfruit has a neutral flavor that can be seasoned with herbs, spices, and sauces.

If you're interested in trying ripe jackfruit, look for it in the produce section of certain grocery stores. It has a flavor that's similar to mango. Enjoy it on its own, but don't try to use it for making vegan meat recipes. It's far too sweet for that.

TIP

When making vegan jackfruit recipes, look for canned green or young jackfruit that's packed in water or brine (not syrup). It's sold in Asian markets, natural grocery stores, Trader Joe's, and online.

TIP

Jackfruit is great when you want a vegan meat with a shredded texture. It's especially common as vegan pulled pork. (For a delicious recipe, check out Chapter 12, where I use it as a topping for Barbecue Jackfruit Nachos.)

Keep in mind that while jackfruit is a popular meat substitute, it's not high in protein like other vegan meats, seitan, tofu, or tempeh. Consider pairing jackfruit dishes with something protein-dense like baked beans, lentil salad, or a cup of split pea soup.

Depending on how it's seasoned, jackfruit can be used in a variety of ways. Some of my favorite uses are in any of the following veganized dishes:

- » Reuben sandwich

- » French dip sandwich

- » Taquitos

>> Carnitas-style tacos

>> Barbecue sandwich

The first time you open a can of green jackfruit, you may be a little surprised that there are pods and firmer parts to the jackfruit. However, all parts of the canned jackfruit are edible.

After draining jackfruit, move it to a colander and rinse it to remove excess brine. Then put it on a clean kitchen towel, roll it up like a Tootsie Roll, and squeeze to remove any brine left inside.

After that, move the jackfruit to a food processor and pulse several times. That way it all gets broken up and looks uniform. (If you don't have a food processor, chop it up or break it apart with a spatula in the pan.) Chopping jackfruit into smaller pieces also means it will absorb the seasonings and sauce better. From there, you can cook it however you like.

Impart smoky flavor with liquid smoke

When people make Southern-style greens, they often add smoked turkey or a ham hock. However, the only reason those animal parts have a smoky flavor is because they were cooked in a smoker.

So instead of using smoked meat to flavor a dish, cut out the middle pig (or turkey) and use liquid smoke.

Liquid smoke adds a wonderful smoky flavor to foods like:

>> Collard greens

>> Split pea soup

>> Vegan bacon

>> Barbecue sauce

>> Corn chowder

>> Baked beans

TECHNICAL STUFF

As you may have guessed from the name, liquid smoke is condensed and liquefied smoke. It's made by heating hickory, mesquite, or apple wood in large chambers. That causes the wood to smolder and release smoke. The gases are then cooled in condensers, which liquefies the smoke. The droplets are collected, and the impurities are filtered and removed.

Look for liquid smoke next to barbecue sauces in most grocery stores, as well as chain stores like Target. Some brands are more potent than others. My preferred choice is Wright's hickory flavor.

TIP

When it comes to liquid smoke, I recommend starting with a small amount and working up. Like truffle oil or sesame oil, it's a strong flavor that can overtake a dish if given the opportunity. Start with ¼ teaspoon and increase the amount from there. You can always add more, but you can't take it out.

Cracking the Code on Egg Substitutes

Have you noticed how plentiful eggs are on cooking shows nowadays? For something to immediately be seen as "elevated," a fried egg with a runny yolk is laid on top of it. It doesn't seem to matter what the dish is — a burger, rice bowl, pasta, salad — when a chef puts an egg on top, everyone acts duly impressed (even though eggs are often one of the first things children are taught to cook). It seems to have overtaken the bacon craze of the 2010s.

It's no wonder eggs are a point of confusion for people considering veganism. What will they eat for breakfast? How will they bake a cake? What will they throw at the houses of their enemies?

Okay, so I can't help you with that last one. However, the other questions are easily remedied. You can either eat something completely different for breakfast (like oatmeal), or if you like eggy flavors, try one of the following ideas.

Adding eggy flavor with kala namak

Kala namak, also known as black salt, is a kiln-fired rock salt with a strong sulfurous scent. It's commonly used in Indian cuisine. The amazing thing about this salt is how it instantly adds eggy flavor to dishes. It pairs especially well with tofu, which is a blank slate for flavor.

TIP

Look for kala namak in Indian grocery stores or online. Be aware that a little goes a long way. Start sparingly — you can always add more.

In addition to using black salt on tofu, you can sprinkle a pinch of it on sliced avocado. Add the seasoned avocado to an Old School Chef Salad (recipe in Chapter 13). It replaces the boiled egg that's usually in a chef salad.

You can even make vegan deviled eggs using baby potatoes instead of eggs. Bake or boil the whole tiny potatoes. Then cut them in half and scoop out a yolk-sized center. Add the scooped potato to a bowl with vegan mayo, stone-ground mustard, paprika, kala namak, and pepper. Then combine and fill the baby potatoes with the mixture using a piping bag.

Replacing eggs with tofu

Tofu is back, and this time it's an egg replacer. Not only does it work well as a binder in baked recipes, but it can also take on the flavor of eggs in savory recipes. It works especially well in tandem with the aforementioned kala namak.

If you're looking for some ways to use tofu as a stand-in for eggs, try these tasty options:

>> **Make Eggy Tofu slices.** Cut super-firm tofu into slices. Then brown it in a skillet with oil, and season with kala namak, nutritional yeast, pepper, and granulated onion. (Get the complete recipe in Chapter 11.) Serve Eggy Tofu with toast or anywhere you'd put a fried egg — like a breakfast sandwich, vegan eggs Benedict, or vegan *shakshuka* (eggs in spicy tomato sauce).

>> **Make Eggy Tofu crumbles.** Instead of cutting the tofu into slices, brown it in crumbled pieces. Once it's brown on all sides, season it the same as above with kala namak, nutritional yeast, and granulated onion. Enjoy crumbled tofu with toast, or use it as a topping on Pineapple Fried Rice (see Chapter 12).

>> **Make a tofu scramble.** Start your day with veggies by making a tofu scramble. It's similar to scrambled eggs, but with tofu and lots of fiber-rich vegetables. Brown crumbled tofu in a skillet with oil. Then add vegetables like onion, bell pepper, and garlic. Sprinkle on seasonings, and finish by incorporating handfuls of baby spinach. Get the recipe for Veggie-Packed Tofu Scramble in Chapter 11.

>> **Enjoy tofu right out of the package.** Don't worry; it's a fully cooked product. Crumble it into a bowl. Then stir in vegan mayo, black pepper, kala namak, stone-ground mustard, and chives for vegan egg salad. Pile it on a sandwich, in a wrap, or on top of crackers as a snack. (For a complete recipe, see the Eggless Egg Salad Wrap in Chapter 13.)

Gathering vegan eggs

You can find loads of store-bought vegan eggs that serve a variety of purposes.

>> **Want vegan fried eggs?** Try JUST Egg, which is made with mung beans. It's sold in two forms — a pourable liquid or ready-to-eat patties.

Use the pourable liquid to make fried vegan egg for breakfast sandwiches, in quiche, as a dipping liquid for French toast, or as a binder for vegan meat loaf. The premade patties are good when you're in a hurry or don't have access to a full kitchen.

>> **Want vegan boiled eggs?** Check out WunderEggs. The white part is made from *agar*, which is a vegan version of gelatin. They can be eaten on their own, added to ramen, made into vegan egg salad, or turned into vegan deviled eggs. WunderEggs come complete with a little package of kala namak for sprinkling on top just before eating.

>> **Want vegan poached or sunny side up eggs?** Try Yo Egg if a runny yolk is what you crave. The poached style is perfect for vegan eggs Benedict. Primarily made of soy and chickpea, Yo Eggs are available in a small selection of stores and restaurants.

>> **Want to use vegan eggs in baked goods?** Head on to the next section!

Binding without eggs

Many baked goods recipes use eggs as a binder. That's what people have gotten used to using, but eggs aren't magic. You can easily substitute other plant-based ingredients instead.

In fact, it's kind of funny when you think about it. Eggs have such a specific flavor. Consider the taste of fried eggs at breakfast. Now can you imagine someone saying, "I just can't have a cupcake without an egg in it?"

Eggs add moisture, *leaven* (raise or lighten) batter and dough, and bind ingredients. However, they can easily be replaced by plant-based ingredients that also do those things.

Here are some options:

>> **Flaxseed or chia seed:** Mix together 1 tablespoon of ground flaxseed and 3 tablespoons of water in a bowl, and wait about 15 minutes. Then stir the mixture again until it's goopy and gelatinous. Now you have a flax egg that can be used in baked goods to replace one egg. (This method also works with whole chia seeds.)

>> **Banana:** Half a banana (or ¼ cup mashed) can replace one egg. Keep in mind that this substitution may give your baked good a banana flavor, though. This is best in dessert breads, muffins, or pancakes.

>> **Applesauce:** Use ¼ cup of applesauce to replace an egg. This replacement has a more neutral flavor than banana, although it does add some sweetness.

Use this for cakes and dessert-style baked goods. If you like, add a pinch of baking powder to help with leavening.

>> **Pumpkin puree:** Use ¼ cup of pumpkin puree to replace an egg. (Remember to use canned pumpkin, not pumpkin pie filling.) This works especially well with fall-inspired ingredients like cinnamon and apples.

>> **Silken tofu:** Replace one egg with ¼ cup of blended silken tofu. Because of its neutral flavor, tofu doesn't draw attention to itself in baked goods. It works especially well for muffins, scones, and quick breads. If you like, add an extra ¼ teaspoon of baking powder to help with leavening.

>> **Aquafaba:** Substitute 3 tablespoons of aquafaba for one egg in your recipe. You may not realize it, but there's a good chance you have some in your pantry! *Aquafaba* is the name for the cooking liquid in a can of beans. (Chickpeas are most commonly used, but any type of bean works.) Aquafaba can be used in place of eggs in cakes and quick breads.

You can use aquafaba along with sugar, cream of tartar, and vanilla to make vegan meringue. You can even use aquafaba to make vegan mayonnaise!

TIP

>> **Vinegar and baking powder:** Mix together 1 teaspoon of baking soda and 1 tablespoon of vinegar to replace one egg. The combination of vinegar and baking powder acts as a leavening agent that makes for light and airy baked goods. The Wacky Cake recipe in Chapter 15 uses this substitute with amazing results.

>> **Nondairy yogurt:** Sub ¼ cup of nondairy yogurt for one egg. Plain unsweetened nondairy yogurt works well in muffins, cupcakes, and cakes.

>> **JUST Egg liquid:** Use 3 tablespoons of JUST Egg in place of one egg for binding veggie burgers or vegan meat loaf, cakes, muffins, breads, cookies, or even boxed cake mixes. It adds fat and structure.

>> **Powdered egg replacers:** Vegan egg substitutes like Ener-G or Bob's Red Mill are made with potato starch, tapioca flour, and baking soda. Just follow the package directions. They work best as a binder in recipes.

Slathering on vegan mayonnaise

One condiment that's usually made with eggs is mayonnaise. It's used as a sandwich spread or as a base for salad dressings, dips, and sauces.

Vegan mayo options are made with oil, vinegar, and soy milk instead of eggs. You can find recipes online to make your own, or you can pick some up at most grocery stores as well as big-box stores.

There are a wide variety of vegan mayo makers. The names of some of them may be familiar, as many egg mayo makers are getting in on the eggless mayo scene. My favorite brand is Vegenaise. Along with their original variety, they have soy-free, avocado oil, grapeseed oil, reduced fat, organic, and chipotle.

TIP

Use vegan mayonnaise 1 to 1 anywhere you would have used mayo made with eggs.

Selecting a Plant-Based Milk

Of all the vegan specialty products on the market, the general public seems to have embraced nondairy milk the most. Even if people have dairy ice cream in their shopping cart, they often have oat or almond milk right beside it.

Whether you choose to make your own nondairy milk from scratch or pick up a container of soy milk at the grocery store, a ton of fabulous options for dairy-free drinking are available.

TIP

When you're veganizing a recipe, cow's milk can be replaced with nondairy milk 1 to 1. For example, if a recipe calls for a cup of cow's milk, simply use 1 cup of cashew, almond, soy, or oat milk.

Experiment with homemade nut milks

One thing that's super handy about being vegan is how easy it is to make staples when you run out. Back when I drank dairy milk, if I ran out, I didn't have a lactating cow in the backyard. But now, if my cereal bowl needs filling, it's super easy to make my own nondairy milk with pantry staples.

Some of the quickest and easiest nondairy milks to make are nut-based. Here are a couple homemade options to try.

>> **Cashew milk:** My favorite nut-based milk is cashew milk, because when you make it with a high-speed blender, you don't have to strain it. You can add more or less water to reach your perfect level of creaminess. It can be really thick like whole milk or coffee creamer, or thinner like skim milk. It all depends on your ratio of water to nuts.

In a high-speed blender such as a Vitamix, blend 1 cup of raw cashews with 4 cups of water, a pinch of salt, and a couple pitted dates (or a teaspoon of your preferred liquid sweetener) for sweetness. For vanilla milk, add a teaspoon of vanilla extract.

TIP

If you have a standard blender, before blending, cover the raw cashew nuts in water to soak overnight. Then drain and blend the soaked nuts with 4 cups of water.

>> **Almond milk:** If you'd prefer, you can follow the same guidelines above for almond milk using raw almonds. However, I like to strain raw almond milk with a nut milk bag or cheesecloth after blending, because it doesn't get quite as smooth and pulp-free thanks to the almonds' tough outer skin.

TIP

Keep experimenting with these easy nondairy milks! You can use the same guidelines and ratios as above with other types of nuts like pistachios or hazelnuts. If you have a nut allergy, try pumpkin seed or sunflower milk — or a combination of the two!

Store homemade nut and seed milks in a sealed jar in the fridge. They'll last 3 to 5 days. If you notice any separation, simply give the milk a stir before drinking.

Opt for store-bought vegan milk

You can find endless types of nondairy milk on the market. You've got milk made from soy, cashews, almonds, oats, hemp, coconut, macadamias, and the list goes on! From there, you can choose from unsweetened and sweetened, flavored and unflavored.

My everyday choice is Silk plain unsweetened cashew milk. It has a neutral flavor that works nicely in coffee as well as recipes. However, it's worth sampling a variety to see what you like best.

TIP

If you're trying to match dairy milk's protein content, soy is the best option. It has a naturally high-protein content, ranging from 7 to 12 grams per cup depending on the brand. (Eden Soy has 12 grams per cup!) Soy milk also has a full-bodied texture and creaminess that's similar to cow's milk, which can make it an easy adjustment from dairy.

If you want to optimize your mineral intake and make sure you're getting a dose of calcium and vitamin D, opt for fortified plant-based milk. Look at the percentage of the daily values on the nutrition facts label, which should indicate that it has calcium and vitamin D (usually 15 to 30 percent of the daily value). Or look at the ingredients label to see if it states that calcium and vitamin D have been added.

TIP

If you try a new brand of nondairy milk and don't love it by the glassful, use it in recipes instead. Then try again with another type until you find one you love. (If you've ever switched from whole milk to skim milk, you know it can take time for your palate to adjust to what you think milk should taste like.)

Making the World a "Butter" Place

Whether you're baking, cooking, making vegan buttercream, or looking for something to spread on toast, you'll find endless nondairy butter options. You have your choice of longtime vegan brands, as well as mainstream dairy brands that have gotten in on the plant-based butter game.

Vegan butter can be used to replace dairy butter in any recipe 1 to 1. It is generally made from a blend of vegetable oils, or ingredients like nuts or seeds.

Miyoko's European-style plant milk butter is a popular option. Available in natural grocery stores and big-box stores like Target, Miyoko's offers vegan butter made from cashew milk or oat milk. It is especially good when you really want to taste the butter — like spread on warm bread or drizzled over popcorn. Plus, Miyoko's doesn't use palm oil, which many vegans avoid because of concerns about palm oil's environmental and social impact, as well as habitat loss for animals like orangutans.

Sample a few of the many nondairy butters on the market, and see what you like best.

TIP

If you'd prefer, you can make your own vegan butter from scratch using refined coconut oil. You can choose from plenty of recipes online.

TIP

If you're simply looking for something to spread on your toast, consider fresh avocado or nut butter. When making avocado toast, finish it with a pinch of salt and a few shakes of nutritional yeast flakes.

Feeling "Grate-ful" for Vegan Cheeses

For many people, the biggest roadblock on the way to veganism is cheese. People are attached, to say the least. Luckily, these days you have a dizzying array of options with vegan cheddar-style cheeses for your tacos, mozzarella for your pizzas, and fancy artisanal cheeses for your vegan cheese board.

In addition to vegan cheeses, you can add cheesy flavor and umami to dishes with nutritional yeast and miso paste.

There's no need to go without cheese in your new vegan life. Just choose cheeses made from a plant-based source.

Get cheesy with nutritional yeast

When you look up vegan cheese recipes, you're almost certain to see one common ingredient: nutritional yeast flakes. They have a scientific-sounding name, but these flakes are a dried inactive yeast that's grown on molasses.

Known informally as *nooch*, nutritional yeast has a cheesy, nutty flavor that's a wonderful addition to sauces, dips, or gravies. Here are some of my favorite ways to use it:

>> Make vegan parmesan and sprinkle it on pasta. (Get the Cashew Parmesan recipe in Chapter 14.)

>> Sprinkle it on popcorn.

>> Add a dash to a vegan-buttered baked potato.

>> Use it in vegan mac and cheese.

>> Make chili cheese dip.

>> Add it to homemade pesto instead of Parmesan.

>> Stir it into grits.

>> Put it in tomato soup for added depth of flavor.

>> Sprinkle it on roasted chickpeas.

>> Use it in the breading mix for appetizers like fried ravioli.

>> Add it to your tofu scramble.

>> Use it in homemade seitan for richness.

>> Incorporate it into both vegan turkey gravy and mashed potatoes at the holidays.

In addition to giving foods a cheesy taste, fortified nutritional yeast is a good source of protein and vitamin B12.

Look for nutritional yeast at natural grocery stores, Trader Joe's, Walmart, or online. It's usually in the natural foods section or near the flour. It's sometimes sold in bulk bins as well.

TIP

Nutritional yeast doesn't need to be refrigerated. It can be stored anywhere cool and dark to preserve its B vitamins. Since it's a dry product, the key is keeping moisture out. If you'd prefer, you can freeze it in a sealed airtight bag. It has a shelf life of 1 to 2 years.

Add umami with miso paste

Miso is a fermented soybean paste that fills homemade vegan cheeses with umami. It's rich in protein and digestive enzymes. Plus, it imparts savory depth and flavor to soups, salad dressings, and marinades.

Look for it in the refrigerated section of the grocery store near the tofu. Of the many different types available, the one I use most often is white miso paste. Here are some of my favorite ways to use it in recipes:

» Add it to cashew cheese spread or vegan queso.

» Incorporate it in tofu ricotta.

» Add it to ramen noodle broth or other soups.

» Spoon a dollop in basil pesto.

Indulge with homemade vegan cheeses

When it comes to making vegan cheeses, some can be whipped up in minutes. Others are more labor-intensive. It all depends on how much time and energy you want to put into the project.

Some of the easiest vegan cheeses to make are vegan parmesan (see Chapter 14), tofu ricotta, and vegan queso with raw cashews. Both vegan parmesan and tofu ricotta just require a quick blend in a food processor. Cashew queso is made by blending raw cashews with a few ingredients in a blender and then thickening the mixture in a pot on the stove. Perfect for nachos!

When I have a little more time, I like to make baked almond feta with blanched almonds, lemon juice, olive brine, extra virgin olive oil, salt, and garlic. (You can find my Cashew Queso, Tofu Ricotta, and Vegan Feta Cheese recipes at https:// cadryskitchen.com/.)

Choose store-bought vegan cheese

There's a vegan cheese for every need. Whether you want something hard and sliceable, melty and gooey, or tangy and soft, you can find a nondairy cheese on the market that fits the bill. Looking for vegan cream cheese? Yep, they've got that too!

Most grocery stores and big-box chains sell common vegan brands like Daiya, Miyoko's, Violife, Field Roast, and Follow Your Heart. Other vegan options aren't as widely available. Find them online, or check out your favorite natural grocer.

Here are some of my go-tos:

>> **Miyoko's Creamery:** Choose an array of nondairy cheeses like Aged Black Ash, European Truffle, and Sharp English Farmhouse for a stunning vegan charcuterie board. Their Savory Scallion Cream Cheese is my favorite for toasted bagels, and Roadhouse Cheddar is delicious spread on crackers.

   Their mozzarella cheeses have amazing meltability for pizzas. Choose either a sliceable plant milk mozzarella, or opt for the pourable variety that goes on like a liquid and solidifies into a gooey cheese when baked.

>> **Follow Your Heart, Daiya,** or **Violife:** For cheddar-style cheese shreds and slices, look for these vegan cheesemakers, which also offer shredded mozzarella. Violife's parmesan wedge is perfect for grating on pasta, and their vegan feta is a standout.

>> **Treeline:** This company offers an artisanal cashew cheese that comes in a variety of flavors like Herb Garlic, Creamy Scallion, and Cracked Pepper. They have both sliceable and spreadable cheeses. Great for a vegan cheese board!

>> **Darë Vegan Cheese:** A small vegan cheesemaker out of Asheville, North Carolina, their wedges of Pepperjack, Balsamic Fig, and Roasted Garlic are outstanding. They're available at Whole Foods in a few states or online. They also make delicious vegan cheesecake.

>> **Rebel Cheese:** This company is based out of Austin, Texas, where they have a deli, and a vegan cheese and wine shop. They also offer dairy-free cheese subscriptions by mail.

Getting Sweet on Vegan Honey

Even people who know that vegans don't consume milk, dairy, or eggs are often surprised by one more thing vegans don't partake of — honey. They become incredulous: "What? You don't even eat honey?"

The reaction always takes me by surprise, because honey was the easiest non-vegan food to give up by far. I was really only in it for the cute squeezable bear bottle. Outside of putting a little squeeze in tea or on top of nut butter sandwiches, I barely (or should that be bear-ly?) even used it.

Honey is bee food — as in food for bees. They make it for themselves, their offspring, and their hive for nutrients and energy. Luckily, you can find plenty of other liquid sweeteners on the market. Replacing honey is a breeze. Some of my favorite options include:

>> **Maple syrup:** You likely already have maple syrup in your refrigerator for pancakes and waffles. Add a drizzle to English breakfast tea or on top of peanut butter and banana toast. It does have more of a maple flavor than honey (for obvious reasons), but it's so delicious, that flavor is more than welcome to me. Replace honey with maple syrup at a 1-to-1 ratio.

>> **Agave syrup:** Also known as *agave nectar,* this sweetener comes from the same plant as tequila. It has a more neutral flavor than maple syrup and a runny consistency very similar to honey. You can choose between light, dark, amber, or raw agave, depending on your preferences. Substitute it 1 to 1 for honey.

>> **Vegan honey:** Most of the vegan honeys on the market are made from apple juice that has been reduced to a syrup. Others are made with monk fruit. Depending on the product, you may need less than you would with honey made by bees.

TIP

You can make your own vegan honey by reducing apple juice in a saucepan with sugar and a squeeze of lemon juice until it becomes a syrup. Amp up the honey flavor by adding bags of chamomile tea.

>> **Date syrup:** This caramel-colored syrup is made from liquefied and concentrated dates. If you like the flavor of dates, you'll love this sweetener. Substitute it 1 to 1 for honey.

By the way, if you'd like to store any of these syrups in a bear-shaped bottle, I support that decision.

Chapter **10**

Enjoying Holidays and Get-Togethers

When you first go vegan, every season brings unique challenges. You're navigating Easter without eggs, and the 4th of July cookout without hamburgers. You're researching vegan candy for trick-or-treaters, and brainstorming a new main course for Thanksgiving dinner.

It can feel a little awkward to do something different. But it can also feel exciting. For maybe the first time, you can think about what really makes holidays meaningful for *you*.

Many of our traditions are based on what someone else chose a long time ago, and everybody just kept doing things that way. But now you can consider what makes a holiday feel special and important, and lean into that instead.

In this chapter, I share how to make your way through the year while staying true to your vegan lifestyle — from holidays and weddings to summer potlucks and cookouts. Some holidays require a few simple swaps or substitutions. Others involve more robust changes. (Keep in mind that I don't cover every holiday in this chapter, just the ones I celebrate with my family. However, I hope my ideas will give you a solid start toward veganizing your own traditions!)

REMEMBER Whatever the holiday, there are no rules. You can do what works for you, and leave behind what doesn't.

Savoring Sweets (and More) with Your Valentine

When stores are filled with flowers, sentimental cards, and heart-shaped candies, you know Valentine's Day is just around the corner.

This romantic holiday is an excuse to treat your sweetheart to a box of chocolates or a romantic dinner. Whether you like to make an elaborate meal or just reservations, you have plenty of vegan options for this lovers' holiday.

Make them melt with chocolates

Did you know that chocolate in and of itself is vegan? It comes from cacao beans, which are grown on cacao trees. It's only what gets added to chocolate that can make it non-vegan.

TIP To find vegan chocolate, it's just a matter of reading ingredients labels. First, look for dark chocolate. Not all dark chocolate is vegan. So next, you need to check that milk, butter, or dairy by-products haven't been added along the way.

If you're used to milk chocolate, dark chocolate may taste a little bitter at first. But once you've adjusted to it, wow! Dark chocolate has such an intense flavor. It really bursts with all that chocolatey goodness.

If you still prefer milk chocolate, you're in luck. All kinds of chocolatiers make vegan milk chocolate with nondairy milks. Browse the chocolate aisle at the grocery store. I think you'll be pleasantly surprised. (Some chocolate makers label the front of the packaging with the type of nondairy milk they use, like oat milk. That's very handy for easy buying.)

Sjaak's and Lagusta's Luscious make outstanding vegan truffles. Even major chocolate brands like Hershey's and Reese's are getting in on the plant-based chocolate game.

REMEMBER If you see cocoa butter on an ingredients list, don't worry. It's vegan, even though butter is in the name. (It's similar to peanut butter that way.) Cocoa butter is made by extracting fat from cacao beans.

Share a romantic dinner

Restaurants are busy, crowded, and expensive on Valentine's Day. So I usually prefer to make a special meal at home. Here are some date-worthy dinner ideas.

Enjoy a vegan cheese board

Vegan cheese boards are super simple to prepare but consistently popular. The array of bright colors and textures on a board makes it instantly eye-catching. It isn't hard to put together an elaborate vegan charcuterie board, but it always impresses. And there's something instantly romantic about nibbling on finger food together while sipping glasses of red wine.

1. Grab a couple store-bought vegan cheeses. Miyoko's, Treeline, Kite Hill, and Nuts For Cheese all have good options.

2. Add vegan deli slices or seitan pepperoni.

3. Put them on a board or platter along with berries, carrot and celery sticks, radishes, sugar snap peas, olives, and crackers.

4. Make a meal of it!

Cook together

Want another fun date-night idea? Look through vegan cookbooks with your sweetheart, and pick out a meal to make together. Planning the menu, going to the grocery store, and preparing the dinner are all part of the fun.

Depending on your mood, you can go with something really ambitious, or choose something low-key and easy. Here are some ideas:

>> Tomato bruschetta (This classic appetizer is often vegan as is.)

>> Seitan bacon-wrapped dates stuffed with spreadable nondairy cheese

>> Vegan crab cakes made with artichoke hearts

>> Vegan chicken piccata with a lemon caper sauce

>> Basil Pesto Pasta with Roasted Chickpeas (Find my recipe in Chapter 12.)

Go out on the town

Prefer to let someone else do the cooking? Start with dinner reservations! If you're not familiar with vegan restaurants in your town, do a quick Google search for "vegan restaurants in my area."

TIP

If you don't have any exclusively vegan restaurants, no worries. Thai, Ethiopian, Mediterranean, and Indian restaurants tend to be vegan-friendly.

For more tips on finding vegan options in restaurants, check out Chapter 18.

Celebrating a Hoppy Easter

Easter is a religious holiday that's often associated with colorful baskets, chocolate bunnies, egg hunts, and a trip to see the Easter Bunny.

Vegans don't have to miss out! Visit your local mall for a photo with everyone's favorite costumed rabbit. Then fill your Easter basket with any of the following:

» Toys or stuffed animals

» Dairy-free chocolate eggs from Chomp!, Moo Free, or Lagusta's Luscious

» Dairy-free chocolate bunnies from Sjaak's, Trupo Treats, No Whey, Vegan Treats, or Lindt

» Seasonal gummy candies from Sour Patch Kids, YumEarth, or Annie's

WARNING

Most gummy candies aren't vegan because they contain gelatin. Gelatin comes from the skin, bones, and connective tissues of animals. Be sure to read that ingredients label!

Dyeing eggs

Many kids get excited about dyeing eggs at Easter. Keep the fun alive with these vegan alternatives:

» **Dyeable plastic eggs:** At some big-box stores you can find plastic eggs that come with dye. They usually cost just a couple of dollars. Plus, kids can play with them as toys for the rest of the year.

» **Ceramic or wooden eggs:** Many craft stores sell ceramic or wooden eggs. Grab some craft supplies, stickers, and paint. Then have the kids decorate to their hearts' content.

» **Refillable plastic eggs:** Any retail store that sells Easter decorations will have refillable plastic eggs in a variety of colors. Fill them with vegan candies, stickers, or small toys. Perfect for Easter baskets and egg hunts.

Serving a bountiful Easter brunch

Easter is closely associated with brunching. Luckily, it's never been easier to make all those egg dishes of yore, but with plant-based ingredients.

TIP

Tofu has long been the go-to option for making an eggy breakfast without eggs. It's packed with filling protein, and it has a neutral flavor that can pick up whatever spices you add to it.

Use tofu to make:

>> Vegan eggs Benedict with a cashew-based hollandaise

>> Vegan *shakshuka* (eggs in tomato sauce) with seasoned tofu rounds instead of poached eggs

>> Breakfast sandwiches

>> Veggie-Packed Tofu Scramble (Get my favorite tofu scramble recipe and more ideas on how to veganize classic brunch dishes in Chapter 11.)

Another vegan egg option is JUST Egg, a store-bought egg alternative made from mung beans. I recommend adding a dash of *kala namak* (black salt), pepper, and nutritional yeast flakes to really take it over the edge.

Use liquid JUST Egg to make:

>> Vegan omelets

>> Vegan quiche

>> French toast (JUST Egg works great as part of the dipping liquid.)

Round out your brunch with country potatoes, veggie sausage, and a fruit salad.

Creating a celebration-worthy Easter dinner

Many folks make ham at Easter. Luckily, you can find plenty of vegan ham alternatives, including a popular option from Tofurky.

Look for vegan ham in the frozen food aisle at natural grocery stores, or order online from companies like Herbivorous Butcher, a fully vegan butcher shop.

Vegan ham is hardly the only way to go, though. Any main course that feels "celebration worthy" works here. Store-bought vegan roasts, vegan turkey, or seitan en croûte (wrapped in dough) are all holiday-appropriate options.

Easter dinner is also a good time to celebrate the arrival of spring produce. Fill the table with raw carrot salad, roasted asparagus, grilled artichokes, Sautéed Kale with Garlic, and Sesame Sugar Snap Peas. (Look for my kale and sugar snap peas recipes in Chapter 14.)

Eat, Drink, and Be Married

There's nothing like watching a couple start their life together. The outfits, flowers, and toasts are enough to make you a little bit misty. And depending on the caterer, it may also make you a little bit hungry!

Weddings are an unusual situation in which someone else is deciding what you'll have for dinner. As a guest, you're not always sure what the vegan options will be, or if you'll even have any.

Plus, once you're at the reception, you're a bit of a captive audience. If there's nothing vegan to eat, it would be rude to dash out in the middle of the couple's first dance. Here are some ways to avoid that eventuality.

Getting a vegan meal

Engaged couples love to talk about their wedding plans. So when a good moment pops up, ask the happy couple about their planned dinner options. You can find out if they'll be having a formal sit-down dinner, a buffet, or something more casual.

That's a good time to gauge if they're planning on having vegan options or if their caterer can handle dietary restrictions.

A formal sit-down dinner is often the best-case scenario in terms of vegan options. When individual meals are being prepared, guests tend to have more of an opportunity to interject their preferences or needs.

TIP

When you receive the RSVP card with dinner options, see if there's a space for listing dietary restrictions, and express your desire for a vegan dinner. If only a vegetarian option is listed, tick that box, and then politely note that you don't eat meat, dairy, or eggs.

Then follow up with the bride or groom to see if that's possible.

Buffets are often trickier. Many times the meat option is the star of the show. Pasta dishes, salads, and sides are often topped with cheese or cream-laden sauces or dressings. Plus, it can be harder to track down people who know the specific ingredients in each dish.

TIP

If you know it's going to be a buffet, eat before you go, and don't arrive too hungry. That way if there happens to be something vegan on the buffet line, terrific. But if not, you won't be ravenous.

If you're certain the wedding you're attending won't have vegan options, do a quick search online to see if there are any vegan or vegan-friendly restaurants in the area. Between the ceremony and reception, grab a quick meal. (If you're going to eat elsewhere, consider giving a heads-up to the spouses-to-be, so they aren't paying for a meal you won't be eating.)

If you don't know the couple well, you may not feel comfortable asking about vegan options. In that case, pack snacks. If there happen to be vegan options, you can save the snacks for another time. If there aren't any, you have a backup plan.

Once the reception is going, no one will be paying attention to what's on your plate. A peanut butter and jelly sandwich or energy bar in your pocket or purse can really save the day.

Planning a vegan wedding

If the wedding in question is yours, congratulations! Laying the groundwork for a wedding is no small task. It can be a lot of fun, but also overwhelming at times.

If you can find a vegan caterer in your area, that's a great place to start, of course. If not, reach out to other caterers and see if they're game to cook for a vegan wedding.

Another option is enlisting the help of your favorite restaurant. Ask the manager at any local vegan or vegan-friendly restaurants or food trucks if they cater events. Mediterranean, Indian, Thai, and Ethiopian cuisines are well suited for a delicious plant-based spread.

If your wedding will be intimate or casual, consider asking friends or family members to help with the food. One of the most memorable and mouthwatering wedding meals I ever ate was prepared by someone's aunt for their backyard nuptials. She made a butternut squash curry that was out of this world. I still think about it to this day.

Create a menu by looking through your cookbooks or favorite blogs for recipes that feel both celebratory and potluck-friendly.

Letting them eat cake

An ornate cake is often the centerpiece of the reception. However, wedding cakes are usually made with eggs, dairy, and butter-packed frosting. Luckily, vegan cakes are becoming more readily available.

Do a simple Google search for a vegan bakery in your area, or reach out to any traditional bakeries to see if they offer egg-free and dairy-free options.

TIP

If you're making your own cake, dairy butter and milk can be swapped out for vegan butter and nondairy milk. Eggs can be replaced with store-bought egg replacer, mashed bananas, applesauce, or a flaxseed gel made with ground flaxseed and water. (For more helpful tips on veganizing recipes, turn to Chapter 9.)

WARNING

If you have a vegan wedding, you may get some pushback from loved ones who are unfamiliar with or resistant to eating a plant-based dinner. Remember that their feelings are for them to manage, and it's just one meal. Your wedding day is a representation of you and your partner, an expression of your love and your values.

With any luck, any resistant family members or friends will come to the reception and be blown away by how delectable a vegan meal can be.

WEDDING PLANNING BEYOND THE FOOD

Use your label-reading skills to make sure other aspects of your wedding are free of animal products.

- Avoid silk in the wedding gown, bridesmaids' dresses, neckties, and bouquet wraps.

- Beware of wool in tuxedos or suits.

- Choose vegan and cruelty-free beauty products.

- Steer clear of leather shoes.

Being the Life of the Dinner Party

Getting together with friends and sharing a meal is one of life's greatest pleasures. After a stressful workweek, it feels good to pop open a bottle of wine and break bread with pals in the comfort of your own home. No reservations needed.

Whenever you're cooking for someone else, it's always a good idea to consider their preferences. If you're going to be the host, here are some things to keep in mind:

>> Do your guests enjoy trying new-to-them cuisines, or do they prefer sticking to the foods they grew up eating?

>> Do they like a bit of heat, or do they consider ketchup spicy?

>> What are their favorite things to order at restaurants?

>> Are there any foods they specifically avoid?

You'll have the highest likelihood of success if you play to your guests' preferences.

TIP

Think about the foods your guests like to eat. If those foods aren't typically vegan, find a way to prepare them with plant-based ingredients. (Flip to Chapter 9 for a lot more about this topic.)

Serving meals everyone can agree on

People are creatures of habit. Many folks prefer to eat the same things again and again, and don't venture far from their usual fare. If you know your guests don't like to veer out of their comfort zone, stick to foods that are familiar to them.

>> If you know your guests are hesitant about plant-based proteins like tempeh or tofu, opt for beans instead.

>> If your guests rarely eat their veggies, consider a meaty veggie burger and fries.

>> If your guests are wary of vegan meats and cheeses, choose recipes that focus on whole plant foods.

It obviously depends on the crowd, but here are some foods that tend to go over well:

>> Chili

>> Soups of all sorts

>> Pasta and rice dishes

>> Vegetable stir-fries

>> Tacos and burritos

>> Mediterranean spread with hummus, pita, and falafel

Accepting a dinner invitation

When a non-vegan friend invites you to their home for dinner, inquire about the menu. If they don't know you're vegan, make sure to mention it then.

REMEMBER

Feel awkward broaching the subject? It's a lot less uncomfortable to talk about it beforehand. After all, you don't want your host to go to a lot of trouble preparing a meal you won't eat.

TIP

Offer to bring a dish to share. If the host says yes, take something that complements their menu. It's especially handy if the dish is substantive enough to be a vegan main course and also works as a side dish for other guests. A filling soup, hearty salad, or cold pasta dish are all solid options.

Firing Up the Grill

Nothing says summer like cookouts, potlucks, and picnics. Everything is better cooked over an open fire. Foods pick up those smoky flavors and get all toasty around the edges. Just the smell of dinner on the grill is enough to make your stomach grumble.

Enjoy a cookout with plant-based foods

Many people associate grilling season with steaks, hot dogs, and burgers. But you have no shortage of vegan options when it comes to cooking out. Here are some plant-based foods for your summer cookout menu:

>> Store-bought veggie burgers (Impossible, Beyond, and Field Roast hold up particularly well on the grill.)

>> Veggie dogs or sausages

- » Seitan steaks or ribs (Herbivorous Butcher makes delicious options!)
- » Marinated tofu slabs
- » Barbecued tempeh
- » Marinated portobello mushroom caps
- » Corn on the cob
- » Veggies like asparagus, zucchini, onions, eggplant, or bell peppers (Remember to use a grill basket!)
- » Mushroom Fajitas (Get the recipe in Chapter 12.)
- » Grilled Vegetable Skewers (Find the recipe in Chapter 14.)
- » Fruit like pineapple, halved bananas (still in the peel), peaches, plums, pears, nectarines, halved avocados (still in the peel), or watermelon

Pack up the basket: Potluck and picnic fare

Of course, all those tasty grilled items are going to need some summery sides to go with them.

TIP

Lots of traditional potluck and picnic side dishes like potato salad or coleslaw can easily be made vegan. You simply have to swap out standard mayonnaise for vegan mayo. (Vegenaise is my favorite!)

Here are some potluck and picnic dishes to whet your appetite:

- » Potato salad (made with vegan mayo)
- » Coleslaw (made with vegan mayo or vinegar)
- » Tomato cucumber salad with a lemon vinaigrette
- » Black bean, corn, and avocado salad with a zesty lime dressing
- » Cold Peanut Noodles (Get the recipe in Chapter 12.)
- » Mediterranean Couscous Salad (Grab the recipe in Chapter 14.)
- » Pasta Salad with Creamy Dressing (Find the recipe in Chapter 14.)
- » Spinach salad with sliced strawberries and balsamic vinaigrette (Find the Balsamic Vinaigrette recipe in Chapter 14.)

Having a Spooktacular Halloween

In recent years, Halloween has increased in popularity. It seems to be creeping up on Christmas in terms of rabid fans. Who can blame them? A holiday that revolves around imaginative costumes, hayrack rides, scary stories, carved pumpkins, and chocolate aplenty is bound to be popular.

Trick-or-treating goes hand in hand with Halloween. That's when children masquerade as their favorite characters, carrying buckets for candy. They go door-to-door in their neighborhoods, asking neighbors to fill their buckets with sweets.

Accidentally vegan candy

If you're looking for Halloween candy options in mainstream grocery stores, you're in luck. You'll find no shortage of options. Here are some conventional candies that happen to be vegan:

>> Charm's Blow Pops

>> Dots

>> Dum-Dums

>> Jolly Ranchers (hard candy and lollipops)

>> Pixy Stix

>> Red Vines

>> Ring Pops

>> Skittles

>> Smarties (only in the U.S.)

>> Sour Patch Kids

>> SweeTarts (Original variety)

>> Twizzlers

WARNING

Ingredients change and can vary from one country to the next. Be sure to read ingredients labels before you buy. Also, be aware that some of these products may contain sugar that was refined with bone char. If that's an issue for you, do some research into the candies before buying. Simply google the product name plus "bone char sugar." (See additional information about sugar refined with bone char in the nearby sidebar.)

When shopping for candy, beware of these non-vegan ingredients:

>> **Carmine:** This is made from the crushed bodies of dried cochineal insects and used for its red color.

>> **Dairy:** This may be listed as casein, butterfat, milk, milkfat, milk powder, or whey.

>> **Eggs:** Look out for eggs, egg whites, or albumen.

>> **Gelatin:** This is made from the skin, bones, and connective tissues of animals and used as a gelling agent.

>> **Shellac or confectioner's glaze:** This is a resin produced by insects and used as a shiny, smooth coating.

IS SUGAR VEGAN?

Sugar usually comes from sugarcane plants or sugar beets. So it seems like sugar should be vegan without question. However, to make sugar pure white in color, *bone char* (burned bones from slaughtered animals, mostly cattle and pigs) is sometimes used as a filtering agent to refine it. (By the way, bone char can be used to refine brown sugar too. Brown sugar is actually refined white sugar, made brown by adding molasses to it.)

Be aware that sugar itself doesn't contain any bone char in the final ingredient. It's only part of the processing.

If you'd like to avoid sugar that was refined with bone char, choose organic sugar instead, which isn't allowed to be filtered with it. Other vegan-friendly options include beet sugar, coconut sugar, or sugars labeled unrefined, raw, or natural. Liquid sweeteners like maple syrup, agave syrup, or date syrup are also free of bone char.

With these vegan-friendly options, it's easy to buy sugar for your own home use. However, if you're buying packaged foods like candies, cookies, or drinks, it's not always possible to tell just by looking at the food label how the sugar in it was refined. The ingredients label often just says "sugar."

Because of this, vegans have varying opinions about how to handle the issue of bone char. Some vegans draw a hard line around sugar refined with bone char. They won't purchase or consume anything made with it, and they'll avoid prepared foods if they don't know with certainty how the sugar in it was processed. They may also write or call companies to inquire about the refining process of the sugar in their packaged foods before buying them.

(continued)

(continued)

Other vegans are more lenient. They point to the original definition of veganism, which was defined as "a way of living that seeks to exclude, *as far as possible and practicable,* all forms of exploitation of, and cruelty to, animals for food, clothing and any other purpose." For these vegans, researching how the sugar was refined in every packaged food they buy is impractical and limiting. They acknowledge that we live in a non-vegan world, and that veganism isn't about personal purity. They do their best with the options they have. Perhaps they'll buy organic sugar for home use, but with packaged goods, let it slide. If a friend bakes them a cake with all plant-based ingredients, they won't quiz the friend about how the sugar they used was refined.

One final thought: Bone char is used for refining because it's readily available and cheap. Hopefully as more people reduce their animal consumption or adopt a fully vegan lifestyle, animal by-products like bone char will be less common and therefore, less of a default for filtering.

Intentionally vegan treats

In addition to mainstream brands, loads of candy options on the market are intentionally vegan. Plus, they often have simpler ingredients lists. In addition, some conventional candymakers are getting in on the plant-based trend and adding vegan options to their line-up. Look for these tasty vegan sweets:

>> Annie's Fruit Snacks

>> Cocomels

>> Eli's Earth chocolate bars (Their Dream Big flavor is my favorite candy!)

>> Hershey's plant-based chocolate bars

>> Justin's Dark Chocolate Peanut Butter Cups

>> Reese's plant-based peanut butter cups

>> Surf Sweets vegan gummies

>> Unreal Dark Chocolate Peanut Butter Cups

>> YumEarth lollipops and hard candies

TIP

You can also think outside the candy box! Individual bags of pretzels, popcorn, potato chips, or juice pouches are crowd-pleasing options.

Kids also love glow bracelets, small toys, stickers, pencils, bubbles, or erasers. Nonfood options have the added benefit of being a stress-free choice for kids who have food allergies.

TIP

Offer nonfood goodies in a teal pumpkin treat bucket, so kids with allergies know you have them in mind. (The Teal Pumpkin Project was started by the Food Allergy Research & Education organization to promote allergy-safe trick-or-treating.) You can find more information by searching for "teal pumpkin project" on their website (www.foodallergy.org). You can even add your address to their interactive map, so that parents can easily locate homes with allergy-safe offerings in their town.

Trick-or-treating for vegan kids

If your vegan child wants to go trick-or-treating with their friends, you may wonder what to do with all that non-vegan candy they bring home.

One popular option is Switch Witch. That's when you and your child go through all their candy after a night of trick-or-treating. They keep the candy that's vegan and set aside what isn't.

Then, after the child has gone to sleep, Switch Witch (also known as Mom or Dad) takes away all the non-vegan candy and replaces it with a special toy, book, or present.

Surviving Your First Vegan Thanksgiving

When we think about traditions, Thanksgiving is often the first holiday that comes to mind. Thanksgiving is a harvest celebration, in which thanks is given for a prosperous farming season.

It's often a big event with extended family (or a large group of friends for Friendsgiving) coming together from all over to share a meal of fall dishes. Year after year, you know the dishes to expect from aunts, uncles, cousins, and parents. The usual suspects include green bean casserole, sweet potatoes, and stuffing. You could almost write out the menu without asking anyone what they're bringing.

That's why it can feel especially daunting to break out of the mold and do something new. But don't worry! After the first year, it gets easier.

Bring a main dish

Thanksgiving for many people is synonymous with turkey. They can hardly imagine the holiday without it. So the first course of action for a vegan Thanksgiving? Get that main course sorted.

You have endless options for a delicious vegan main course that's worthy of sharing.

First of all, grocery stores carry loads of vegan turkey alternatives this time of year. It's a very handy option, because the hard work is already done. Just thaw, heat, and eat!

My favorites are:

>> Field Roast Hazelnut & Cranberry Plant-Based Roast

>> Gardein Plant-Based Turk'y Roast

>> Trader Joe's Breaded Turkey-Less Stuffed Roast

My extended family Thanksgiving is held at a banquet hall. I know the oven will be packed with other people's dishes. So I like to bring along my air fryer. Then I can heat my store-bought holiday roast without worrying about the oven being set at the wrong temperature or some turkey drippings falling onto it.

Another of my favorite main course options is homemade potpie. Potpie is festive, warming, and holiday-appropriate. Plus, if anyone would like to share, potpie is immediately recognizable to non-vegan family members.

I fill my potpie with potatoes, carrots, celery, onions, and garlic, and envelope those veggies in a creamy sauce made from cashews. While non-vegans usually make potpie with chicken or turkey, I add vegan turkey, seitan, or chickpeas.

If I feel like a project, I make my own pie dough. If I don't, I buy frozen pie crust. Many of them are vegan. You just have to read the ingredients labels.

Potpie is a satiating dish. Plus, it works well with the traditional side dishes on offer. (You can find my favorite potpie recipe at https://cadryskitchen.com/vegan-pot-pie.)

TIP

Potpie also travels well! If you're taking potpie to someone else's home, pop it in an insulated carrier before you go. The warm sauce inside the pie helps it hold its temperature for transporting.

Make a meal of side dishes

You can easily forgo the main course and make a meal of sides. Think mashed potatoes with gravy, salads, green beans, and Brussels sprouts. Many people love the sides at Thanksgiving the most anyway!

Oftentimes the sides at your average holiday feast aren't vegan. However, they're easy to prepare that way with a few simple swaps!

>> Anywhere you would've used dairy butter or dairy milk (like mashed potatoes), use vegan butter and vegan milk.

>> If you would've used chicken or turkey broth (like in gravy), replace it with vegetable broth.

>> If you loved sweet potatoes with marshmallows, use gelatin-free vegan marshmallows instead. (Dandies is my favorite brand.)

>> For salads, replace mayo-based dressing with a dressing made with eggless mayo. Or make a balsamic vinaigrette instead.

Sweet endings: Don't forget dessert

Vegans definitely don't have to do without when it comes to dessert. While many dessert recipes call for dairy butter, cow's milk, and eggs, it's easy to make desserts without them.

You can try veganizing your favorite family recipes with the plant-based version of the usual ingredients. Or you can do a simple Google search to find recipes for treats like vegan pumpkin pie, apple crisp, or nondairy cheesecake. If you can dream it, most likely someone has created a recipe for it.

Once your dessert is complete, you'll find lots of whipped topping options to adorn it.

Check out the refrigerated or freezer section of the grocery store for one of these vegan whipped toppings:

>> 365 by Whole Foods Market Non-Dairy Plant-Based Whipped Topping

>> Reddi-wip Non-Dairy Whipped Topping (with almond or coconut milk)

>> So Delicious Dairy Free CocoWhip Coconut Whipped Topping

>> Truwhip Vegan Plant-Based Whipped Topping

Alternatively, you can make your own whipped cream using canned full-fat coconut milk or coconut cream. (It won't work with coconut milk sold in boxed cartons for drinking.)

Here's how to do it:

1. **Refrigerate canned full-fat coconut milk or coconut cream overnight.** As it cools, the cream will rise to the top. (Be sure not to shake the can or it will reincorporate.)

2. **Open the can and skim the thickened cream off the top.** Leave behind the water underneath. (You can use the leftover coconut water for other purposes, like smoothies.)

3. **Put the cream in a chilled mixing bowl and beat with an electric beater for 30 seconds to a minute, until soft peaks form.**

4. **Add ½ teaspoon vanilla extract and ½ cup organic powdered sugar. Mix until creamy, about 30 seconds.**

5. **Use immediately or refrigerate for later use.**

Share the load

Like they say, many hands make light work. So now that you know many dishes require only a few simple substitutions to be vegan, consider asking your family members if they'd be willing to tweak their recipes.

Obviously, if you don't know the host or other guests well, this may be outside your comfort zone. But if you're celebrating with family members or close friends, they may be happy to do it!

TIP

Many times people don't mind making a simple adjustment. You just have to reach out to them well before the holiday. If they don't have nondairy butter or plant-based milk on hand, offer to pick some up for them or share yours.

At our family Thanksgiving, my mom is in charge of the mashed potatoes and gravy. She isn't vegan, but she uses cashew milk and vegan butter for all of her mashed potatoes. They taste just as light, airy, and delicious as always, and that's what matters to most people.

She then makes multiple kinds of gravy, including one vegan batch with vegetable broth and nondairy butter. Once you add in herbs like thyme, parsley, and rosemary, no one can tell the difference.

My niece makes a platter of homemade cookies, similar to Oreo chocolate sandwich cookies. (I gave her a vegan cookie cookbook about 10 years ago, and it's the gift that keeps on giving!) They're a huge hit, and everyone requests them year after year.

My sister-in-law makes the most delectable salads with lots of fall ingredients like roasted apples and candied pecans. Then she either leaves off any dairy-based cheese or serves it on the side.

Not only does it mean I have to prepare fewer dishes, but it also makes me feel loved, considered, and accepted. If your family members are willing to make a few tweaks in your honor, let them, and then thank them for it.

Don't overextend yourself; it's just one day. If you'll be the only vegan at the dinner table, don't feel like you have to prepare every dish that ever graced an issue of *Thanksgiving Monthly*. Think about what makes Thanksgiving special to you, and cook only those dishes. Do the things that bring you joy and let go of the rest.

GIVE THE HOLIDAY NEW MEANING

According to the United States Department of Agriculture (USDA), 46 million turkeys are killed every year in the name of Thanksgiving. The number is sobering, and honestly, it can be super depressing. In the days leading up to the holiday, you see trucks of turkeys stacked in cages on the highway, and you know where they're going.

That's why it can be a salve for the soul to go visit turkeys who escaped the animal industry. Many people across the globe rescue turkeys and give them forever homes at animal sanctuaries.

Visit an animal sanctuary in your area. Many of these sanctuaries have meet and greets in the weeks leading up to Thanksgiving. Instead of eating a turkey, you can watch turkeys have a feast of their own. Plus, while you're there, you can spend time with others who share your values and mindset.

If you don't have a sanctuary in your area, consider making a donation to one instead. Farm Sanctuary has a yearly adopt-a-turkey program. From their website (www.farmsanctuary.org), you can browse pictures of the turkeys who live at the sanctuary. Pick out one you'd like to sponsor. Then if you want, print out their picture or share it on Instagram.

Preparing a Magical Christmas from Head to Mistletoe

For many people, Christmas is the most wonderful time of the year, with its twinkling lights, greeting cards in the mailbox, nostalgic movies on TV, and carols playing on the radio. Plus, the cold weather outside makes a very compelling case for staying inside with your nearest and dearest, and eating something cozy.

On Christmas morning, I like to enjoy a vegan frittata that I've made the day before. After all, when presents are waiting to be unwrapped, who wants to be in the kitchen cooking over a hot stove? Vegan frittata can be eaten cold, enjoyed at room temperature, or quickly warmed in the oven or microwave.

Here are some more Christmas breakfast ideas:

>> Baked donuts

>> Vegan French toast (Use vegan eggnog as the dipping liquid.)

>> Bagels and nondairy cream cheese

>> Sheet Pan Potato Hash (Get the recipe in Chapter 11.)

The foods served at Christmas lunch or dinner often share a lot of overlap with Thanksgiving. There's an eye-catching main course, stuffing, mashed potatoes, green beans, and pie for dessert.

Look over the "Surviving Your First Vegan Thanksgiving" section earlier in this chapter to get ideas for a vegan holiday roast, seitan turkey, and veganized versions of classic side dishes.

Other holiday-worthy main courses include:

>> Dairy-free mushroom risotto

>> Vegetable lasagna

>> Stuffed peppers

>> Cauliflower steaks

Soups that "sleigh"

Perhaps you keep Christmas casual, like my family does. We often have a potluck, and everybody brings whatever they want. There are usually slow cookers going all day long, so people can eat when they get hungry.

Slow cookers were basically made for soups. You can set them on "Warm" and have soup at the ready for whenever hunger strikes. Soups are an especially good dish to serve non-vegans, because they feel very familiar. Plus, people don't have built-in expectations that soup has to be loaded with meat.

Here are some of my favorite soups to serve a crowd:

» Creamy potato soup

» Wild rice soup

» Sweet potato peanut stew

» Split pea soup

» Corn chowder

» Tortilla soup

» Ultimate Homemade Chili (Find the recipe in Chapter 12.)

» Vegan Chicken Noodle Soup (Look for the recipe in Chapter 12.)

Vegan eggnog: All it's cracked up to be

In December, a lot of people like to enjoy a glass of eggnog (either with or without a shot of brandy). If you're an eggnog fan, you'll be happy to hear you can choose from a variety of eggless nogs on the market. (And really, other than Rocky, who wants to drink raw eggs anyway?)

Vegan eggnog is sold in the refrigerated section in mainstream big-box stores, as well as in grocery stores.

Look for the following brands:

» Almond Breeze Almondmilk Nog

» So Delicious Coconutmilk Holiday Nog

» Target Good & Gather Oatmilk Holiday Nog

» Trader Joe's O'Nog Non-Dairy Oat Beverage

How to handle non-vegan gifts

At the holidays, you may find yourself on the receiving end of a gift that doesn't fit your compassionate lifestyle. It may be a gift card to a steakhouse, a pair of leather gloves, a wool sweater, or a beeswax candle.

The situation is a tricky one, because most likely, the gift giver was trying to express their affection and make a connection. They wanted to give you something you'd enjoy.

You don't want to hurt their feelings, but you also don't want them to keep giving you gifts that make you feel uncomfortable or sad. It's a delicate balance between expressing your needs to your loved ones, being conscious of their feelings, and honoring your own feelings too.

If you receive a non-vegan gift, here are some ways to handle it:

» **The most obvious solution is to talk to the gift giver about it.** I recommend not doing it on Christmas Day when there are a lot of people around. You don't want to embarrass them. However, you can broach the subject at a time when it's just the two of you.

» **If the item came with a receipt, take it back to the store.** On December 26, malls are full of people returning presents for a variety of reasons. Maybe the item was too big, too small, or just not their style. You'll hardly be alone, even if your reason is different from theirs.

» **If the item didn't come with a receipt, ask the gift giver for one.** Pair the request with a compliment. Say something like "Thank you so much for the bag. You really pegged my style! Unfortunately, I noticed that it's made with leather, which I don't use since I'm vegan. I want to see if the store has this style made with cloth instead."

» **Donate the item to your preferred charity.** Unwanted shoes and clothing can be taken to shelters for people who are facing homelessness, domestic violence, or other crisis situations. Consider donating toys to a children's hospital. Donate unopened packages of food to your local food bank.

Set your loved ones up for success

The kindest thing you can do is set your loved ones up for success well before the holidays or other gift-giving occasions. Help them out by making your needs known.

>> **Clarify to your family members and friends what it means to be vegan.** Many people know that being vegan means avoiding animal products like meat, dairy, eggs, and honey. But they may not be aware it also extends to avoiding fur, wool, leather, silk, feathers, bone china, and pearls.

>> **Teach by example.** If you're on a shopping trip with a loved one, don't hide the fact that you're checking labels on sweaters, shoes, jackets, and pillows (to make sure they aren't filled with feathers). If they know you always read labels, they'll likely do it too before they buy you a gift.

>> **Make a list.** In my extended family, we always draw names. Then we share a list of five things we'd like to receive. You can send a website link to specific items you'd enjoy or give general ideas like "non-leather running shoes." If your loved ones have a handy list of things you'd like to receive, they're less likely to give you something made with animal products.

For more tips on navigating tricky social situations as a vegan, be sure to check out Chapter 20.

4

Tasting Is Believing: Vegan Recipes

Chapter **11**

Breakfasts

A good breakfast sets the tone for the day. Starting the morning with something satiating and healthy keeps you feeling energized, steady, and ready to face the world. Eating a solid breakfast has many benefits, such as:

» Replenishing stores of glucose, which boosts your energy levels and helps control your appetite

» Improving concentration and metabolism (Children who eat breakfast regularly tend to do better academically than those who don't.)

» Potentially lowering your risk of type 2 diabetes and heart disease

» Contributing to your overall nutrient intake for the day (People who eat breakfast are more likely to meet their Recommended Dietary Allowance of vitamins and minerals.)

Whether you prefer a lighter breakfast or a full-blown brunch, you have several options to choose from in this chapter.

You find meals you can take on the go, like recipes for a Peanut Butter Banana Smoothie or Avocado Toast with Baked Tofu. You also find recipes for sit-down fare like a breakfast bowl, oatmeal, or tofu scramble.

Many people aren't all that hungry when they wake up, so smoothies can be a good drinkable option. They're like a whole foods version of those old-school instant breakfast drinks, and they're a surefire way to front-load nutrient-packed produce into your day. Plus, you can easily sip them on your commute.

TIP

Whenever I make smoothies, I like to add ground flaxseed or chia seeds for an extra boost of fiber and omega-3 fatty acids. Plus, these seeds add a wonderful whippy texture to smoothies that makes them very full-bodied.

Avocado toast is also a cinch to prepare and easy to eat on the go. It can be deliciously simple with smashed avocado, a sprinkling of nutritional yeast flakes, and a dusting of salt. Or you can load it up with baked tofu, browned seitan bacon, or an assortment of veggies. See what looks good in your fridge, and let that lead the way!

While many non-vegans opt for eggs at breakfast, vegans often choose tofu instead. Tofu is a blank canvas for flavor. Plus, it's packed with satiating protein, which is great for keeping you full until lunchtime!

I often make Eggy Tofu by browning tofu slices in a skillet along with a few seasonings. Eggy Tofu is terrific with toast. It's also wonderful in a breakfast sandwich on toasted bread with nondairy cheese and browned seitan bacon.

When you have time for a more elaborate brunch, a tofu scramble is the way to go. Scrambles are hearty, and you can cram a lot of vegetables into them. Enjoy a tofu scramble on its own, or stuff it into a breakfast burrito along with potato hash.

REMEMBER

By the way, even though this section is labeled "breakfasts," these dishes can be delicious snacks or meals any time of the day! Plus, who doesn't love breakfast for dinner?

Peanut Butter Banana Smoothie

PREP TIME: 5 MIN	COOK TIME: 0 MIN	YIELD: 1 OR 2 SERVINGS

INGREDIENTS

1 cup plain or vanilla cashew milk (or your preferred nondairy milk)

2 bananas, peeled and frozen in chunks

¼ cup natural peanut butter

2 tablespoons ground flaxseed

DIRECTIONS

1 Put all the ingredients in a blender, and blend until smooth.

2 Pour into two small glasses or one tall glass and serve.

PER SERVING: Calories 332 (From Fat 187); Fat 21g (Saturated 4g); Cholesterol 0mg; Sodium 151mg; Carbohydrate 32g (Dietary Fiber 7g); Protein 11g.

VARY IT! Try this smoothie with a different type of nut or seed butter like cashew, almond, walnut, or sunflower seed butter. Ground flaxseed can be replaced with chia seeds.

NOTE: I prefer unsweetened nondairy milk, but if you like a sweeter smoothie, sweetened nondairy milk is fine. For the creamiest texture, use frozen bananas for this recipe. Peel ripe bananas, break them into chunks, and then freeze the chunks in a freezer bag until you're ready to use them. For the best flavor and nutrition, use peanut butter that has just two ingredients — peanuts and salt.

Avocado Toast with Baked Tofu

PREP TIME: 2 MIN	COOK TIME: 3 MIN	YIELD: 4 SERVINGS

INGREDIENTS

4 slices whole wheat bread

2 avocados, halved and sliced

½ teaspoon nutritional yeast flakes, divided

Pinch of salt

7 ounces baked tofu, thinly sliced (teriyaki-flavored or your preferred flavor)

DIRECTIONS

1 Toast the bread in a toaster.

2 Top each slice of toast with half an avocado, and smash it onto the bread with a fork.

3 Sprinkle ⅛ teaspoon of nutritional yeast flakes on top of the avocado on each piece of toast, along with a sprinkle of salt.

4 Top each avocado toast with a few thin slices of tofu and serve.

PER SERVING: *Calories 259 (From Fat 150); Fat 17g (Saturated 2g); Cholesterol 0mg; Sodium 212mg; Carbohydrate 22g (Dietary Fiber 8g); Protein 9g.*

TIP: If you prefer heated tofu, warm the whole tofu slabs in an air fryer at 400 degrees for 5 minutes, stopping once to flip. If you don't have an air fryer, warm the tofu in a skillet for a few minutes on each side. Or you can use Eggy Tofu slices (see the next recipe).

VARY IT! Vary your avocado toast by adding Everything But the Bagel seasoning instead of salt and/or substituting fried JUST Egg for the tofu. You can also add other toppings like browned seitan bacon, pickled red onions, microgreens, arugula, sliced tomato, minced chives, chopped cilantro, chopped dill, or thinly sliced radishes. If you like, add a squeeze of lemon or lime to the avocado for tang.

NOTE: You can find packaged baked tofu in a variety of flavors from Trader Joe's, Wildwood, Nasoya, Hodo, and more. The tofu has already been marinated, and it's ready to eat right out of the package. I usually buy teriyaki flavor. Sriracha flavored is nice if you like a little heat. Depending on how loaded you like your toast, you may have leftover tofu.

TIP: Be sure to use a sturdy whole grain bread that doesn't include animal products like dairy or honey. I especially like Silver Hills sprouted bread, Dave's Killer Bread, and Alvarado Street Bakery. If you prefer drier breads, try Food For Life.

Eggy Tofu

PREP TIME: 2 MIN | COOK TIME: 7 MIN | YIELD: 4 OR 5 SERVINGS

INGREDIENTS

1 (16-ounce) vacuum-packed (NOT water-packed) block super-firm tofu

1 teaspoon avocado oil (or your preferred neutral-flavored cooking oil)

1 teaspoon nutritional yeast flakes, divided

1 teaspoon granulated onion, divided

1 teaspoon kala namak (black salt), divided (see Note)

Freshly ground black pepper, to taste

DIRECTIONS

1 Blot the tofu block dry with a clean kitchen towel. (Wet tofu doesn't brown nicely.) Cut the block widthwise into 9 or 10 equal slices, approximately ¼ to ½ inch thick.

2 Add oil to a large nonstick skillet over medium heat.

3 Once the oil is warm, put the tofu slices into the skillet. (If your skillet is too small, you may have to cook the tofu in batches.) Allow the tofu slices to brown on one side. It will take 3 to 4 minutes. Then use a spatula to flip all the tofu slices over.

4 Sprinkle all the tofu slices evenly across the skillet with ½ teaspoon nutritional yeast flakes, ½ teaspoon granulated onion, ½ teaspoon kala namak, and a generous dash of black pepper.

5 Use a spatula to flip the tofu slices and allow the other side to brown for a couple minutes. While the second side is browning, sprinkle all the tofu evenly with the remaining ½ teaspoon nutritional yeast flakes, ½ teaspoon granulated onion, ½ teaspoon kala namak, and another generous dash of black pepper.

6 Flip the tofu slices one more time for 30 seconds to seal in the seasonings.

7 Remove the slices from the skillet and serve with toast, veggie sausage, fruit, and/or hash browns.

PER SERVING: Calories 74 (From Fat 30); Fat 3g (Saturated 0g); Cholesterol 0mg; Sodium 232mg; Carbohydrate 3g (Dietary Fiber 0g); Protein 9g.

NOTE: Kala namak (also known as black salt) is a sulfurous salt that you can find in Indian grocery stores or online. It's essential for adding eggy flavor to this dish.

TIP: Eggy Tofu is terrific on its own or added to a breakfast sandwich along with seitan bacon or veggie sausage, and a slice of vegan cheese. Make a toasted sandwich with regular bread, or use a bagel.

Grits Breakfast Bowl

PREP TIME: 10 MIN   COOK TIME: 30 MIN   YIELD: 4 SERVINGS

INGREDIENTS

2 teaspoons avocado oil (or your preferred neutral-flavored cooking oil), divided

14 ounces Brussels sprouts, ends removed and thinly sliced

Pinch of salt, plus more as needed

4 vegan breakfast sausage patties

2 cloves garlic, minced

3 cups water

½ teaspoon Vegetarian Better Than Bouillon No Chicken Base

1 cup corn grits (see Note)

Dash of freshly ground black pepper

¼ cup nutritional yeast flakes

¼ cup plain unsweetened nondairy milk

Vegan butter (optional)

DIRECTIONS

1   Put 1 teaspoon of the oil in a large nonstick skillet over medium or medium-high heat.

2   Once the oil is warm, put an even layer of thinly sliced Brussels sprouts across the skillet along with a pinch of salt. Don't move the sprouts until they begin to get nice and toasty brown on the bottom. Toss them with a spatula and continue cooking until the other side is brown as well. (If you move them too much, they won't get the lovely dark color that's desired.)

3   Once the Brussels sprouts are browned on both sides, turn the heat to low. Keep cooking and occasionally flipping them for about 10 minutes, or until they're tender. Taste and add more salt, if needed. When the sprouts are done, remove them from the heat and cover the skillet with a lid to keep them warm.

4   Put ½ teaspoon of the oil in a medium-sized nonstick skillet. Bring to a medium heat, and add the vegan breakfast sausage patties. Cook on one side until brown, about 3 minutes. Then flip them with a spatula and brown the other side about 2 minutes more. Once they're browned and heated through-out, remove them from the heat, and cover the skillet with a lid to keep the patties warm while you cook the grits.

5   Put the remaining ½ teaspoon of oil in a medium-sized pot over medium heat. Add the minced garlic and sauté for a couple minutes, until fragrant.

6   Add the water to the pot along with the Vegetarian Better Than Bouillon and stir to dissolve. Bring to a simmer.

7   Slowly pour in the corn grits while stirring constantly to prevent clumping. Add a pinch of salt and dash of pepper. Lower the heat so the grits don't splatter.

8   Cook, stirring frequently, for about 6 minutes, until the grits start to thicken and pull from the edges of the pot when stirred.

9 Once the grits are fairly thick, add the nutritional yeast flakes and nondairy milk. Stir to evenly incorporate all the ingredients. Continue cooking uncovered, stirring frequently, until the grits reach your desired consistency. (Depending on the heat, it may take 4 or 5 minutes longer.) If the grits get too thick, add more milk. If they're too runny, keep cooking until they condense to your preferred thickness.

10 Remove them from the heat and allow the grits to cool for a couple minutes. They will continue to thicken as they cool.

11 Serve the grits in four bowls. If you like, top the grits with a pat of nondairy butter. Then top each bowl with a vegan sausage patty and a generous spoonful of Brussels sprouts.

PER SERVING: *Calories 328 (From Fat 60); Fat 7g (Saturated 0g); Cholesterol 0mg; Sodium 387mg; Carbohydrate 51g (Dietary Fiber 9g); Protein 18g.*

NOTE: I like Bob's Red Mill Organic Corn Grits. Don't use quick-cooking, instant, or white hominy-style grits.

VARY IT! The water and bouillon can be replaced with 3 cups of vegetable broth. For spicier grits, add chopped jalapeños at the same time as the minced garlic. For cheesier grits, add a handful of shredded nondairy cheese at the same time as the nutritional yeast. The Brussels sprouts can be replaced with Sautéed Kale with Garlic (see Chapter 14 for the recipe).

TIP: For the vegan sausage, I like to use either Beyond Breakfast Sausage patties or links, or Field Roast apple and maple breakfast sausage links. If you use links, I recommend two per person. Also, the Field Roast apple and maple sausages are especially nice with a drizzle of maple syrup on top, once plated on the grits.

TIP: If you're making Beyond Breakfast Sausage patties, you may wish to cook them in an air fryer. It's one less skillet to watch! Air fry the frozen patties at 400 degrees for 8 minutes, stopping once halfway through to flip. (You don't need to add any extra oil. The sausages have enough on their own.)

Veggie-Packed Tofu Scramble

| PREP TIME: 10 MIN | COOK TIME: 15 MIN | YIELD: 4 SERVINGS |

INGREDIENTS

1½ teaspoons avocado oil (or other neutral-flavored cooking oil), divided

1 (16-ounce) vacuum-packed (NOT water-packed) block super-firm tofu

½ cup chopped onions

½ cup chopped red bell peppers

1 clove garlic, minced

1 teaspoon ground cumin

1 teaspoon ancho chili powder

½ teaspoon granulated onion

½ teaspoon paprika

Pinch of salt

2 tablespoons water

2 big handfuls baby spinach

2 tablespoons nutritional yeast flakes

¼ teaspoon kala namak (black salt)

1 avocado, sliced

DIRECTIONS

1 Put 1 teaspoon of oil in a medium or large nonstick skillet over medium heat.

2 Blot the tofu block dry with a clean kitchen towel. (Wet tofu doesn't brown nicely.) Use your hands to crumble the tofu block into the skillet. (I like to crumble it in larger chunks, but if you prefer a smaller crumble, that's fine too.) Scatter it evenly across the skillet and don't move it for about 4 minutes so it can get nice and brown. Then flip the tofu with a spatula, and let it sit for about 3 more minutes so it continues to brown.

3 Move the browned tofu to one side of the skillet. Drizzle the remaining ½ teaspoon of oil onto the empty side of the skillet. Add the onions, bell peppers, and garlic to the empty spot. Sauté for a couple minutes. Then incorporate the veggies with the tofu and sauté for 1 or 2 minutes, until the onions are fragrant and softened.

4 Add the ground cumin, ancho chili powder, granulated onion, paprika, and salt to the pan. Combine with a spatula, moving the mixture around the pan to distribute the spices evenly. Add the water to help incorporate the spices.

5 Add the baby spinach, nutritional yeast flakes, and kala namak. Stir to combine. Continue cooking until the spinach has wilted and the nutritional yeast is evenly incorporated.

6 Divide the tofu scramble equally between four plates. Top each portion with sliced avocado. Finish with another pinch of salt, if you like.

PER SERVING: *Calories 198 (From Fat 108); Fat 12g (Saturated 2g); Cholesterol 0mg; Sodium 111mg; Carbohydrate 11g (Dietary Fiber 5g); Protein 13g.*

NOTE: Kala namak gives the dish an eggy, sulfurous flavor. If you don't have black salt, regular table salt can be used instead.

VARY IT! Try this recipe with broccoli, browned vegan sausage, mushrooms, or kale.

Blueberry Banana Oatmeal

PREP TIME: 2 MIN | COOK TIME: 20 MIN | YIELD: 2 SERVINGS

INGREDIENTS

2 cups water

Pinch of salt

1 cup rolled oats (old fashioned oats)

1 banana, sliced or broken into chunks

½ cup blueberries (fresh or frozen)

1 teaspoon maple syrup

¼ teaspoon vanilla extract

Dash of ground cinnamon

DIRECTIONS

1 In a small to medium-sized pot, bring the water to a boil with a pinch of salt.

2 Stir in the rolled oats. Reduce the heat to a low simmer. Stir occasionally for 10 to 20 minutes, until the oatmeal has thickened.

3 During the last 5 minutes of cooking, stir in the banana, blueberries, maple syrup, vanilla extract, and cinnamon.

4 Once the oatmeal has reached your desired thickness, remove from heat, cover, and let stand 2 minutes before serving.

5 Spoon the oatmeal into two bowls and serve.

PER SERVING: *Calories 228 (From Fat 26); Fat 3g (Saturated 1g); Cholesterol 0mg; Sodium 81mg; Carbohydrate 47g (Dietary Fiber 6g); Protein 6g.*

NOTE: Leftovers will keep in the fridge for 3 to 5 days. To reheat, add a splash of water or non-dairy milk. Stir and reheat in the microwave.

VARY IT! If you like, add a splash of nondairy milk to the bowl just before serving. For peanut butter and banana oatmeal, replace the blueberries with 1 to 2 tablespoons of peanut butter. For pumpkin oatmeal, leave out the banana and blueberries, and add ¼ cup of canned pumpkin. Serve with a handful of candied pecans on top.

Sheet Pan Potato Hash

PREP TIME: 10 MIN | COOK TIME: 30 MIN | YIELD: 4 SERVINGS

INGREDIENTS

1 small red bell pepper, chopped

1 small yellow onion, chopped

2 medium-sized russet potatoes, chopped

2 teaspoons avocado oil (or your preferred neutral-flavored cooking oil)

Pinch of salt

Dash of freshly ground pepper

Handful of chives, finely chopped

DIRECTIONS

1 Preheat the oven to 400 degrees. Line a baking sheet with parchment paper. (If your baking sheets are small, use two of them. For proper browning, it's important to spread out the ingredients.)

2 Put the chopped bell pepper, onion, and potatoes on the lined baking sheet. Toss with the avocado oil. Sprinkle with a pinch of salt and dash of pepper. Spread the mixture evenly across the baking sheet in a single layer, being careful that the vegetables don't overlap.

3 Roast in the oven for 20 minutes.

4 Remove the baking sheet from the oven. Toss the vegetables with a spatula. Spread them across the baking sheet again, and cook for 10 more minutes.

5 Remove the hash from the oven and add more salt and pepper, if necessary.

6 Divide the hash onto four plates and sprinkle with chopped chives before serving.

PER SERVING: *Calories 136 (From Fat 22); Fat 2g (Saturated 0g); Cholesterol 0mg; Sodium 51mg; Carbohydrate 27g (Dietary Fiber 3g); Protein 3g.*

VARY IT! Try a different type of potato like red skin or Yukon Gold, shallots instead of onions, or a different colored bell pepper. If you like, add granulated garlic, granulated onion, and a pinch of paprika for color.

TIP: For even cooking, cut all the vegetables in medium, equal-sized pieces. If you need the hash to cook faster, cut the potatoes, onions, and peppers in smaller pieces.

IN THIS CHAPTER

» Getting cozy with chili and soup

» Indulging in burgers, tacos, and nachos

» Making flavorful rice and noodle dishes

Chapter **12**

Main Courses

When many people think of vegan meals, they imagine an endless array of salads, and not much else. Now, I love salads, and I eat a big meal-sized one every day. However, that's not the only thing I eat — by far.

Vegan meals can be just as filling, satisfying, and decadent as their non-vegan counterparts. Whatever you're craving, there's a vegan version out there.

In this chapter, you find a lot of stick-to-your-ribs comfort foods that are full-flavored and easy to prepare. I include something for every palate — from warming chili to veggie-laden fried rice.

These dishes may require a few different ingredients than you typically use, but the same spices, seasonings, and flavors are all there.

» Craving meaty foods you can sink your teeth into? Head toward the aforementioned Ultimate Homemade Chili or Classic Vegan Cheeseburger.

» All about indulgence? Try out Barbecue Jackfruit Nachos or Black Bean Tacos.

» Is colorful produce what you crave? Veer toward Mushroom Fajitas, Cold Peanut Noodles, Pineapple Fried Rice, or Basil Pesto Pasta with Roasted Chickpeas. (Pesto is a great way to squeeze leafy greens into your diet. The sauce is positively packed with nutrient-rich basil.)

I also include one of my husband's all-time favorite recipes, Vegan Chicken Noodle Soup. It's just what you need when there's a chill in the air or a scratch in your throat. Serve it with buttery round crackers and feel like a kid all over again.

Repurposing Leftovers

When people switch over to a vegan diet, they're often surprised at how much their time in the kitchen increases. The plus side is, you can control the ingredients and tweak dishes to suit your tastes. The downside is, the extra kitchen time may be an adjustment for folks who aren't used to cooking.

To avoid burnout, consider making double batches, and then repurposing leftovers throughout the week.

>> Enjoy chili by the bowlful one night. Then repurpose it into chili cheese fries, burritos, or as a topping on nachos or grilled veggie dogs.

>> Use leftover barbecue jackfruit from the nachos as a sandwich filling. Finish it with a heaping helping of vegan coleslaw. (Simply combine shredded cabbage mix with some of the Ranch Dressing in Chapter 14 for the coleslaw.)

>> If you have leftover black bean taco mixture, use it in taco salads, burritos, burrito bowls, and taco pizza.

>> Use leftover fajita vegetables as a topping on the jackfruit nachos or as a tasty addition to burrito bowls with rice.

>> Use leftover pesto from the pasta recipe as a sandwich spread, toss it with roasted vegetables, or add it to roasted or mashed potatoes.

When you repurpose leftovers, you get all the joys of a home-cooked meal, along with the welcome variety of a changing menu.

Ultimate Homemade Chili

PREP TIME: 5 MIN	COOK TIME: 22 MIN	YIELD: 5 SERVINGS

INGREDIENTS

1 teaspoon avocado oil (or your preferred neutral-flavored cooking oil)

½ medium onion, chopped

2 cloves garlic, minced

1 (12-ounce) package soy chorizo, removed from plastic casing

1 teaspoon ground coriander

1 teaspoon ground cumin

1 teaspoon ancho chili powder

1 teaspoon granulated onion

1½ cups water plus more, if needed

1 (14½-ounce) can fire roasted diced tomatoes with juices

1 (15-ounce) can black beans, drained and rinsed

1 (15-ounce) can pinto beans, drained and rinsed

½ teaspoon stone-ground mustard

1 teaspoon hot sauce (optional)

DIRECTIONS

1 Put the oil in a soup pot over medium heat. Add the onion and garlic, and sauté for 3 to 5 minutes, until fragrant and translucent.

2 Add the soy chorizo and cook a couple more minutes. Add the ground coriander, ground cumin, ancho chili powder, and granulated onion to the pot and combine.

3 Add the water, fire roasted diced tomatoes with juices, black beans, pinto beans, stone-ground mustard, and hot sauce (if desired).

4 Bring the chili to a simmer. Cook for 10 to 15 minutes, allowing the flavors to meld and the chili to thicken. (If the chili gets too thick, add more water to thin it out to your preferred consistency.)

5 Ladle the chili into bowls and serve.

PER SERVING: *Calories 286 (From Fat 52); Fat 6g (Saturated 1g); Cholesterol 0mg; Sodium 982mg; Carbohydrate 35g (Dietary Fiber 13g); Protein 24g.*

NOTE: I like to use Trader Joe's soy chorizo. It's sold in the refrigerated section and packaged in a long plastic tube. Be sure to remove it from its plastic casing before using. While this chili is delicious on its own, you can take the fun up a notch by adding your choice of toppings like pickled red onions, sliced scallions, shredded vegan cheddar cheese, vegan sour cream, chopped cilantro, crackers, and/or tortilla chips.

VARY IT! Soy chorizo can be replaced with another can of beans in a different variety or cooked brown lentils. If you're replacing the highly seasoned soy chorizo with canned beans or cooked lentils, double the amount of ground coriander, cumin, and ancho chili powder. Soy chorizo is also salty enough that additional salt isn't required. However, if you replace it with beans or lentils, add ½ teaspoon of salt or to taste.

Vegan Chicken Noodle Soup

PREP TIME: 10 MIN	COOK TIME: 20 MIN	YIELD: 4 SERVINGS

INGREDIENTS

1 teaspoon avocado oil (or your preferred neutral-flavored cooking oil)

1 cup chopped yellow onions

¾ cup sliced celery

1 cup sliced carrots

3 cloves garlic, minced

Pinch of salt

1 teaspoon dried parsley

1 teaspoon dried thyme

1 teaspoon dried basil

Generous dash of freshly ground pepper

7 cups water

1½ tablespoons Vegetarian Better Than Bouillon No Chicken Base

2 bay leaves

3 cups short pasta (about 6 ounces; see Note)

1 (8-ounce) package Tofurky Plant-Based Lightly Seasoned Chick'n (or your preferred vegan chicken), chopped

DIRECTIONS

1 Put the oil in a large soup pot over medium heat. Add the chopped onions, celery, carrots, garlic, and salt. Sauté for 3 to 5 minutes, until the onions are translucent and fragrant.

2 Add the dried parsley, dried thyme, dried basil, and pepper. Fully combine the seasonings with the veggies.

3 Add the water, Vegetarian Better Than Bouillon No Chicken Base, and bay leaves. Stir and bring to a boil.

4 Once the mixture is boiling, add the pasta and vegan chicken. Boil until the pasta is al dente. That's usually about a minute short of what's listed on the package instructions. (If you're using Great Value egg-free ribbons, boil for about 5 minutes.)

5 When the noodles are al dente, lower the heat and cook for a couple minutes more. You want to allow time for the flavors to meld and the soup to come to a reasonable eating temperature.

6 Remove the bay leaves. Then ladle into bowls and serve.

PER SERVING: *Calories 415 (From Fat 50); Fat 6g (Saturated 0g); Cholesterol 0mg; Sodium 1049mg; Carbohydrate 68g (Dietary Fiber 8g); Protein 22g.*

VARY IT! Replace the vegan chicken with 1½ cups of seitan (chopped) or a can of chickpeas, cannellini beans, or great northern beans (drained and rinsed). Vegan chicken and seitan are salty; if you're using beans, you may need to increase the salt and/or Better Than Bouillon.

NOTE: Chicken noodle soup is usually made with egg noodles. Walmart sells egg-free noodles from Great Value that work well here. Or you can use any short pasta you enjoy, like farfalle or fusilli.

Classic Vegan Cheeseburger

PREP TIME: 6 MIN | COOK TIME: 10 MIN | YIELD: 3 SERVINGS

INGREDIENTS

1 (12-ounce) package Impossible Beef (or your preferred vegan ground beef; see Note)

½ teaspoon granulated onion

¼ teaspoon granulated garlic

Pinch of salt

Dash of freshly ground pepper

1 teaspoon avocado oil (or your preferred neutral-flavored cooking oil), divided

3 vegan cheddar cheese slices

3 hamburger buns, toasted if preferred

Ketchup, mustard, and/or vegan mayonnaise, for topping (optional)

3 green leaf lettuce leaves

½ yellow onion, thinly sliced

6 sandwich pickle slices

DIRECTIONS

1 In a mixing bowl, use your hands to combine the Impossible Beef, granulated onion, granulated garlic, salt, and pepper. Separate the burger mixture into three equal balls.

2 Put the oil in a large nonstick skillet over medium-high heat. Flatten the balls into burger shapes, and add them to the skillet.

3 Cook about 4 minutes on one side, or until the burgers have a nice crusty bottom. Use a thin wide spatula to flip the burgers. (You want to get underneath the burgers and not lose any of the crispy browned crust from where the burger meets the skillet.)

4 Add a slice of vegan cheddar cheese to each burger. Lower the heat and cover the skillet with a lid to allow the cheese to melt. Cook for about 4 more minutes, or until the cheese has melted.

5 Slather the buns with ketchup, mustard, and/or vegan mayonnaise, if you like. Add the cheeseburgers to the buns. Finish with green leaf lettuce, sliced onion, and two sandwich pickle slices per burger before serving.

PER SERVING: *Calories 332 (From Fat 95); Fat 11g (Saturated 5g); Cholesterol 0mg; Sodium 1221mg; Carbohydrate 34g (Dietary Fiber 7g); Protein 25g.*

VARY IT! These burgers are also great on the grill. Bring an outdoor grill to a medium-high heat. Lightly oil the burgers or put them on an oiled grill grate to prevent them from sticking. Grill for about 4 minutes on each side, or until they have reached your preferred level of doneness. After flipping the burgers, add the cheese slices and close the grill lid to allow the cheese to melt.

NOTE: You can find many different types of vegan ground beef. For this recipe, you want the kind that's packaged like ground beef, like Impossible or Beyond Beef. Vegan ground beef that's packaged in crumbles won't work for this recipe, because it won't hold together in a burger shape.

This makes burgers that are done medium. If you prefer them less well-done, shorten the cooking time slightly. If you prefer them more well-done, cook longer. Be sure that the internal temperature reaches 160 degrees so they're safe to eat.

Barbecue Jackfruit Nachos

PREP TIME: 15 MIN   COOK TIME: 20 MIN   YIELD: 4 TO 6 SERVINGS

INGREDIENTS

1 (20-ounce) can green or young jackfruit, packed in water or brine (see Note)

2 teaspoons avocado oil (or your preferred neutral-flavored oil), divided

½ cup chopped onions

1 clove garlic, minced

½ teaspoon ground cumin

½ teaspoon ancho chili powder

½ teaspoon ground coriander

¼ teaspoon salt, or to taste

2 teaspoons tahini

½ cup barbecue sauce, divided

8 to 10 ounces tortilla chips

½ cup corn, thawed from frozen or drained from can

1 cup shredded vegan cheddar cheese

¼ cup sliced scallions

¼ cup chopped red, orange, or yellow bell peppers

1 avocado, diced in chunks

Drizzles of vegan ranch dressing (see Chapter 14; optional but recommended)

DIRECTIONS

1 Preheat the oven to 400 degrees.

2 Drain the jackfruit in a colander. Rinse well with water.

3 Place the rinsed jackfruit on a clean, dry kitchen towel. Dry the jackfruit with the towel, and then wrap it like a Tootsie Roll and wring it dry until all the water or brine comes out.

4 Move the dried-off jackfruit to a food processor. Pulse several times until it's fully broken up and shredded. (All parts of the canned jackfruit are edible — including pods and firmer pieces. The food processor completely breaks those up, so they're easy and pleasant to chew. If you don't have a food processor, just chop the jackfruit with a knife; see the Note below.)

5 Put 1 teaspoon of the oil in a large nonstick skillet over medium heat. Spread the jackfruit across the skillet. Allow it to brown for about 4 or 5 minutes. Flip it once it has browned on one side.

6 Move the jackfruit to one side of the skillet. Then put the remaining teaspoon of oil on the empty side of the skillet. Add the onions and garlic. Sauté for a minute or two, until fragrant. Then mix the onions and garlic with the jackfruit using a spatula.

7 Season the jackfruit with the ground cumin, ancho chili powder, ground coriander, and salt. Fully incorporate the seasonings with the jackfruit, and cook for about a minute. Then add the tahini; it makes the jackfruit stickier (like pulled pork) and adds protein and fat.

8 Add 6 tablespoons of the barbecue sauce to the jackfruit mixture, and fully incorporate it. Cook about a minute longer, until the barbecue sauce is warmed.

9 Line a baking sheet with tortilla chips. Top with spoonfuls of barbecue jackfruit and corn. Sprinkle on the vegan cheddar cheese. Drizzle the 2 remaining tablespoons of barbecue sauce over the chips.

10 Place the nachos in the oven and bake for about 8 to 10 minutes, or until the cheese has melted. (Be careful not to overbake and burn the chips.)

11 Remove from the oven. Finish with sliced scallions, bell peppers, avocado, and a few drizzles of vegan ranch dressing, if you like. Pass around plates and serve the warm nachos from the baking sheet.

PER SERVING: *Calories 465 (From Fat 219); Fat 24g (Saturated 2g); Cholesterol 0mg; Sodium 1734mg; Carbohydrate 58g (Dietary Fiber 13g); Protein 7g.*

VARY IT! If you like, add one shredded carrot to the jackfruit mixture in the skillet right after adding the spices. You'll likely need more barbecue sauce. Continue cooking until the carrot has reached your preferred level of softness. If you like a spicier filling, add a dash of hot sauce along with the barbecue sauce. You can also add pickled jalapeños to the finished nachos. If you can find frozen fire roasted corn, it's especially delicious on these nachos. The nachos are also tasty topped with a sprinkling of chopped cilantro. For an even more filling platter, consider making a double batch of the barbecued jackfruit.

NOTE: *Don't* use fresh ripe jackfruit or canned jackfruit packed in syrup. They are much too sweet for this recipe. If you don't have a food processor, that's not an issue. After you wring the water or brine out of the jackfruit in a towel, you can either give it a rough chop or break it up with your fingers and put it into the warm oiled skillet. As you cook the jackfruit, break it up further with your spatula.

Black Bean Tacos

PREP TIME: 7 MIN | COOK TIME: 13 MIN | YIELD: 6 TACOS

INGREDIENTS

1 teaspoon avocado oil (or your preferred neutral-flavored cooking oil)

½ yellow onion, chopped

2 cloves garlic, minced

1 (15-ounce) can black beans, drained and rinsed

1 teaspoon ancho chili powder (see Note)

1 teaspoon ground cumin

½ teaspoon paprika

Pinch of salt, or more to taste

1 tablespoon freshly squeezed lime juice

¼ cup water, or more if needed

6 crunchy corn taco shells

½ cup chopped tomatoes

1 cup romaine lettuce, roughly chopped

1 avocado, sliced

Handful of cilantro, roughly chopped, for garnish

DIRECTIONS

1 Preheat the oven to 425 degrees.

2 Put the oil in a large nonstick skillet over medium heat. Add the onion and garlic. Sauté a few minutes, until fragrant and translucent.

3 Add the drained black beans, ancho chili powder, ground cumin, paprika, and salt. Combine. Then add the lime juice and water. Combine and cook for 10 minutes, until heated through.

4 Once the black bean mixture has warmed and excess liquid has cooked off, taste for salt and add more, if needed. (The beans should be saucy but not soupy. If there's too much liquid, keep cooking. If there's not enough, add a tablespoon or two of water.)

5 Put the crunchy corn taco shells on a baking sheet. Bake for 2 to 3 minutes, until warm.

6 Remove the shells from the oven. Stuff each taco shell with two or three spoonfuls of black bean mixture, chopped tomatoes, romaine lettuce, and avocado. Finish with a sprinkling of cilantro and serve.

PER SERVING: *Calories 216 (From Fat 91); Fat 10g (Saturated 2g); Cholesterol 0mg; Sodium 181mg; Carbohydrate 27g (Dietary Fiber 7g); Protein 6g.*

NOTE: Ancho chili powder is different from standard chili powder, which tends to be a mix of spices. Ancho chili powder has just one ingredient: dried ancho chili peppers. If you use a chili powder blend, it may include cayenne pepper, which will change the spiciness of this dish. Adjust accordingly.

VARY IT! Instead of black beans, use pinto beans. Instead of crunchy taco shells, use soft corn or flour tortillas. Romaine lettuce can be replaced with shredded cabbage mix. Avocado can be replaced with guacamole. Add any other toppings you enjoy like shredded vegan cheddar cheese, nondairy sour cream, pickled red onions, and/or jalapeños.

Basil Pesto Pasta with Roasted Chickpeas

PREP TIME: 5 MIN   COOK TIME: 10 MIN   YIELD: 4 SERVINGS

INGREDIENTS

3 cups fresh basil leaves, lightly packed

2 cloves garlic, minced

1 tablespoon freshly squeezed lemon juice

1 teaspoon white miso paste

1 tablespoon nutritional yeast flakes

¼ cup shelled roasted pistachios, salted or unsalted

Pinch of salt

¼ cup extra-virgin olive oil

8 ounces short pasta (like penne or farfalle), whole wheat or white

3 cups broccoli florets

1 batch roasted chickpeas (see Chapter 14)

DIRECTIONS

1 Place the basil leaves, minced garlic, lemon juice, white miso paste, nutritional yeast flakes, roasted pistachios, and salt in a food processor.

2 Set the food processor to Low. While it's running, pour the extra-virgin olive oil down the food processor chute. Stop and scrape down the sides, as needed, and continue processing until the pesto is mostly smooth.

3 Cook the pasta according to the package directions, until al dente.

4 During the last 6 minutes of cooking the pasta, put the broccoli florets in a bamboo or metal steamer insert with lid over the boiling pasta. Steam 5 to 6 minutes, or until bright green and tender. (You should be able to easily pierce it with a fork.) Finish with a pinch of salt and set aside.

5 After the pasta has finished cooking, drain it in a colander.

6 Move the pasta to a large mixing bowl. Spoon the pesto over the pasta, and toss until evenly combined. Taste and add more salt if needed. Top with the roasted chickpeas and steamed broccoli, and serve.

PER SERVING: *Calories 551 (From Fat 197); Fat 22g (Saturated 3g); Cholesterol 0mg; Sodium 428mg; Carbohydrate 72g (Dietary Fiber 11g); Protein 19g.*

TIP: If you don't have a steamer insert that fits over a pot, you can steam the broccoli separately using a metal folding steamer basket that opens up like a flower. Put about an inch of water into a separate pot, and add the insert. Bring the water to a boil. Add the broccoli florets, cover with a lid, and steam for 5 to 6 minutes or until bright green and tender. If you don't have any type of steamer insert, you can boil the broccoli in water instead for 2 to 3 minutes, or until tender. Then drain.

Mushroom Fajitas

| PREP TIME: 10 MIN | COOK TIME: 20 MIN | YIELD: 3 TO 4 SERVINGS |

INGREDIENTS

1 red bell pepper, cut into ½-inch strips

1 yellow onion, cut into ¼- to ½-inch slices

8 ounces cremini or white button mushrooms, cut into ½-inch slices

1 tablespoon freshly squeezed lime juice

1 tablespoon avocado oil (or your preferred neutral-flavored cooking oil)

1 teaspoon ancho chili powder

1 teaspoon ground cumin

1 teaspoon paprika

½ teaspoon salt

6 to 8 small corn tortillas

2 avocados, sliced

Handful of cilantro, roughly chopped, for garnish

DIRECTIONS

1 Preheat the oven to 425 degrees. Line two baking sheets with parchment paper, and set aside. (See the sidebar if you prefer to grill the vegetables.)

2 In a large mixing bowl, combine the red bell pepper, onion, and mushrooms. Add the lime juice, oil, ancho chili powder, ground cumin, paprika, and salt. Toss until the vegetables are evenly coated. Set aside and let the vegetables marinate while the oven heats.

3 Divide the vegetable mixture evenly between the two baking sheets, and spread the veggies across them, being careful not to overcrowd. If they overlap, the vegetables will steam instead of roast.

4 Roast the vegetables for 15 to 20 minutes, stopping once about halfway through to toss the vegetables with a spatula.

5 While the vegetables finish roasting, bring a skillet to medium heat. Warm each tortilla in the skillet for a couple minutes on each side. Then move them to a plate and cover with a clean kitchen towel to keep warm while you continue warming the remaining tortillas.

6 When the vegetables are done, remove them from the oven. To serve, fill each tortilla with a couple spoonfuls of fajita vegetables. Top with the avocado slices and garnish with the cilantro.

PER SERVING: *Calories 230 (From Fat 129); Fat 14g (Saturated 2g); Cholesterol 0mg; Sodium 316mg; Carbohydrate 25g (Dietary Fiber 8g); Protein 5g.*

VARY IT! The vegetables can be replaced with a roughly equal amount of any vegetables you enjoy, like zucchini or yellow summer squash. Just remember that heartier vegetables like cauliflower or broccoli may need more time to cook.

TIP: I recommend serving these fajitas with something filling and protein-dense like refried pinto or black beans.

GRILLING DIRECTIONS

If you'd prefer to cook the fajitas on an outdoor grill, bring the grill to 500 degrees. Spritz a grill basket with oil if it's prone to sticking. Place the marinated vegetables in the grill basket. Depending on the size of your basket, you may need to work in batches. Don't overcrowd.

Grill for 15 to 20 minutes, tossing occasionally for even browning. Grill the corn tortillas on the grill grate for about 3 minutes on each side, until they soften and develop brown grill marks. Then fill the warmed corn tortillas with the fajita vegetables, avocado slices, and cilantro garnish.

Cold Peanut Noodles

PREP TIME: 10 MIN	COOK TIME: 10 MIN	YIELD: 6 SERVINGS

INGREDIENTS

8 ounces spaghetti, whole wheat or white

6 to 7 tablespoons natural peanut butter, creamy or crunchy

2 tablespoons tamari

2 tablespoons rice vinegar

¼ cup water

½ teaspoon sriracha, or to taste

1 clove garlic, minced

¼ teaspoon toasted sesame oil

4 radishes, thinly sliced

2 small carrots, thinly sliced or shredded

¼ cup chopped scallions

½ red bell pepper, chopped

½ cup chopped cilantro

Handful of roasted peanuts, whole or coarsely chopped, for garnish

DIRECTIONS

1 Cook the spaghetti according to the package instructions, until al dente. Drain the spaghetti in a colander, rinse in very cold water, and drain again. Set aside.

2 In a medium-sized bowl, combine 6 tablespoons of natural peanut butter, tamari, rice vinegar, water, sriracha, garlic, and toasted sesame oil with a fork or whisk. The sauce should have the texture of a thick ranch dressing.

Peanut butter thickness varies by brand. If your sauce is too thin, incorporate the remaining 1 tablespoon of peanut butter into the sauce. If it's too thick, add another splash of water.

3 Put the drained noodles into a large mixing bowl along with the radishes, carrots, scallions, red bell peppers, and cilantro.

4 Pour the peanut sauce over the noodles and vegetables and use a serving spoon to fully combine. Garnish with the roasted peanuts. Serve right away or refrigerate until time to eat.

PER SERVING: *Calories 250 (From Fat 79); Fat 9g (Saturated 2g); Cholesterol 0mg; Sodium 355mg; Carbohydrate 34g (Dietary Fiber 3g); Protein 10g.*

VARY IT! Swap out any of the vegetables for sugar snap peas, pea shoots, shredded cabbage, or cucumber. If you like, top this dish with cubed baked teriyaki-flavored tofu.

NOTE: Cold peanut noodles will stay perfectly creamy in the refrigerator for a day or two. However, if the noodles dry out over time, freshen them with a splash of tamari, rice vinegar, sriracha, and/or water. Add a pinch of salt, if needed, and stir before serving.

TIP: Look for peanut butter with just two ingredients — peanuts and salt. If you like some texture in your peanut sauce, use the crunchy variety. If you prefer it totally smooth, use creamy peanut butter.

Pineapple Fried Rice

PREP TIME: 10 MIN	COOK TIME: 15 MIN	YIELD: 4 SERVINGS

INGREDIENTS

1½ tablespoons tamari

¼ teaspoon toasted sesame oil

1 teaspoon sriracha, or more if desired

1½ teaspoons avocado oil (or your preferred neutral-flavored cooking oil), divided

½ cup chopped yellow onions

½ red bell pepper, chopped

1 carrot, chopped

2 cloves garlic, minced

2½ cups cold brown rice (fully cooked)

½ cup chopped pineapple, preferably fresh

¼ cup peas, fresh or frozen

Handful of cilantro, chopped, for topping

Handful of whole roasted cashews, salted, for topping

Pinch of salt (optional)

DIRECTIONS

1 In a small bowl, combine the tamari, toasted sesame oil, and sriracha with a fork or whisk until blended. Set aside.

2 Put 1 teaspoon of avocado oil in a large nonstick skillet over medium heat. Add the onions, bell pepper, and carrot. Sauté for about 5 minutes, until the carrot has softened but still have some bite.

3 Push the vegetables to one side of the skillet, and add the remaining ½ teaspoon of avocado oil to the empty side. Add the garlic and sauté for about 30 seconds, until the garlic is fragrant.

4 Combine the garlic and vegetables in the skillet. Then add the cold cooked rice. Allow it to toast a bit and then fully combine with the vegetables.

5 Add the pineapple, peas, and tamari mixture to the rice. Once the pineapple and peas are warmed through, top with a handful of chopped cilantro, and roasted cashews. Taste for salt, and add a pinch if needed. For extra spice, drizzle more sriracha across the top and serve.

PER SERVING: Calories 294 (From Fat 98); Fat 11g (Saturated 2g); Cholesterol 0mg; Sodium 493mg; Carbohydrate 43g (Dietary Fiber 5g); Protein 8g.

NOTE: Using cold rice is essential for this recipe. Otherwise, the rice will clump, and the seasonings won't get evenly combined. I recommend putting frozen rice in the refrigerator the day before to thaw. (I always get frozen organic brown rice at Trader Joe's.) If you're in a pinch, you can cook rice from scratch. Then spread it on a baking sheet, and move it to the freezer to cool for about 15 minutes. If you don't have fresh pineapple, canned will work; although, the texture isn't as firm. Be sure to drain it first.

VARY IT! For more spice, add up to a teaspoon of curry powder with the tamari mixture and/or sauté chopped jalapeño and grated ginger with the garlic.

TIP: For an extra bump of protein, add cubed tofu that's been marinated in tamari, rice vinegar, and sesame oil and browned in a skillet with a little oil. This fried rice is also delicious with browned JUST Egg. For the best texture, fully cook the vegan egg separately, break it into bite-sized pieces, and then add it to the fried rice at the end.

Chapter **13**

Kid- and Dorm-Friendly Dishes

For many parents, getting their kids to eat vegetables is a struggle. If the kids were in charge, every meal would be shaped like a nugget or french fry.

If you've faced similar troubles, take heart. You're not alone. According to a 2021 report from the Centers for Disease Control and Prevention, nearly one-third of children ages 1 to 5 don't eat a daily fruit. Even more surprising, almost 50 percent don't eat a daily vegetable.

TIP

Here are a few ways to get kids on board with eating more fruits and vegetables:

» Get them involved in meal planning. Offer some suggestions, and ask which meals sound good to them.

» Take them to the grocery store or farmers market with you. Talk about what's there, and allow them to have a hand in picking a fruit and vegetable to try.

>> Offer fruits and vegetables with every meal. Invite them to smell, touch, and, of course, taste, but keep the pressure low.

>> Talk with them in age-appropriate language about all the ways fruits and veggies help in growth, nutrition, and energy. Reaffirm why they're a valuable part of mealtime.

>> Make foods that are easy to hold in little hands.

>> Don't forget the allure of a good dipping sauce! It can make all the difference in snacking on baby carrots, cauliflower, and sugar snap peas.

In this chapter, you find kid-friendly recipes that are great for getting children involved in food preparation. Depending on their age, they may be able to sprinkle on toppings, roll pinwheels or crescent rolls, or prepare the dishes from beginning to end.

I also include recipes for college students. Whether you're cooking in a dorm or your first apartment, you're set with easy and inexpensive meal options like bagel sandwiches and that college classic, ramen.

Getting Kids Involved at Dinnertime

TIP

When parents teach their kids how to cook and give them room to prepare their own meals, it helps children to become self-sufficient. Cooking is an important lifelong skill that continues to pay dividends — in health and in saving money down the road.

For Tortilla Pinwheels, offer hummus (flavored or plain) or vegan cream cheese as the base spread. Then kids can choose the veggies for filling options. Romaine, cilantro, and shredded carrots are my favorite.

In addition to being a kid-friendly dinner, Pizza Bagels are a fun recipe for the whole family. Put out a variety of topping options, and let everyone compile their ideal pizza.

>> Go classic with vegan pepperoni, onions, and bell peppers.

>> Make a taco-style pizza with soy chorizo, and then finish the cooked pizza with chopped tomatoes, lettuce, and cilantro.

>> Have a Hawaiian-inspired pizza with vegan ham and pineapple.

>> Think Mediterranean with artichoke hearts, olives, and spinach.

The only limit is your imagination!

Kids also enjoy rolling up vegan hot dogs in store-bought crescent dough to make Happy Pigs in a Blanket. This tasty recipe can be made in either the oven or the air fryer. It's a delicious appetizer, snack, or lunch when served with a salad or vegetable side dish. I recommend adding a tasty dipping sauce like mustard, ketchup, or Vegan Ranch Dressing (see Chapter 14).

Preparing College-Friendly Cuisine

College is an exciting time in the lives of many young people. No longer under their parents' roof, they can decide for themselves what to make at mealtimes. With busy schedules, lean wallets, limited cooking equipment and space, students often require recipes that are quick, easy, and won't break the bank.

Dressed Up Ramen Noodles elevates that old stand-by into a full and satiating lunch. It's finished with your choice of vegetables and baked tofu for added protein and nutrients.

Have limited cooking equipment in your dorm room? Make Eggless Egg Salad Wraps or Chicken-Free Salad Sandwiches. In addition to filling wraps and sandwiches, these tasty salads are great with crackers for noshing during study sessions.

When you can't stomach another pizza delivery, make a hearty Old School Chef Salad or Hummus Bagel Sandwich. They're packed with good-for-you vegetables, plus plant protein that will fuel your on-the-go lifestyle.

REMEMBER

Even though this chapter is for kids and college students, anyone can make and enjoy these dishes.

Pizza Bagels

PREP TIME: 3 MIN	COOK TIME: 10 MIN	YIELD: 4 SERVINGS

INGREDIENTS

4 bagels, sliced in half
(see Note)

½ cup marinara plus more
if needed

24 slices vegan pepperoni

¼ cup chopped bell peppers

¼ cup chopped yellow onions

½ cup shredded vegan
mozzarella cheese

DIRECTIONS

1 Preheat the oven to 425 degrees. (If using an air fryer, see the sidebar.)

2 Place the sliced bagels cut side up on a baking sheet. Top each bagel half with equal amounts of marinara, vegan pepperoni, bell peppers, onions, and vegan mozzarella cheese.

3 Bake for 10 minutes, or until the cheese has melted.

4 Remove the bagels from the oven. They will be quite hot, so allow them to cool a couple minutes before serving.

PER SERVING: *Calories 330 (From Fat 75); Fat 8g (Saturated 0g); Cholesterol 0mg; Sodium 867mg; Carbohydrate 51g (Dietary Fiber 3g); Protein 12g.*

VARY IT! Try different topping options such as browned vegan sausage, pineapple, olives, tomatoes, mushrooms, seitan bacon, browned vegan ground beef, jalapeños, artichoke hearts, or spinach. Finish with a sprinkling of vegan parmesan cheese. (Get the vegan parmesan recipe in Chapter 14.)

NOTE: Read the bagel ingredients list to make sure they don't include eggs or dairy. Bagels vary in size, so adjust the toppings accordingly. Plain, sun-dried tomato, everything, rosemary olive oil, and onion bagels are all good flavor options for a pizza bagel.

AIR FRYER INSTRUCTIONS

Prefer to use an air fryer? Put the bagel halves, cut side up, in the air fryer basket. (Depending on the size of your air fryer, you likely need to work in batches.) Toast them without toppings at 370 degrees for 2 minutes. Remove the bagel halves from the air fryer. Top each bagel half with equal amounts of marinara, vegan pepperoni, chopped bell peppers and onions, and vegan mozzarella cheese. Return the bagel halves to the air fryer. Air fry at 370 degrees for 4 to 5 minutes, until the cheese has melted.

Tortilla Pinwheels

INGREDIENTS

¾ cup homemade or store-bought hummus or vegan cream cheese

4 (8-inch) flour tortillas, whole wheat or white (see Tip)

1 cup chopped romaine lettuce

½ cup shredded carrots

¼ cup chopped cilantro

DIRECTIONS

1 Spread a layer of hummus onto each tortilla. Make sure to go all the way to the edges. (I use about 3 tablespoons per tortilla, but amounts will vary depending on the size of the tortilla.)

2 On each tortilla, sprinkle about ¼ cup of chopped romaine lettuce, 2 tablespoons of shredded carrots, and 1 tablespoon of cilantro. For easiest rolling, leave about an inch gap around the edge of the tortilla, and don't overfill.

3 Roll the tortillas as tightly as you can. If you want to serve the pinwheels right away, use a serrated knife to evenly cut the rolled tortillas into pinwheels, roughly 2 inches in length. Place the pinwheels on a platter to serve. See the Note for storing before serving.

PER SERVING: *Calories 172 (From Fat 38); Fat 4g (Saturated 1g); Cholesterol 0mg; Sodium 342mg; Carbohydrate 28g (Dietary Fiber 2g); Protein 5g.*

VARY IT! Veggie combinations in pinwheels are endless: sliced olives, cucumber, marinated artichoke hearts, red bell pepper, spinach, or chives. Instead of plain hummus or vegan cream cheese, try a flavored variety.

NOTE: If you plan to serve the pinwheels later, wait to cut them. You don't want the fillings to get dried out. Wrap the individual tortilla roll-ups in cling wrap, store them in the fridge, and cut them just before serving.

TIP: If your tortillas are on the dry side, warm them in a dry skillet or microwave to make them more pliable before filling and rolling.

Happy Pigs in a Blanket

PREP TIME: 10 MIN	COOK TIME: 15 MIN	YIELD: 8 SERVINGS

INGREDIENTS

1 (8-ounce) refrigerated tube crescent rolls (see Note)

1 (8-count) package vegan hot dogs (standard-sized)

1 teaspoon sesame seeds or Everything But the Bagel seasoning

DIRECTIONS

1 Preheat the oven to 375 degrees. Line a baking sheet with parchment paper. (If using an air fryer, see the sidebar.)

2 Unroll the crescent dough onto a cutting board and separate it into eight large triangles. Use a knife to cut each triangle in half into skinnier triangles.

3 Cut the hot dogs in half.

4 Put each hot dog piece onto the widest part of a crescent roll triangle. Then roll it up. Continue until you have rolled all the hot dog pieces in dough.

5 Place the wrapped crescent dogs on the lined baking sheet, leaving at least an inch of space between them. Sprinkle with the sesame seeds or Everything But the Bagel seasoning.

6 Bake for 12 to 15 minutes, until golden brown and cooked through. Use a spatula to transfer to a serving platter.

PER SERVING: *Calories 142 (From Fat 29); Fat 3g (Saturated 0g); Cholesterol 0mg; Sodium 516mg; Carbohydrate 16g (Dietary Fiber 1g); Protein 11g.*

NOTE: Many brands of crescent rolls are accidentally vegan. Trader Joe's, Annie's, Immaculate Baking Company, and the classic Pillsbury crescent rolls are all free of animal products. Formulations change, so read the ingredients label to be sure. If you can only find long, stadium-sized vegan hot dogs, cut them into 2-inch pieces.

AIR FRYER INSTRUCTIONS

Prefer to use an air fryer? Follow Steps 2 through 4. Then put the crescent dogs into the air fryer basket, leaving space in between them. (Don't overcrowd. Depending on the size of your air fryer, you may need to cook in batches. Subsequent batches may cook faster.) Air fry at 390 degrees for 5 minutes. Use a spatula or fork to gently turn each one over. Then air fry for 2 minutes, or until golden brown and cooked through.

Eggless Egg Salad Wrap

INGREDIENTS

1 (16-ounce) vacuum-packed (NOT water-packed) block super-firm tofu (see Tip)

2 tablespoons chopped chives

½ cup vegan mayonnaise

1 teaspoon stone-ground mustard

¾ teaspoon kala namak (black salt; see Note)

Generous dash of freshly ground black pepper

⅛ teaspoon turmeric

4 (8-inch) whole wheat tortillas

4 romaine lettuce leaves

Shredded carrots, thinly sliced onion, sliced avocado, and/or shelled pumpkin seeds, for topping (optional)

DIRECTIONS

1 Crumble the tofu into a large mixing bowl with your fingers. Add the chopped chives, vegan mayonnaise, stone-ground mustard, kala namak, pepper, and turmeric.

2 Combine the filling ingredients with a fork, mashing some of the tofu. But don't make it a puree — you want it to still have some texture.

3 Taste for any adjustments. Add more mayo, stone-ground mustard, kala namak, or pepper, if you like.

4 Top each tortilla with a romaine lettuce leaf. Then add several generous spoonfuls of the tofu mixture. If you like, add optional toppings like shredded carrots, thinly sliced onion, sliced avocado, and/or shelled pumpkin seeds. Roll each tortilla like a burrito and serve.

PER SERVING: *Calories 405 (From Fat 228); Fat 25g (Saturated 4g); Cholesterol 0mg; Sodium 520mg; Carbohydrate 32g (Dietary Fiber 5g); Protein 17g.*

VARY IT! Instead of serving eggless egg salad in a wrap, spoon it on sandwich bread or a toasted bagel. It's also a delicious snack dolloped onto crackers or eaten in lettuce cups.

NOTE: Kala namak (also known as black salt) is essential in this dish. Look for it at Indian grocery stores or online. The eggy flavor fades in the dish over time. So if you're eating leftovers, I recommend adding another sprinkle of kala namak just before serving.

TIP: The handy thing about vacuum-packed tofu is that you don't have to press the water out before using it. You can find vacuum-packed tofu in the refrigerated section of many grocery stores and Trader Joe's. If you only have water-packed tofu, you'll need to press it first. See Chapter 9 for instructions. Water-packed tofu usually comes in 14-ounce packages, but that includes water weight. In that case, you'll need two packages of drained and pressed tofu for this recipe.

Dressed Up Ramen Noodles

PREP TIME: 5 MIN	COOK TIME: 4 MIN	YIELD: 1 SERVING

INGREDIENTS

1½ cups water plus more if desired

1 (60-gram) package vegan ramen with seasoning packet (see Note)

1 teaspoon tahini

½ teaspoon tamari (or your preferred soy sauce)

¼ teaspoon rice vinegar

½ cup chopped vegetables of your choice, raw or cooked

1½ to 2 ounces thinly sliced baked tofu (see Tip)

DIRECTIONS

1 Bring 1½ cups of water to a boil with the ramen seasoning packet in a small or medium saucepan. Once the broth is boiling, add the ramen noodles. Cook about 4 minutes (or the time listed in the package instructions), until the noodles are softened to your liking.

2 Stir in the tahini, tamari, and rice vinegar until fully dissolved. If you like a brothier soup, add another ¼ cup of water or more.

3 Pour the noodles and broth into a large soup bowl. Top with your choice of vegetables and baked tofu slices before serving.

PER SERVING: *Calories 179 (From Fat 40); Fat 4g (Saturated 1g); Cholesterol 0mg; Sodium 592mg; Carbohydrate 27g (Dietary Fiber 3g); Protein 8g.*

VARY IT! For this recipe, choose from raw veggies like shredded cabbage mix, cilantro, chopped bell pepper, thinly sliced radishes, scallions, jalapeños, or pickled red onions. Or add cooked veggies like sautéed mushrooms, steamed sugar snap peas, steamed broccoli, sautéed bok choy, green peas, or corn.

TIP: You can find several vegan ramen noodle brands on the market. I often choose Koyo shiitake mushroom or garlic pepper flavor. For the tofu, look for packages of baked tofu that are fully seasoned. They come in a variety of flavors from Trader Joe's, Wildwood, Nasoya, Hodo, and more. They're ready to eat right out of the package, or you can briefly warm them before serving. I usually buy teriyaki flavor, but sriracha flavor is also good here.

NOTE: If your seasoning packet is especially salty or strongly flavored, you may want to add only a portion of the packet. Or you can omit the seasoning packet completely and use vegetable broth instead of water or ½ teaspoon of Vegetarian Better Than Bouillon No Chicken Base.

Chicken-Free Salad Sandwich

PREP TIME: 15 MIN | COOK TIME: 0 MIN | YIELD: 4 SERVINGS

INGREDIENTS

8 ounces chicken-style seitan or vegan chicken

2 tablespoons diced dill pickles

3 tablespoons sliced celery

1 tablespoon diced onions

2 tablespoons vegan mayonnaise plus more as needed

¼ teaspoon stone-ground mustard

⅛ teaspoon dried thyme

⅛ teaspoon dried dill

⅛ teaspoon granulated onion

Dash of freshly ground pepper

4 burger buns

4 romaine or green leaf lettuce leaves

DIRECTIONS

1 Put the chicken-style seitan, dill pickles, celery, onions, vegan mayonnaise, stone-ground mustard, dried thyme, dried dill, granulated onion, and pepper into a food processor. (If you don't have a food processor, see the Note.)

2 Process on Low, until everything is in small pieces. Stop once to scrape down the sides, so all the ingredients are incorporated.

3 Put a thin slathering of vegan mayonnaise onto the cut side of each burger bun if desired. Scoop the seitan mixture onto the buns, along with a leaf of romaine, and serve.

PER SERVING: *Calories 242 (From Fat 83); Fat 9g (Saturated 1g); Cholesterol 0mg; Sodium 505mg; Carbohydrate 26g (Dietary Fiber 7g); Protein 16g.*

VARY IT! Omit the dill pickles and stir in sliced grapes for a sweeter take on this sandwich. For a creamier filling, add more mayo to taste. Burger buns can be replaced with sandwich bread or bagels, or use a tortilla or pita for a wrap.

NOTE: If you don't have a food processor, simply chop the seitan into bite-sized pieces. Then combine it with the remaining vegan chicken salad ingredients in a bowl with a spoon.

TIP: You can use homemade or store-bought seitan or vegan chicken. For store-bought, Upton's Naturals traditional style, Herbivorous Butcher chicken, or Tofurky Plant-Based Lightly Seasoned Chick'n are good choices. If you make your own seitan, use 1 cup of bite-sized seitan pieces.

Old School Chef Salad

INGREDIENTS

3 cups chopped romaine lettuce

2 medium tomatoes, sliced in wedges

½ cup sliced cucumber

2 slices vegan cheddar cheese, diced

½ cup chopped vegan deli slices or vegan chicken

1 avocado, sliced

Pinch of kala namak (black salt), optional (see Note)

½ cup Vegan Ranch Dressing (see Chapter 14)

Freshly ground black pepper, for serving

DIRECTIONS

1 Fill a large salad bowl with the romaine lettuce. Top the lettuce with distinct rows of the tomato wedges, cucumber slices, diced vegan cheddar cheese, chopped vegan deli slices.

2 Place the avocado slices on top of the salad. If you like, sprinkle a tiny amount of kala namak over the avocado for an eggy flavor.

3 Serve the salad with the vegan ranch dressing on the side (see the Tip). When ready to serve, the salad can be divided into meal-sized portions or sides and then dressed as desired. Finish each serving with a sprinkle of pepper.

PER SERVING: *Calories 254 (From Fat 210); Fat 23g (Saturated 5g); Cholesterol 0mg; Sodium 503mg; Carbohydrate 11g (Dietary Fiber 5g); Protein 5g.*

VARY IT! If you're short on time, replace the homemade vegan ranch dressing with store-bought vegan ranch dressing like Follow Your Heart brand. The vegan deli slices or vegan chicken can be replaced with seitan or cubes of baked tofu. The avocado and kala namak can be replaced with WunderEggs, vegan hard-boiled eggs sold in stores like Whole Foods or online.

NOTE: Chef salads are typically made with hard-boiled eggs, not avocado. If you'd like your avocado to have some eggy flavor, sprinkle it with kala namak (also known as black salt). It's amazing how much it tastes like you've added egg to this vegan dish. You can find kala namak at Indian grocery stores or online. For the cheese, use your favorite vegan cheddar slices, or dice a vegan cheddar block. (Two slices are about 1½ ounces.)

TIP: This salad keeps best when it hasn't been tossed with salad dressing. If you're making the salad ahead of time, store the dressing separately from the salad, and to avoid browning, don't cut or add the avocado until serving.

Hummus Bagel Sandwich

PREP TIME: 5 MIN	COOK TIME: 2 MIN	YIELD: 1 SERVING

INGREDIENTS

1 bagel, sliced in half (see Note)

2 tablespoons homemade or store-bought hummus

1 radish, thinly sliced

1 tablespoon chopped onions

2 tomato slices

4 to 5 thin slices red bell pepper

2 leaves green leaf lettuce (or several baby spinach leaves)

DIRECTIONS

1 Toast the bagel in a toaster or toaster oven on the Bagel setting.

2 Slather the hummus on each toasted bagel half.

3 Top one bagel half with the thinly sliced radish, onions, tomato slices, red bell pepper slices, and green leaf lettuce leaves. Then top with the other bagel half and serve.

PER SERVING: *Calories 253 (From Fat 35); Fat 4g (Saturated 4g); Cholesterol 0mg; Sodium 386mg; Carbohydrate 45g (Dietary Fiber 4g); Protein 9g.*

VARY IT! Replace the plain hummus with a flavored hummus, vegan cheese spread, smashed avocado, or nondairy cream cheese. Replace any of the vegetables with sliced cucumber, pickles, sliced olives, sauerkraut, pickled jalapeños, cilantro, arugula, microgreens, or shredded carrot. Instead of a bagel, use sandwich bread, sourdough, or baguette. To turn it into a wrap, use a tortilla or pita.

NOTE: Read the bagel ingredients list to make sure they don't include eggs or dairy. Flavors that are especially nice for a sandwich include: rosemary olive oil, onion, poppy, sesame, everything, or sun-dried tomato.

Chapter **14**

Side Dishes, Dressings, and Toppings

The U.S. Department of Agriculture (USDA) recommends eating at least 2½ cups of veggies a day, but most folks are falling short. In fact, according to the Centers for Disease Control and Prevention (CDC), only one in ten American adults meets the recommended amounts of vegetables every day.

You're in luck, though! Vegans are uniquely positioned to meet that daily goal, because they don't have animal products like meat and eggs displacing produce in their diet. More of the plate is available for antioxidant-packed fruits and vegetables.

In this chapter, you find recipes for dishes that will help you meet the USDA's produce targets, like Sesame Sugar Snap Peas and Sautéed Kale with Garlic. These staples come together lightning fast, which is super handy if your main course is more labor-intensive.

You also get recipes for crowd-friendly sides for summer potlucks and cookouts, like Grilled Vegetable Skewers, Mediterranean Couscous Salad, and Pasta Salad with Creamy Dressing. Outside of picnic season, these substantive salads make excellent packed lunches!

Taking Your Salads to the Next Level

When it comes to eating your leafy greens, having the right dressing makes all the difference. This chapter includes recipes for dressings that will suit a variety of needs.

>> Tahini dressing is a tasty all-purpose dressing that works for lighter greens just as well as hearty kale. It's also very multipurpose. Remember it for drizzling on rice bowls, adding to wraps, or dipping into with falafel.

>> Balsamic vinaigrette is a nice choice for lighter greens like spinach. It also works as a marinade for vegetables, or you can toss it with noodles and veggies for a summery pasta salad.

>> Ranch dressing is my one true love and obsession. It performs best on romaine or green leaf lettuce, where it can be the star of the show. Drizzle it on Barbecue Jackfruit Nachos from Chapter 12. It's also an excellent dipping sauce for carrots, celery, cauliflower, and broccoli. (Yes, it's amazing for dipping french fries and vegan chick'n strips too!)

Roasted chickpeas add crispy texture and staying power when sprinkled on top of salads. I discovered them when I first went vegan, and I haven't stopped eating them ever since. I still make them multiple times a week. They're extremely versatile! In addition to topping salads, they offer a bump of protein when used as a topping on Basil Pesto Pasta (see Chapter 12). They can also be enjoyed by the handful, like a beany popcorn.

Speaking of popcorn, don't miss my cashew parmesan recipe at the end of this chapter. It's a tasty popcorn topping, as well as a mouthwatering finish for pasta with marinara or pizza by the slice. I recommend keeping a shaker full of it in the refrigerator at all times.

CREATING A SALAD YOU'LL CRAVE

I aim to eat at least one meal-sized salad every day. Salads are ideal for getting fiber, phytonutrients, folate, and immune-boosting vitamins into your diet. Here are my top tips for keeping salads exciting:

- **Variety:** Try a variety of greens for the base, like kale, romaine, green leaf lettuce, or spinach. Then add a smorgasbord of veggies for a rainbow of colors. Throw in a handful of cherry tomatoes, cucumbers, bell peppers, celery, broccoli, cauliflower, sugar snap peas, and radishes. Chop up the ingredients, so you get different tastes in every bite.

- **Bold flavors:** Incorporate bold, pungent flavors with olives, stuffed grape leaves, jarred artichoke hearts, sauerkraut, pepperoncini peppers, or vegan feta cheese.

- **Texture:** Salads are best when they have a mixture of chewy, creamy, and crunchy textures. For crunch, add nuts, seeds, croutons, or a side of crusty garlic bread.

- **Substance:** Turn your salad into a meal by including a hearty element that will really stick with you. Go for roasted chickpeas, beans, seitan, browned cubes of tofu, chopped vegan deli meat, or vegan chick'n strips.

- **Fat:** Adding some fat makes your salad more filling and satisfying. It also helps with the absorption of certain nutrients, like alpha- and beta-carotene, lycopene, lutein, and vitamins A, D, E, and K. Boost the healthy fat content with avocado or the afore-mentioned olives, nuts, or seeds. Finish with a creamy dressing or tart vinaigrette.

Sesame Sugar Snap Peas

PREP TIME: 10 MIN	COOK TIME: 8 MIN	YIELD: 4 SERVINGS

INGREDIENTS

1 pound (16 ounces) sugar snap peas

1¾ teaspoons tamari (or your preferred soy sauce) plus more to taste (see Note)

1¾ teaspoons rice vinegar

½ teaspoon toasted sesame oil

½ teaspoon maple syrup

1 teaspoon avocado oil (or your preferred neutral-flavored cooking oil)

3 cloves garlic, minced

Pinch of salt

2 teaspoons sesame seeds

DIRECTIONS

1 Rinse the sugar snap peas in a colander and dry. If necessary, remove the stems and strings. (See the tip for more information.)

2 In a small bowl, combine tamari, rice vinegar, toasted sesame oil, and maple syrup with a spoon. Set aside.

3 Put the oil in a large skillet over medium heat. Add the garlic and sauté for a couple minutes, until fragrant.

4 Add the sugar snap peas to the skillet. Use a spatula to fully incorporate them with the garlic. Sauté for about 3 minutes, until the sugar snap peas are warmed through.

5 Add the tamari and rice vinegar mixture to the skillet. Use a spatula to fully combine the mixture with the sugar snap peas, making sure everything gets coated. Cook another minute or two longer.

6 Add salt to taste, plus two or three more dashes of tamari, if desired.

7 Sprinkle with the sesame seeds before serving.

PER SERVING: *Calories 77 (From Fat 25); Fat 3g (Saturated 0g); Cholesterol 0mg; Sodium 153mg; Carbohydrate 9g (Dietary Fiber 3g); Protein 4g.*

TIP: To save time, I recommend buying sugar snap peas that are trimmed and stringless. If they're packaged in plastic bags, they're usually prepped. And on the bag it often says, "Ready to eat." Then you can just rinse them with water, and they're ready to use. If you bought the kind with stems and/or strings, snap off the stems and pull back to remove the strings before cooking.

NOTE: If you need this dish to be gluten-free, be sure to use gluten-free tamari. To reduce the amount of sodium, use reduced-sodium tamari.

Sautéed Kale with Garlic

PREP TIME: 5 MIN	COOK TIME: 10 MIN	YIELD: 4 SERVINGS

INGREDIENTS

½ teaspoon avocado oil (or your preferred neutral-flavored cooking oil)

2 cloves garlic, minced

1 bunch curly kale, removed from ribs and roughly chopped (see Note)

1 to 2 tablespoons water plus more, if needed

⅛ teaspoon Vegetarian Better Than Bouillon No Chicken Base (optional)

Pinch of salt

DIRECTIONS

1 Put oil in a skillet or pot over medium heat. Add the garlic and sauté until fragrant, about a minute or so.

2 Add the kale. If the bunch of kale is on the small side, add 1 tablespoon of water. If the bunch is larger, add 2 tablespoons of water.

3 Stir in the Vegetarian Better Than Bouillon No Chicken Base, if using. Then add the salt.

4 Continue cooking the kale, stirring occasionally, until it's wilted and soft. For bright green steamed kale, cook for 2 to 3 minutes. For softer kale that's deeper in color, turn the heat to low and cover with a lid. Cook for about 10 minutes, until all the liquid cooks off. (If the water cooks off before the kale is fully tender, add another splash.)

5 Taste for salt and add more, if needed, and then serve.

PER SERVING: *Calories 30 (From Fat 8); Fat 1g (Saturated 0g); Cholesterol 0mg; Sodium 60mg; Carbohydrate 5g (Dietary Fiber 1g); Protein 2g.*

VARY IT! Curly kale can be replaced with any type of kale, like lacinato or purple.

NOTE: Although kale stems can be eaten, I prefer this dish without them. While you're washing the kale, pull the leaves off the stems with your hands. Then chop the leaves.

Grilled Vegetable Skewers

PREP TIME: 10 MIN PLUS 30 MIN FOR MARINATING	COOK TIME: 10 MIN	YIELD: 4 SERVINGS

INGREDIENTS

2 tablespoons avocado oil (or your preferred neutral-flavored cooking oil) plus more if needed

2 teaspoons balsamic vinegar

1 clove garlic, finely grated or minced

½ teaspoon dried parsley

½ teaspoon dried basil

½ teaspoon dried oregano

Generous pinch of salt

Dash of freshly ground pepper

½ red bell pepper, cut in medium to large chunks

6 white button mushrooms

14 grape tomatoes

1 small zucchini, cut in ¾-inch pieces

DIRECTIONS

1 In a mixing bowl, use a fork or whisk to combine the oil, balsamic vinegar, garlic, dried parsley, dried basil, dried oregano, salt, and pepper.

2 Add the red bell peppers, white button mushrooms, grape tomatoes, and zucchini to the mixing bowl. Use your hands to make sure the vegetables get evenly coated on all sides with the marinade. (If it looks like there's not quite enough oil for the vegetables, add more to make sure all the spices are evenly dispersed.)

3 Put the bowl of vegetables into the refrigerator. Let them marinate for 30 minutes to an hour.

4 Once the vegetables have marinated, spear them onto metal skewers. Depending on the size of your skewers, you likely need three or four of them. (If you're using an indoor grill pan, make sure to use skewers that will fit on it.)

5 Bring an outdoor grill or indoor grill pan to a medium–high heat.

6 Put the vegetable skewers on the outdoor grill or indoor grill pan. Grill the skewers for 8 to 10 minutes, rotating a few times with tongs to evenly brown the veggies on all sides. When the skewers are done, remove them from the heat and serve.

PER SERVING: *Calories 90 (From Fat 66); Fat 7g (Saturated 1g); Cholesterol 0mg; Sodium 47mg; Carbohydrate 6g (Dietary Fiber 2g); Protein 2g.*

VARY IT! Make this recipe your own by varying the vegetables. Ultimately, you want 4 heaping cups of sturdy veggies. Try it with chunks of onions, sliced rounds of corn on the cob, steamed baby potatoes, pieces of eggplant, or chunks of yellow summer squash. Remember, some veggies take longer to cook than others.

NOTE: If you don't have skewers, this dish also works well in an outdoor grill basket. You likely need a couple of baskets, or plan to work in batches. Food grills best when it isn't overcrowded and has plenty of room to brown.

Mediterranean Couscous Salad

INGREDIENTS

1¼ cups water

Pinch of salt plus more to taste

1 cup pearl couscous (or Israeli couscous; see Note)

½ medium cucumber, sliced and quartered

½ cup cherry tomatoes, halved

1 scallion, thinly sliced

½ cup marinated artichoke hearts, drained from jar and chopped

¼ cup pitted kalamata olives, sliced

1 small clove garlic, finely grated or minced

¼ cup fresh basil, roughly chopped

1½ teaspoons balsamic vinegar

1½ teaspoons extra-virgin olive oil

Freshly ground pepper, to taste

DIRECTIONS

1   Bring salted water to a boil in a pot. Add the pearl couscous, cover, and lower the heat to a simmer for 8 to 10 minutes, stirring occasionally, until al dente. If there's any water left in the pot, drain with a fine-mesh sieve.

2   In a large mixing bowl, use a spoon to combine the cooked pearl couscous, cucumber, cherry tomatoes, scallion, marinated artichoke hearts, kalamata olives, garlic, basil, balsamic vinegar, and extra-virgin olive oil. Add salt and pepper to taste.

3   After the salad is fully combined, taste for seasonings. If you'd like, add more balsamic vinegar, extra-virgin olive oil, salt, and pepper. Serve right away, or cover and store in the refrigerator until serving time.

PER SERVING: *Calories 207 (From Fat 26); Fat 3g (Saturated 0g); Cholesterol 0mg; Sodium 164mg; Carbohydrate 38g (Dietary Fiber 4g); Protein 7g.*

TIP: If you're serving the salad cold from the refrigerator, taste and add another splash of balsamic vinegar, extra virgin olive oil, salt, and pepper, if necessary. The salad has a way of soaking up flavors. Give it a little refresh before serving.

NOTE: Pearl couscous is bigger than standard Moroccan couscous. The regular kind is small and grainy, while pearl couscous is pea-sized. Don't replace the pearl couscous with the standard variety for this recipe.

Pasta Salad with Creamy Dressing

PREP TIME: 15 MIN	COOK TIME: 10 MIN	YIELD: 10 SERVINGS

INGREDIENTS

16 ounces fusilli pasta (gluten-free, if necessary)

Pinch of salt plus more to taste

1 cup vegan mayonnaise

1 teaspoon apple cider vinegar

½ teaspoon lemon juice

2 tablespoons nondairy milk

1 teaspoon dried parsley

1 teaspoon dried basil

1 teaspoon granulated onion

2 cloves garlic, minced

Dash of freshly ground pepper

4 carrots, thinly sliced

4 Persian or mini cucumbers, thinly sliced (see Note)

16 radishes, thinly sliced

1 cup chopped bell peppers (red, yellow, or orange)

DIRECTIONS

1 In a pot, cook the pasta in salted boiling water according to the package directions. Once the pasta is al dente, drain and rinse with cold water. Set aside.

2 To make the dressing, combine the vegan mayonnaise, apple cider vinegar, lemon juice, nondairy milk, dried parsley, dried basil, granulated onion, garlic, a pinch of salt, and pepper in a bowl with a spoon.

3 Put the drained pasta into a large mixing bowl. Add the carrots, Persian cucumbers, radishes, and bell peppers.

4 Pour the dressing over the pasta and vegetables. Use a spoon to combine everything evenly. Taste for salt and add more if necessary. If you'd like a tangier pasta salad, add another splash of apple cider vinegar.

5 Eat right away, or for best results, move the pasta salad to a covered container and refrigerate for several hours. The vegetables will soften and flavors will meld over time.

PER SERVING: *Calories 319 (From Fat 138); Fat 15g (Saturated 3g); Cholesterol 0mg; Sodium 151mg; Carbohydrate 39g (Dietary Fiber 3g); Protein 7g.*

VARY IT! Any short pasta works for this recipe. Replace fusilli with your choice of penne, rotini, farfalle, or shell pasta. If you prefer, you can use fresh basil and parsley instead of dried. Replace 1 teaspoon of dried herbs with 1 tablespoon of freshly chopped herbs.

NOTE: Persian cucumbers are skinnier and shorter than the garden variety. (They're usually just 5 or 6 inches long.) If you're swapping them out for standard cucumbers, keep that in mind and use fewer.

Easy Tahini Dressing

PREP TIME: 3 MIN | COOK TIME: 0 MIN | YIELD: 4 SERVINGS

INGREDIENTS

3 tablespoons tahini

2 to 3 tablespoons water plus more as needed

2 to 3 teaspoons lemon juice

Pinch of salt

DIRECTIONS

1 In a small or medium-sized bowl, combine the tahini, 2 tablespoons of water, 2 teaspoons of lemon juice, and the salt with a spoon or whisk. At first the tahini will seize up and look very thick. That's normal.

2 Slowly stir in up to another tablespoon of water until the mixture has the consistency of a thick ranch dressing. (If necessary, add more water, a small splash at a time.)

3 Add more lemon juice or salt to taste. For a more lemony dressing, add another ½ to 1 teaspoon of lemon juice. If it needs more salt, add another pinch.

4 Store the dressing in a covered container in the refrigerator until ready to use.

PER SERVING: *Calories 68 (From Fat 54); Fat 6g (Saturated 1g); Cholesterol 0mg; Sodium 32mg; Carbohydrate 3g (Dietary Fiber 1g); Protein 2g.*

TIP: This simple dressing is great on salads, bowls, wraps, or falafel.

VARY IT! If you'd like, add a squeeze of maple syrup for sweetness, minced garlic for bite, and a few drops of toasted sesame oil for nuttiness.

NOTE: The consistency of tahini varies both by brand and by how well you stirred it when you first opened the jar. Depending on these factors, the amount of water you need in the dressing will vary slightly.

TIP: The dressing will thicken as it cools in the refrigerator. When you're ready to use it, add another splash of water or lemon juice, and stir until the texture and consistency is just right. Add another pinch of salt, if needed.

Balsamic Vinaigrette

PREP TIME: 3 MIN	COOK TIME: 0 MIN	YIELD: 6 SERVINGS

INGREDIENTS

¼ cup extra-virgin olive oil

2 tablespoons balsamic vinegar

¼ teaspoon stone-ground mustard

½ teaspoon maple syrup

Pinch of salt

DIRECTIONS

1 Put the extra-virgin olive oil, balsamic vinegar, stone-ground mustard, maple syrup, and salt into a small bowl. Combine with a fork or whisk until it's thick and emulsified.

2 Serve right away, or store for later use in a covered container. If the oil separates from the vinegar, just give it a good shake or whisk.

PER SERVING: *Calories 86 (From Fat 81); Fat 9g (Saturated 1g); Cholesterol 0mg; Sodium 17mg; Carbohydrate 1g (Dietary Fiber 0g); Protein 0g.*

VARY IT! This dressing is easy to adjust to suit your preferences. If you want more tartness, add more vinegar. If you want a more muted flavor, add more oil. If you like more tang, increase the mustard. If you prefer a sweeter dressing, increase the maple syrup.

Vegan Ranch Dressing

PREP TIME: 5 MIN	COOK TIME: 0 MIN	YIELD: 6 SERVINGS

INGREDIENTS

¾ cup Vegenaise or your preferred vegan mayonnaise

½ teaspoon apple cider vinegar

½ teaspoon lemon juice

4 teaspoons nondairy milk

½ teaspoon dried parsley

½ teaspoon dried basil

½ teaspoon dried dill

1 teaspoon granulated onion

½ teaspoon granulated garlic

1 clove garlic, finely grated or minced

Generous pinch of salt

DIRECTIONS

1 In a medium-sized bowl, combine all the ingredients with a spoon.

2 Check the dressing to see if it's the thickness you prefer. Some mayonnaise brands are thicker than others, and that will affect the thickness of the dressing. If you like your dressing thinner and more pourable, add another splash of nondairy milk, and stir it in completely. If you like your dressing thicker, add another spoonful of vegan mayonnaise, and stir it in completely.

3 Taste for salt and add more if needed. Store in a covered container in the refrigerator until ready for use.

PER SERVING: Calories 163 (From Fat 163); Fat 18g (Saturated 3g); Cholesterol 0mg; Sodium 169mg; Carbohydrate 0g (Dietary Fiber 0g); Protein 0g.

TIP: I recommend using a Microplane zester to finely grate the fresh garlic into a paste. If you don't have one, mincing works.

NOTE: The dressing will thicken in the refrigerator. If it gets too thick, add another splash of nondairy milk and stir or shake.

Roasted Chickpeas

INGREDIENTS

1 (15-ounce) can chickpeas

1 teaspoon avocado oil (or your preferred neutral-flavored cooking oil)

2 teaspoons nutritional yeast flakes

½ teaspoon granulated onion

Pinch of salt

DIRECTIONS

1 Preheat the oven to 400 degrees. Line a baking sheet with parchment paper. Drain and rinse the chickpeas. Then completely dry them on a clean kitchen towel. (Wet chickpeas won't brown as nicely.)

2 Put the chickpeas on the lined baking sheet. Drizzle them with the oil. Use your hands or a spoon to toss the chickpeas, making sure they're evenly coated.

3 Sprinkle the nutritional yeast flakes, granulated onion, and salt over the chickpeas. Then combine with a spoon, making sure the chickpeas are evenly coated, and spread them across the baking sheet.

4 Put the chickpeas in the oven and roast for 20 minutes, stopping once or twice to shake the pan for even browning. If you like them browner and crispier, continue cooking for 5 minutes, or until they reach your desired level of crispiness. Remove from the oven and serve.

PER SERVING: *Calories 131 (From Fat 29); Fat 3g (Saturated 0g); Cholesterol 0mg; Sodium 220mg; Carbohydrate 20g (Dietary Fiber 6g); Protein 6g.*

VARY IT! Vary the seasonings: Add ⅛ to ¼ teaspoon of granulated garlic, dried parsley, dried dill, dried oregano, cumin, smoked paprika, or curry powder.

TIP: Roasted chickpeas are great eaten by the handful as a snack, used as a salad topping, or added to a bowl of pesto pasta.

AIR FRYER INSTRUCTIONS

Prefer to use the air fryer? Put the drained chickpeas into the air fryer basket. (No need to dry them on a kitchen towel, because the hot blowing air in the air fryer will take care of that.) Cook the plain chickpeas at 400 degrees for 5 minutes. Then move them to a mixing bowl. Add the oil and combine with a spoon. Then sprinkle on the nutritional yeast flakes, granulated onion, and salt and combine with the spoon. Return the seasoned chickpeas to the air fryer basket. Cook at 400 degrees for 7 minutes, or until your desired level of crispiness.

Cashew Parmesan

PREP TIME: 5 MIN	COOK TIME: 0 MIN	YIELD: 12 SERVINGS

INGREDIENTS

½ cup raw cashews

¼ cup nutritional yeast flakes

¼ teaspoon dried basil

¼ teaspoon dried oregano

¼ teaspoon granulated onion

¼ teaspoon granulated garlic

½ teaspoon salt

DIRECTIONS

1 Put all the ingredients into the food processor. Process on High for about 20 seconds, or until the cashews have broken down into fine pieces. Don't over blend. You want it to be the texture of Parmesan cheese, not cashew butter.

2 Move the cashew parmesan into a covered jar or shaker. Store in the refrigerator (or freezer for longer storage). Cashew parmesan will keep in a covered container in the refrigerator for several weeks. In the freezer, it will last up to 3 months.

PER SERVING: *Calories 38 (From Fat 22); Fat 2g (Saturated 0g); Cholesterol 0mg; Sodium 101mg; Carbohydrate 3g (Dietary Fiber 1g); Protein 2g.*

VARY IT! If you like, replace the raw cashews in all or in part with hemp hearts, walnuts, almonds, pine nuts, sunflower seeds, or *pepitas* (shelled pumpkin seeds). The dried basil, dried oregano, granulated onion, and granulated garlic can be replaced with ¾ teaspoon of your favorite Italian spice blend. I don't recommend making this recipe without the nutritional yeast flakes. It's the dominant flavor and main source of cheesiness.

TIP: Use cashew parmesan on pasta with marinara, on top of pizza, in pesto for added cheesiness, or as a topping for roasted vegetables or popcorn.

Chapter **15**

Desserts

Here's the scoop on vegan desserts — they're amazing! Entire cookbooks are devoted to decadent vegan treats, so this chapter offers just a sampling of what's possible. You find easy warm-weather delights, childhood favorites, and simple recipes that get dessert on the table ASAP.

Included in this chapter is my mom's recipe for Wacky Cake, the cake I grew up eating at birthday parties and special events. Although we didn't have a vegan household, the cake recipe my mom turned to again and again just happened to be plant-based!

According to its origin story, Wacky Cake was invented during the Great Depression, when dairy milk, butter, and eggs were expensive or hard to come by. Endless variations of the recipe have been passed down, but I'm partial to the one in my mom's handwriting.

This pantry-friendly cake is economical and delicious! Finish it with a sprinkling of powdered sugar, or go all out with a layer of chocolate frosting. (I've tweaked the cake ingredients slightly to use avocado oil, which is my current go-to oil. And for the chocolate frosting adorning the cake, these days my mom uses vegan butter and nondairy milk instead of dairy whenever she makes it for me.)

Outside of the recipes here, I encourage you to try your hand at veganizing your favorite traditional dessert recipes like my mom does with her chocolate frosting. It usually isn't hard to do. It just requires a few simple swaps.

» Swap out eggs for applesauce, ground flaxseed and water, banana, or store-bought vegan egg replacer.

» Replace dairy butter with an equal amount of vegan butter.

» Ditch dairy milk for cashew, almond, oat, or soy milk.

» Trade out standard marshmallows (made with gelatin) for vegan marshmallows.

See Chapter 9 for information about plant-based substitutions that will keep beloved family recipes on your vegan table.

Chocolate Banana Nice Cream

INGREDIENTS

¼ to ½ cup cashew milk (or your preferred nondairy milk)

2 tablespoons cocoa powder

3 ripe bananas, peeled and frozen in chunks (see Note)

DIRECTIONS

1 Blend ¼ cup nondairy milk, cocoa powder, and frozen bananas in a blender until smooth but still thick. (If you have a Vitamix, use your tamper to help push the bananas down.) If the nice cream isn't blending well enough, add up to another ¼ cup of nondairy milk. Remember not to add too much. You want the mixture to blend, but not become thin like a smoothie.

2 Serve the nice cream in two bowls.

PER SERVING: *Calories 174 (From Fat 15); Fat 2g (Saturated 1g); Cholesterol 0mg; Sodium 3mg; Carbohydrate 44g (Dietary Fiber 7g); Protein 3g.*

TIP: Garnish your nice cream with a grated chocolate chip or maraschino cherries. You can find nondairy semi-sweet or dark chocolate chips in most grocery stores. Just read the ingredients label.

NOTE: It's essential that the bananas are frozen for this recipe. That's what makes this dessert so creamy. Peel ripe bananas, break them into chunks, and then freeze the chunks in a freezer bag until you're ready to use them.

Strawberry Crispy Rice Treats

PREP TIME: 5 MIN	COOK TIME: 3 MIN	YIELD: 12 SERVINGS

INGREDIENTS

½ teaspoon avocado oil (or other neutral-flavored oil) plus more if needed

1 (1- or 1.2-ounce) package freeze-dried strawberries

1 (10-ounce) package vegan marshmallows (see Note)

3 tablespoons nondairy butter

5 cups crisp rice cereal

DIRECTIONS

1 Lightly grease an 8- or 9-inch square baking dish with the oil. Set aside. (If you'd rather, you can line the dish with parchment paper.)

2 In a food processor, grind the freeze-dried strawberries for about 20 seconds on Low, or until they are mostly powder. (A few chunks are fine.) If you don't have a food processor, use a clean coffee grinder, crumble the dried strawberries with your hands, or leave them whole.

3 Cut or tear the marshmallows into quarters using kitchen shears or your fingers.

4 Put the nondairy butter and quartered marshmallows in a large glass mixing bowl. Microwave for 80 seconds, stopping every 30 seconds to stir for even melting. Microwaves vary from one to the next. You know the marshmallows are ready when they soften, lose most of their shape, and look somewhat wet.

5 Stir in the rice cereal and the strawberry powder with a spoon or rubber spatula until completely coated.

6 Pour the marshmallow and cereal mixture into the oiled dish and press it evenly across the dish. Allow the treats to cool completely for easiest cutting.

7 Cut into squares and serve.

PER SERVING: *Calories 229 (From Fat 26); Fat 3g (Saturated 2g); Cholesterol 0mg; Sodium 124mg; Carbohydrate 50g (Dietary Fiber 0g); Protein 1g.*

VARY IT! You can vary the type of freeze-dried fruit with dried raspberries or dried blueberries. If you prefer plain treats, omit the freeze-dried strawberries; the rest of the recipe stays the same. If you like, add other mix-ins like chocolate pieces, pretzels, or crushed sandwich cookies. If you'd prefer to skip the marshmallow-cutting step, full-sized marshmallows can be replaced with an equal amount of mini vegan marshmallows.

NOTE: Standard marshmallows contain gelatin, which is made from animal skin, bones, and ligaments. Instead, I recommend Dandies or Trader Joe's vegan marshmallows. For the cereal, choose one that isn't fortified with vitamin D3, which usually isn't vegan because it's derived from sheep's wool. I recommend Trader Joe's or Nature's Path rice cereal.

STOVETOP DIRECTIONS

Prefer to make crispy rice treats on the stovetop instead of the microwave? Follow Steps 1 through 3. Then add the nondairy butter to a large pot over low heat. Once the butter has melted, add the quartered marshmallows. Stir until the marshmallows become warm and soft. Remove from the heat, and stir the rice cereal and strawberry powder into the pot. Evenly incorporate with a spoon or rubber spatula. Continue with Step 6.

Puffy Banana Bread Cookies

INGREDIENTS

1 cup all-purpose flour

½ teaspoon baking soda

1 teaspoon baking powder

½ medium-sized ripe banana

2 tablespoons agave syrup or maple syrup

3 tablespoons applesauce

1 teaspoon vanilla extract

2 tablespoons avocado oil

¼ cup vegan semi-sweet or dark chocolate chips (see Note)

DIRECTIONS

1 Preheat the oven to 350 degrees. Line two baking sheets with parchment paper and set aside.

2 In a large mixing bowl, combine the all-purpose flour, baking soda, and baking powder with a fork.

3 In a separate bowl, smash the banana with a fork until mostly smooth. Add the agave syrup, applesauce, vanilla extract, and avocado oil. Combine with a spoon.

4 Add the wet ingredients to the dry ingredients. Gently mix together until the mixture becomes a dough. (If necessary, use your hands.) Be careful not to overwork it. Add the chocolate chips and combine with a spoon.

5 Use a tablespoon to scoop the dough onto the lined baking sheets. Lightly press on each cookie to flatten it slightly. (If your fingers stick to the dough, lightly moisten your hands with water or oil.)

6 Bake for 10 minutes until puffy. Remove the baking sheets from the oven, and use a spatula to carefully transfer the cookies onto a cooling rack. You can enjoy the cookies warm, or allow them to cool 10 minutes before serving.

PER SERVING: *Calories 92 (From Fat 34); Fat 4g (Saturated 1g); Cholesterol 0mg; Sodium 87mg; Carbohydrate 13g (Dietary Fiber 0g); Protein 1g.*

TIP: The applesauce can be replaced with a flax egg. Whisk 3 tablespoons of water with 1 tablespoon of ground flaxseed. Let the mixture sit for 5 minutes until it becomes thick and gooey. Then add it to the wet ingredients.

NOTE: Vegan semi-sweet or dark chocolate chips are easy to find. Just read the ingredients labels. I usually buy them from Trader Joe's.

Wacky Cake with Chocolate Frosting

| PREP TIME: 15 MIN | COOK TIME: 35 MIN | YIELD: 12 TO 15 SERVINGS |

INGREDIENTS

3 cups all-purpose flour

2 cups organic cane sugar

¼ cup cocoa powder

2 teaspoons baking soda

1 teaspoon salt

2 cups water

⅔ cup avocado oil (or your preferred neutral-flavored cooking oil)

2 tablespoons white vinegar

2 teaspoons vanilla extract

Chocolate Frosting (see the following recipe)

DIRECTIONS

1 Preheat the oven to 375 degrees.

2 In a large mixing bowl, use a spoon to combine the all-purpose flour, cane sugar, the cocoa powder, baking soda, and salt.

3 Add the water, oil, white vinegar, and vanilla extract. Combine with a spoon until you don't see any dry flour.

4 Pour the batter into an ungreased 9-x-13-inch metal or glass baking dish.

5 Bake 30 to 35 minutes. Test at 30 minutes to see if the cake is done by sticking a toothpick into it. If the toothpick comes out clean, the cake is done. If not, bake the remaining 5 minutes.

6 Remove from the oven. Allow the cake to cool completely (at least an hour) before frosting.

7 Once the cake has cooled, spread frosting evenly over the top. Cut into squares to serve.

Chocolate Frosting

½ cup (1 stick) nondairy butter

¼ teaspoon vanilla extract

1 (16-ounce) bag organic powdered sugar

¼ cup nondairy milk plus more if needed

½ cup cocoa powder plus more if desired

1 In a large mixing bowl, use a beater on a medium setting to beat the nondairy butter and the vanilla until light and fluffy, about 3 minutes.

(continued)

2 Turn the beater to Low, and slowly add the powdered sugar. The mixture will become very thick. (If it gets too thick, move the beater back up to medium speed, if necessary.) Slowly add the nondairy milk. If you like fluffier frosting, add a few drops of milk at a time until it's the consistency you want.

3 Beat in the cocoa powder. If you like a darker chocolate flavor/color, sprinkle in a little more cocoa powder and beat (or use a spoon to stir) until it's incorporated.

PER SERVING: *Calories 455 (From Fat 142); Fat 16g (Saturated 6g); Cholesterol 0mg; Sodium 360mg; Carbohydrate 78g (Dietary Fiber 2g); Protein 3g.*

VARY IT! For plain buttercream frosting, omit the cocoa powder. If you prefer, leave off the frosting and sprinkle the cake with powdered sugar to finish.

5

Vegan in the Outside World

Understand the many ethical reasons behind going vegan.

Determine what you need to avoid when buying clothes, cosmetics, and home goods.

Find and order plant-based meals at restaurants.

Enjoy an amazing road trip, hotel stay, plane ride, or campout while staying true to your vegan values.

Make the best of sticky social situations and maneuver expertly through uncomfortable interactions.

IN THIS CHAPTER

» Looking at what happens to animals in factory farms

» Exploring the fishing industry

» Understanding the impact of honeybees on the environment

» Knowing about animals in captivity

» Weighing the environmental impact of animal products

Chapter **16**

The Ethics Behind Veganism

Many of us think of ourselves as animal lovers. We spend our lives with cats and dogs. We cuddle them on the couch. We take them on walks. We even buy them gifts at the holidays.

A study in *Science* (2015) found that when humans and dogs looked into each other's eyes, both had increased levels of oxytocin, the same hormone that's released when a parent looks at their newborn child.

Humans and companion animals develop deep and meaningful bonds. When cats and dogs pass, we mourn their absence. It feels like part of our home and our heart is missing. In fact, many people say they mourn harder and longer for their cats and dogs than for other humans.

But with other animals, we find ways to compartmentalize them. We may enjoy petting goats, seeing cows in a field, or feeding ducks at a pond. But most of us try not to think too hard about the step in between pasture and plate. We find ways to rationalize it away. We teach children to be kind and gentle with animals, but we also teach them animals are here to serve us.

In this chapter, I cover some of the many ways that animals like cows, pigs, chickens, and turkeys are used in animal agriculture. I offer information about the fishing industry and clarify why honey isn't vegan. Finally, I give a glimpse of the many environmental concerns with modern day farming.

Considering Our Two- and Four-Legged Friends

People are eating meat in larger amounts than ever before in human history. In the U.S., meat consumption has doubled in the last century. An estimated 92.2 billion land animals are killed every year for meat, according to the Food and Agriculture Organization of the United Nations (FAO). When you include sea creatures, it's trillions more.

The numbers are staggering, and almost impossible to wrap your head around. To understand the magnitude, we can look at the lives of some of the animals most commonly used in animal agriculture: cows, pigs, chickens, and turkeys. Keep in mind, this only scratches the surface of the types and ways that animals are used.

TIP

If you're looking for a good place to begin on your vegan journey, I can't think of a better place to start than dairy.

Cows

In the town where I grew up, the local dairy features a statue of a mama cow and her calf by their production facilities. I passed by it every day on my way to school. It seemed kind of sweet — a mama and her baby.

What I didn't realize is that I was being marketed to. I was being sold an image of innocence and Americana, and I wasn't alone.

Dairy cows and veal

Most of us are taught from a young age that consuming dairy is essential for strong bones. Not only that, we're given the impression that dairy farming is quaint and wholesome. Like the statues on display at my hometown's dairy, we imagine a mama cow out in a field with her offspring. The idea seems very picturesque.

Seems is the operative word here. Roughly 9 million cows are used for dairy in the U.S., according to the Humane Society of the United States. And dairy cows spend most or all of their lives indoors or in dirt feedlots. (The cows you see in fields are usually beef cattle.)

Like all mammals, cows produce milk only as a result of being pregnant. After they're impregnated by artificial insemination, they're pregnant about the same length of time as humans — roughly 9 months.

After they've given birth, their offspring are taken from them so that humans can have their milk instead. Calves are generally separated from their mothers within their first 24 hours of life. Some mama cows bellow for their calf for days, and have been known to chase after the trailer carrying their baby away.

REMEMBER

Many people say about dairy cows, "But you have to milk them! Otherwise, they're in pain." But think about that. Why would cows need humans to milk them? In nature, wouldn't someone else be doing the milking? Yes. Their calf. Of course, their calf. But their calf has been taken from them.

Milking cows isn't a kindness. It's a commodity.

If the calf is a girl, she becomes a dairy cow like her mother. If the calf is a boy, either he is used for veal and spends his short life in a tiny crate, stall, or hutch; or he lives a little longer and is used for meat as beef.

According to the U.S. Department of Agriculture, "Male dairy calves are used in the veal industry. Dairy cows must give birth to continue producing milk, but male dairy calves are of little or no value to the dairy farmer."

REMEMBER

The dairy industry is the main source of veal calves. The industries are two sides of the same coin. When you support one, you support the other.

Veal calves are kept in small spaces and often fed an inadequate diet so that their meat is tender. But it means in their short lives, they are trapped with nothing that qualifies as a quality existence. Some veal calves live just hours or days; others live 4 to 6 months.

Like humans, cows don't keep producing milk forever. Cows are repeatedly impregnated and give birth so that they produce milk again and again. Cows can live as long as 20 years. However, once a dairy cow has had a few pregnancies, she's considered "spent." Milk production declines with age. It's less profitable to keep spending money on a cow's feed when her output slows. So she's sent to the same slaughterhouse as the beef cows, usually at around 4 or 5 years old.

According to a 2021 article published in the *Journal of Animal Science,* "More than 3 million head of dairy cows enter the food supply chain in the U.S. every year." The authors note that, "Meat production from dairy cows is a significant component of beef production, accounting for almost 10 percent of U.S. commercial beef production."

Is drinking cow's milk necessary? Humans are the only animal that drinks the milk of another species. We're also the only animal that continues to drink milk past the age of weaning. Once other animals can eat solids, they move on from breast milk. And even humans don't keep drinking human breast milk into adulthood.

Instead of drinking milk that was meant for a calf, we can get calcium from plants. Turn to Chapter 6 to get more information about vegan sources of calcium.

Beef cattle

Cattle raised for beef stay with their mothers for a longer time than veal calves. They are allowed to be together for 6 to 8 months until the calves are weaned and they're separated. Like with veal calves, after separation the mother cows and their offspring have been known to call out to each other for days.

Cattle used for beef have their own painful experiences. Many are branded with a hot iron, causing third-degree burns. Their horns are removed by gouging or burning, and they are *castrated* (their testicles are removed). These procedures are all done without painkillers or anesthetic.

These gentle, social animals are raised on feedlots, where they're fed grain and corn to quicken their weight gain. Because this isn't a natural diet for them, it can cause stomach pains. They are given regular doses of drugs like antibiotics, which can contribute to the spread of drug-resistant bacteria. Cattle are also given hormones to accelerate their growth. Most are slaughtered once they've lived about a year and a half.

Pigs

In the state where I live, pigs outnumber humans by more than seven to one. That comes out to 23 million pigs in just one state. Driving across endless farmland, though, you'd never know it. You can go for miles and miles and never see a pig. The only time many people encounter pigs is at a fair or when passing them in large semitrucks as the pigs are on their way to slaughter. So where are all these pigs?

On modern farms, pigs spend their entire lives confined to warehouses, standing on concrete. Pigs are known to be intelligent — smarter than dogs or even 3-year-old children. In nature, they love taking mud baths, sunbathing, forming family bonds, and foraging for food by rooting with their snouts. However, in factory farms, their lives are spent without anything that's natural or important to them.

Mother pigs are impregnated through artificial insemination. They spend their lives in gestation crates, giving birth to litters of up to 12 piglets at a time.

In nature, mother pigs nurture their piglets by building them a nest, and taking care of them until they're 10 to 17 weeks old. However, in factory farms, their time together is surrounded by metal, in spaces so small the mother can barely turn around.

Piglets are separated from their mothers after about 3 weeks. Their mother continues being impregnated and giving birth to more litters until her body wears out, and she is slaughtered.

Standard industry procedures for pigs include chopping off their tails, snapping off teeth, and for males, castration, all without anesthetic or any painkillers. Although, pigs can live as long as 15 to 20 years, most pigs are slaughtered after 5½ to 6 months.

At the end of their lives, pigs are forced onto transport trucks. In the sweltering heat of summer and bitter cold of winter, they go past on highways with their snouts sticking out of open holes. Some die before they get to the slaughterhouse. Industry reports show that more than a million pigs die in transport every year. Tens of thousands more are injured before they arrive at the slaughterhouse.

Chickens

Chickens are used in two main ways in animal agriculture: They are killed for meat or used for their eggs. (Egg-laying hens are eventually killed for food too.)

According to the Humane Society of the United States (HSUS), more than 9 billion chickens are killed for their meat every year in the U.S. The USDA National Agricultural Statistics Service reported that 372 million chickens were used for eggs in 2022.

In nature, these birds are known to be social. They enjoy having dust baths, roosting in trees, building nests, and scratching for food. However, that's not the life they live in factory farming. Most chickens spend their entire life in total confinement, without any protection from humane treatment laws. (All farmed birds are exempt from the Humane Methods of Slaughter Act as well. See the sidebar for more information about the act and what it covers.)

Egg-laying hens

Hens lay eggs as a regular part of their monthly reproductive cycle, similar to a human's menstrual cycle. If the egg has been fertilized, it will form an embryo inside. Unfertilized eggs are the ones you see in the grocery store.

THE HUMANE METHODS OF SLAUGHTER ACT

The Humane Methods of Slaughter Act (HMSA) was originally passed in 1958. The purpose of the act was to require a quick and effective death to animals at slaughterhouses. HMSA covers all land animals raised for food, except poultry like chickens, turkeys, and ducks.

Although it's difficult to rationalize how the words "humane" and "slaughter" go together, this is how the USDA National Agricultural Library defines it: "In the case of cattle, calves, horses, mules, sheep, swine, and other livestock, all animals are rendered insensible to pain by a single blow or gunshot or an electrical, chemical or other means that is rapid and effective, before being shackled, hoisted, thrown cast, or cut."

Other regulations include that electric prods should be "used as little as possible to minimize excitement or injury," and that electric prods should be "reduced by a transformer to the lowest effective voltage not to exceed 50 volts AC."

While farmed birds aren't included in the Humane Methods of Slaughter Act, they are covered by the Poultry Products of Inspection Act of 1957 (PPIA). However, PPIA mostly focuses on making sure poultry isn't misbranded, and that the slaughter conditions are sanitary. The welfare of the birds isn't the main priority. PPIA does note that birds must be dead before scalding, and that if birds are injured, it disqualifies them from being sold.

According to a 2017 article about PPIA on the Modern Farming website, "The actual enforceable laws are incredibly limited, and while the USDA does have guidelines that go into more depth, the poultry industry is not legally compelled to follow them."

Egg-laying chickens come from hatcheries. In these hatcheries, male chicks are useless because laying chickens are bred to be smaller than chickens used for meat. Obviously, male chicks don't lay eggs. So that means male chicks are killed at birth by being *macerated* (ground in a machine) or thrown into dumpsters, still alive, and then suffocated and crushed by other chicks on top of them.

According to a 2021 article on Vox.com, 300 million chicks are killed this way every year. Globally that number reaches up to 7 billion, according to a 2018 article in the journal *Poultry Science*.

In a 2021 press release, the United Egg Producers (UEP) provided an update about ending this practice. It said, "In 2016, UEP's Board called for the elimination in the laying industry of day-old male chick culling after hatch. Since that time our members have supported and strongly advocated for the research of methods and the adoption of new technologies to end male chick culling at hatcheries — this is a priority and is the right thing to do."

Although "chick culling" has been banned in a handful of countries, as of 2023, it's still legal and standard practice in the United States.

As for the females, most egg-laying chickens spend their lives in cages stacked on top of each other with little to no access to the outdoors. The chickens are packed in spaces so small that they can't spread a wing. In nature, hens produce about 12 to 20 eggs a year. However, in factory farms, chickens are bred to lay 250 to 300 eggs per year. As a result, laying chickens lose a tremendous amount of nutrients and calcium, often developing weak bones.

This environment is understandably stressful for the birds. To keep the birds from pecking each other, they are *debeaked* (their beaks are cut off with a scissor-like machine or a hot blade). Because the beak is a highly sensitive part of the animal, debeaking is similar to cutting off the end of your finger. Plus, it affects how well the birds can drink and eat, since they typically eat by pecking.

After about two years, the chickens are weak, sick, and/or not producing eggs so they're slaughtered. According to a 2019 article on The Poultry Site, most egg laying hens are killed and rendered into protein meal for feed or turned into pet food. The article notes, "Hens that are at the end of their laying life are considered a by-product of the egg industry, unlike broilers that are reared for meat and are a valuable food product." For laying chickens that are used in human food products, they are usually used in soups, stock, or stews. The article continues, "Other birds are simply composted or just buried after being euthanized because of their low market value."

REMEMBER

Some people opt for cage-free or free-range eggs, assuming this means a better life for the chickens. More than anything, these are marketing terms. They can mean as little as there's a window or door in the shed where the animals live. These terms are not legal definitions, and therefore are not regulated or enforced.

Plus, cage-free and free-range chickens are still killed when their egg production declines. Most of the time, they go to the same slaughterhouses as factory-farmed chickens. These marketing terms give the buyer a false sense of complacency about eating animals. They remove some guilt, but do very little for the chickens.

To find plant-based alternatives to eggs, check out Chapter 9.

Broiler chickens

Chickens raised for meat are known as *broilers*. They spend their lives in sheds with concrete floors. They are bred to grow as big as possible, as quickly as possible. When they are 6 to 7 weeks old, they're slaughtered.

REMEMBER

What about organic chicken? When people buy organic chicken, what they may not realize is that *organic* doesn't mean an improved life for the chickens. It only refers to the feed the animals consumed. It means no pesticides were used on that feed.

Turkeys

If you ever get a chance to spend time with turkeys at a sanctuary, you'll realize they are a joy. They love to be petted, and if you find the right spot, they will trill or purr. In nature, they can fly short distances, run, and live up to 10 years.

On factory farms, however, turkeys are killed when they're just 3 to 5 months old. The birds live their short lives in sheds with thousands of others. They know nothing of the natural world of grass, sun, or fresh air. To be profitable, they are bred to grow as big as possible in the least amount of time. Each bird gets about 3½ square feet of space.

All turkeys raised on factory farms are created by artificial insemination. Turkeys have been bred to grow larger and faster than they would in the wild, and that excessive size prevents them from reproducing naturally. They grow up to 35 pounds in their short lives. In fact, farmed turkeys are twice as heavy as they were 60 years ago, and they gain that weight in half the time.

Because they're crowded in sheds and unable to display any of their natural behaviors, turkeys can act out. To minimize the damage the birds can do, it's standard procedure to cut off parts of their beaks, toes, and snoods on the males. (The *snood* is the flap of skin under the chin.) This is done without any pain relief or anesthesia.

According to the USDA, 219 million turkeys were raised for food in 2023. Turkeys are not protected under most states' anti-cruelty laws and are exempt from the federal Humane Methods of Slaughter Act. When you consider Thanksgiving and Christmas alone, about 68 million turkeys are killed for holiday dinners, according to a 2018 article on Food Business News.

CONSIDERING LOCAL FARMS

In Chapter 9, I note that people sometimes use the place they're from as an excuse not to go vegan. They might say things like, "I'm from Philly — I can't live without cheesesteaks." Or "I was raised in the Midwest — I have to eat pork."

And yet, when people hear about terrible things that happen to animals in agriculture, they sometimes make themselves feel better by saying, "Oh, but that doesn't happen here."

It's interesting how they simultaneously excuse themselves from going vegan because meat eating is so ingrained where they live. And yet, they also think that where they live is one place where bad things don't happen to animals.

Unfortunately, factory farms are all over the place. A status report for 2022 from the United States Environmental Protection Agency (EPA) showed that there are only four states in the U.S. without *CAFO*s (concentrated animal feeding operations — another word for factory farm). Iowa had the most CAFOs with 4,203.

According to a 2019 article by the Sentience Institute, 99 percent of farmed animals in the U.S. are living on factory farms. So that means your local farm may also be a factory farm, and that factory farmed meat is what's most prevalent by far.

You may be asking yourself, "But what about that 1 percent of farms that are small?" Regardless of farm size, many of the ways animals are treated are industry standards. Castration and/or dehorning without anesthetic, branding, ear notching, tail chopping, and killing piglets because they are "runts" and won't meet the desired weight by slaughter date, can all be done on small farms too. No matter the farm size, dairies separate mother cows from their babies, and sell the cows' male offspring for veal or beef. Small farms often get their egg-laying chickens from hatcheries, where the male chicks are killed in mass. And when dairy cows and egg laying chickens have outlived their usefulness on small farms, they aren't sent to a lovely retirement community.

Some people who want to eat meat but also care how animals are treated choose meat that's marketed as "humane" or "ethically raised." But these terms aren't legally defined by the USDA or FDA. These marketing terms may make buyers feel better, but they don't guarantee anything about the ways the animals are treated.

Finally, farms are for-profit businesses. People in the business of selling meat can't do that without killing animals. So when the time comes, the animals raised on small farms usually go to the same slaughterhouses as animals raised on factory farms. And there's no way to kindly kill a healthy, young animal who wants to live.

While it can be comforting to think that sad things don't happen to animals where you live, I encourage you to ask yourself why you think that (if you do), and spend some time examining if that's true or wishful thinking.

Contemplating Sea Creatures

More than any other animal, fish are killed for food in the highest numbers. According to a 2017 article on Forbes.com, it's estimated that up to 2.7 trillion fish are caught and killed in the wild each year worldwide, and that number doesn't include the billions of farmed fish.

About half of the fish killed for food are raised on aquafarms. These aquafarms can be housed on land in raised pools, ponds, or concrete tanks. Or they can be alongside the ocean, adjacent to the shoreline. The fish that are most commonly farmed are tilapia, trout, bass, and salmon.

In the wild, salmon prefer a solitary life. They can travel more than a thousand miles in their lifetime in order to spawn and feed. However, on aquafarms, they spend their lives in overcrowded tanks, where they are susceptible to *necrotic* (flesh-killing) diseases.

Fish that are caught in the wild meet their death on the surface of boats, where they suffocate or die crushed underneath the animals above them. Their gills are severed while they are still alive, and their subsequent death can take as long as 40 minutes.

REMEMBER

People sometimes discount the pain that fish feel, because they seem so dissimilar to humans. However, many studies have shown that fish feel pain. Plus, there are no welfare laws to protect fish.

In addition to fish, many more animals are killed collectively as *bycatch* (when unwanted marine life is caught and discarded during commercial fishing). Animals like seals, birds, whales, dolphins, sea turtles, and sharks die when they are caught in fishing nets or dragged on lines. When the bycatch is thrown back into the water, the animals are often dying or already dead. *Trawling* (fishing with a net) also destroys seabeds and corals, which are home to millions of marine animals and support a healthy ocean.

Looking Out for Bees

Of all the animal products out there, people are most confused about the vegan status of honey. But there should be no doubt about it: Honey — and other bee products like beeswax — is made by bees for bees. Since vegans don't eat or use animal products, that means honey isn't vegan.

In a honeybee's lifetime, they produce $\frac{1}{12}$ teaspoon of honey. They use it for their food and nutrients, and store it for cold months when they can't leave the hive or flowers aren't in bloom. It also keeps the colony in balance.

Here's a look at how honey is made:

1. Honeybees visit flowers, and collect nectar by sucking it out with their *proboscises* (or tongues).

2. They ingest the nectar and store it in a second stomach, where enzymes start breaking it down into simple sugars. After they've filled that stomach, they return to the hive.

3. Back at the hive, they *regurgitate* (bring swallowed food back up to the mouth) the honey into the mouths of other bees. Those bees chew on the nectar for about half an hour before passing it to other bees. After the honey is passed from one bee mouth to another, it becomes a thin honey.

4. The bees store it in honeycomb, where they flap their wings to make the honey thicker and more syrupy.

5. Once the honey has reached the right consistency, the bees seal the honey-comb cell.

When you know how honey is made, it seems very odd that humans think of it as food at all.

(*Note:* Honeycomb is also made by bees. Worker bees eat honey and then secrete wax scales through glands in their abdomens. The bees gather the scales and chew them until soft and malleable, build them into combs, and attach them together. It takes the hive anywhere from 2 weeks to 2 months to produce the honeycomb alone.)

REMEMBER

Some people argue that humans are just taking "extra" honey from the bees. But who decides what is "extra"? The bees? Of course not. According to the National Beekeeping Trust in the United Kingdom, honeybees don't overproduce honey. It's supposed to be in their hive for times of scarcity.

A 2021 study in *Proceedings of the National Academy of Sciences of the United States* notes that when conventional beekeepers remove honey from the hive, they often swap it out with a sugar substitute for the bees, which lacks important nutrients. That makes the bees more susceptible to disease.

Some beekeepers clip the queen bee's wings to easily identify her, to prevent swarming, and to keep her from flying away and taking her colony with her. However, it can also affect her balance and her health.

Once winter comes, some beekeepers kill off their entire hive (20,000 to 80,000 honeybees) so they don't have the expense of taking care of the bees all winter long.

Finally, the presence of honeybees being bred in mass can disrupt native bees and pollinators. Native bees are different from honeybees, and native bees are in trouble. They are dwindling in number because of pesticides, disease, climate change, and habitat loss. Additionally, they are competing with honeybees for pollen and nectar, and honeybees can pass diseases on to them.

REMEMBER

In simple terms, bees make honey for themselves, not for humans. Plus, there are loads of delicious alternatives to honey like maple syrup or agave nectar. To read about the many alternatives to honey, be sure to check out "Getting Sweet on Vegan Honey" in Chapter 9.

TIP

If you want to help bees, grow native flowering plants, and don't use pesticides.

Using Animals for Entertainment

Animals kept in captivity for the entertainment of humans are deprived of their quality of life, freedom, natural habitat, and natural social structure. This includes settings like circuses, zoos, aquariums, and marine parks. The amount of room they have to move around and the stimulation they receive from their surroundings varies. They're prone to becoming depressed and bored.

In marine parks and aquariums, dolphins swim in tanks that are a tiny fraction of the area they'd swim in a single day in the ocean. Instead of expressing their normal behaviors, they're forced to do tricks, and they die before their natural life expectancy.

TIP

For more on this topic, I recommend the documentaries *The Cove* and *Blackfish*.

More than 40 countries worldwide, 8 U.S. states, and a variety of individual cities have passed restrictions or bans on the use of wild animals in circuses. However, there are still circuses operating in the U.S. that use wildlife. In circuses, animals are forced to engage in behaviors that they wouldn't naturally perform, and in environments that are alien to their nature. Animals used in circuses are often confined, beaten, and trained with abusive techniques.

Some people say that we need circuses, zoos, and the like so that children can gain an appreciation for animals. But really, what are we teaching kids by taking them to these places? We're saying that it's okay to take animals from their homes, lock them up, and then force them to live out their lives on display. We're teaching children that our temporary pleasure trumps an animal's agency to live freely.

TIP

Instead of visiting zoos, circuses, marine parks, or aquariums consider the following:

» Watch documentaries about animals living in the wild.

» Visit national parks and wildlife areas. Appreciate the animals who live there (from a safe and appropriate distance).

» Visit animal sanctuaries, where animals have been rescued from factory farms, hoarding situations, and abuse.

» Attend shows like Cirque du Soleil that have human acrobat artists instead of animal acts.

Addressing Environmental Concerns

Climate change is a looming and growing concern. While many folks think of transportation emissions as being the major issue, the leading contributor is closer to home. It's in the refrigerator and on the stove.

According to the United Nations (UN), animal agriculture is the leading contributor to the climate crisis we are facing. They report, "Meat and dairy provide just 18 percent of calories consumed, but use 83 percent of global farmland and are responsible for 60 percent of agriculture's greenhouse gas emissions."

The UN notes that animal-based foods like red meat, dairy, and farmed shrimp are to blame for the highest greenhouse gas emissions. However, powerful lobbying groups in the U.S. work diligently to make sure the public doesn't become too focused on the climate-related effects of the livestock industries they represent.

Cattle farming in particular is the largest driver of global deforestation. Animal agriculture is also known for:

>> Overusing antibiotics

>> Spreading infectious diseases

>> Increasing water scarcity

>> Driving biodiversity loss

>> Inefficient land use

According to Our World in Data, "The land use of livestock is so large because it takes around 100 times as much land to produce a kilocalorie of beef or lamb versus plant-based alternatives." They continue, "The same is also true for protein – it takes almost 100 times as much land to produce a gram of protein from beef or lamb, versus peas or tofu."

Consider the carbon footprint of certain animal products. According to the UN, these are the kilograms of greenhouse gas emissions per kilogram of food:

>> Beef — 70.6

>> Lamb — 39.7

>> Shellfish — 26.9

>> Cheese — 23.9

Weigh that against these plant-based foods:

>> Legumes — 2

>> Breads and pasta — 1.6

>> Fruits — 0.9

>> Vegetables — 0.7

>> Nuts — 0.4

The UN notes, "A diet that is higher in plant-based foods, such as vegetables, fruits, whole grains, legumes, nuts, and seeds, and lower in animal-based foods, has a lower environmental impact (greenhouse gas emissions and energy, land, and water use)."

This line of thinking is backed up by the British Dietetic Association, which says, "In the UK, it is estimated that well-planned, completely plant-based or vegan diets need just one third of the fertile land, fresh water, and energy of the typical British 'meat-and-dairy' based diet. Reducing animal-derived foods and choosing a range of plant foods can be beneficial to the planet, animals, and our health."

To bring it full circle, factory farm *runoff* (water that moves contaminants into local streams, rivers, and groundwater) is one of the biggest causes of pollution in our rivers and lakes. The bacteria and viruses in animal waste also contaminate the groundwater.

According to the EPA, "Agricultural runoff is the leading cause of water quality impacts to rivers and streams, the third leading source for lakes, and the second largest source of impairments to wetlands." They note that, "About a half million tons of pesticides, 12 million tons of nitrogen, and 4 million tons of phosphorus fertilizer are applied annually to crops in the continental United States. Soil erosion, nutrient loss, bacteria from livestock manure, and pesticides constitutes the primary stressors to water quality." The EPA warns that pesticide runoff can pose risks for drinking water supplies.

Plus, people who live near factory farms have been shown to have higher rates of neurological diseases and respiratory conditions, an issue that affects poor and marginalized people more acutely.

Chapter **17**

Embracing the Whole Vegan Lifestyle: Beyond Food

Being vegan means avoiding animal products in all aspects of your life. You aren't just reading nutrition labels at the grocery store. You're also checking sweaters for wool, making sure there's no shellac in nail polish, and flipping over bowls at the home goods store to see if they're made of bone china.

As with other parts of a vegan lifestyle, the longer you're vegan, the more you'll know what to look for and what to avoid. In this chapter, I lead you through how to read labels on clothing, cosmetics, and cleaning liquids, and steer clear of animal products and by-products. Then I guide you toward cruelty-free items you can choose instead.

Deciphering Product Labels

The first thing to do when seeking out vegan clothing and household products is to look at the object closely, and read the label. Check for any of these materials:

>> Angora (wool from angora rabbits)

>> Cashmere (wool from cashmere goats)

>> Feathers or down

>> Fur

>> Leather or suede

>> Mohair (wool from angora goats)

>> Shearling (sheep's wool with the skin still attached — both leather and wool)

>> Silk

>> Wool

TIP

If you don't recognize some of the words on the label, pull out your phone, and do a search to find out more.

REMEMBER

While you're looking at the item, check for any trimming or ornamentation that may not be noted on the label, like leather patches, leather zipper pulls, or pearl buttons. (Not all countries require that ornamentation be labeled, including the U.S. and Canada.) If you're unsure, reach out to the specific brand for clarification.

Avoiding Animal Products

Non-vegan products and by-products can go by many names. In this section, I cover some of the biggies you should look out for and avoid when buying clothes, accessories, and home goods.

Keep in mind that finding out what humans do to animals at such an enormous scale can be very depressing. While it can be hard to face these ugly realities, it can also spur positive lifelong changes. Throughout this chapter, I share suggestions for cruelty-free materials to choose instead.

Leather or suede

Leather is made from the skin of animals — cows, pigs, goats, kangaroos, snakes, crocodiles, and more. While leather is made from the outer side of an animal's skin, suede is made with the side facing the flesh. Suede is typically made from sheepskin, but it can also be made with the skin of cows, goats, deer, or pigs.

Many people think of leather as "natural," or even a useful by-product of the meat industry. Some folks rationalize wearing leather by saying, "Hey, if animals are going to be killed for food anyway, it's better that nothing goes to waste."

Make no mistake about it. Leather production isn't altruism. It isn't done out of respect for the animal. It's done out of respect for profit. By selling leather, ranchers boost profit margins. This is about protecting one thing: their bottom line.

REMEMBER

Leather isn't a by-product of the meat industry. It's a valuable coproduct. According to Fortune Business Insights, in 2022 the global leather goods market was valued at $440.64 billion, and by 2030 it's expected to grow to $738.61 billion. Buying leather supports slaughter industries.

Most leather comes from animals who have been raised on factory farms. After suffering things like castration and branding (without anesthetic), the animals are trucked to slaughter. Sadly, the softest leather comes from baby animals like calves and lambs, and even from unborn calves whose mothers have been slaughtered.

Leather is bad for the environment. If left to its own devices, animal skin would decompose naturally. For obvious reasons, that won't work for a purse, wallet, or couch.

Chromium, formaldehyde, arsenic, and other carcinogenic chemicals are used in tanneries to keep the animal skins from breaking down. That's part of why leather is one of the worst environmental offenders. According to The Ecologist, "Tanning is one of the most toxic industries in the world because of the chemicals involved."

Unsurprisingly, the environmental fallout is felt most acutely in developing countries, where untreated waste from tanneries is released into the groundwater and surface water, and child labor is common. The waste from tanning pollutes waterways, which harms the people who live in those communities and rely on that water.

In terms of water use, deforestation, biodiversity loss, and greenhouse gas emissions, leather is catastrophic. According to a 2021 study in *Global Environmental Change*, cattle ranching for beef and leather is responsible for 80 percent of the deforestation in the Amazon rainforest. (Once areas are deforested, the remnants are burned, and the soil is treated to make way for grass and cattle.)

Leather alternatives

When you know the costs of the leather industry, it makes sense to choose compassionate alternatives. Stay away from leather, suede, leather trim, and leather patches. Choose cars that have fabric or synthetic seats, steering wheels, and gear shifts.

TIP

To avoid leather, check labels on purses, belts, shoes, jewelry, wallets, coats, furniture, and luggage. Instead of leather, look for words like cotton, man-made, synthetic, or vegan leather.

Vegan leather is made from a variety of alternative fabrics, including the following:

>> *Piñatex* is made from pineapple leaves. It's a by-product of pineapple farming, and a good secondary income source for farmers.

>> Cork leather is made from cork oak trees.

>> Wine leather or grape leather is made from waste in wine production.

>> Mushroom leather is made from the roots of the mushroom plant.

>> Leaf leather is made from teak leaves.

>> Polyurethane is a plastic-based leather product. (It's also known as PU leather.)

As you can see, there are many different types of options here, and each have their own environmental footprint. Obviously, plastic-based leather like PU has its environmental drawbacks. Still, according to the Higgs Materials Sustainability Index, the environmental impact of plastic leather is a quarter of the environmental impact of leather made from cow skins. Animal-based leather contributes more to global warming, water depletion and pollution, and greenhouse-gas emissions than any synthetic or plant-based leather. And let's not forget about the loss of life for the animals whose skins are used.

Depending on your budget and concerns, pick the vegan leather that meets your needs, or choose other types of animal-free fabrics.

Wool or cashmere

Many people assume that the process of wool removal is a simple haircut. However, the removal process is often done with an emphasis on quickness over compassion. Rather than earning an hourly wage, workers are paid to *shear* (or cut) the wool off as many sheep as they can, which inevitably leads to injuries along the way. (Ninety percent of the world's wool supply comes from sheep. The remaining 10 percent comes mostly from goats, alpacas, and rabbits.)

Some people argue that sheep have to be shorn, almost as if it's a kindness. But it's important to remember that sheep have been bred specifically with extra wrinkly skin to produce more wool and to grow wool all year round. That's what keeps the industry profitable. When the wool production of sheep declines, they are sent to slaughter.

Sheep farming often includes painful procedures like tail docking and mulesing. Do you remember that extra wrinkly skin sheep were bred to have? Well, flies can lay eggs inside those skinfolds and cause a condition called *flystrike*. Once the eggs hatch into larvae, they feed off the flesh of the sheep. To prevent flystrike, ranchers slice off strips of the wrinkly flesh near a lamb's hindquarters, often without anesthetic or painkillers. This procedure called *mulesing* is excruciatingly painful, and many sheep don't survive it. Usually, mulesing is done when lambs are just 2 to 10 weeks old.

Similarly, many sheep have their tails *docked* (cut off or seared) to further reduce the chances of flystrike. In addition to being very painful, docking may cause *rectal prolapse* (a condition in which part of the rectum protrudes outside the anus) if not done properly.

Australia is the largest wool producer. Once wool production declines and the sheep have ceased to be "useful," they are put onboard boats in Australia heading to the Middle East and North Africa. The multitiered boats carry up to 85,000 sheep. Approximately 3 million sheep are sent across the ocean every year as live exports. After their long journey, they are slaughtered.

Wool alternatives

To avoid animals' hair in clothing, stay away from cashmere, pashmina, mohair, angora, camel hair, and shearling.

TIP

Check the labels of sweaters, scarves, suits, mittens, socks, and coats. You usually find the label either at the back of the neck or alongside the body of the clothing. Felt can be made with either synthetic materials or wool. Just check the label before buying. You'll also want to steer clear of wool rugs.

When buying clothes, choose cotton, hemp, linen, flannel, polyester, acrylic, or synthetic material. If you knit, choose acrylic yarn.

REMEMBER

Fur

On January 1, 2023, California became the first state in the U.S. to ban the sale of new animal fur products — either through brick-and-mortar stores or online. In addition, more than 20 countries have passed laws to limit or ban fur farming, including Israel — the first country to prohibit the sale of fur products.

That's good news, because fur is brutal. If you've ever seen behind-the-scenes pictures, you know it's impossible to witness animals spending their tortured lives in cages and not feel sad about it. Fur comes from animals like rabbits, minks, chinchillas, raccoon dogs, and foxes who were raised, trapped, and killed for their pelts.

Eight-five percent of fur comes from animals on fur factory farms, which can house thousands of animals. After spending their lives in cages, they are killed with gruesome methods like suffocation, gas, poison, or electrocution, none of which are prohibited by animal welfare laws or humane slaughter laws.

Like the animal skin used in the leather industry, fur would decompose if left on its own. To make fur last, it's treated with toxic chemicals to preserve and dye it. This pollution (along with the standard pollution involved in all factory farming) is terrible for the environment.

Fur alternatives

TIP

If you want to buy fake fur, look for words like faux, polyester, and acrylic. It should be noted, however, that while faux fur exists, many vegans avoid wearing it, because they don't feel comfortable in something that may be mistaken for animal fur. Plus, there have been cases where fur was marked as fake, but turned out to be real animal fur.

Silk

Silk comes from silkworms (actually caterpillars). They weave fiber to make their cocoons. In the silk industry, before they are able to turn into moths, silkworms are baked, steamed, or boiled alive in their cocoons so that growers can obtain the silk. Billions of silkworms are killed every year to make silk.

Without human involvement, the insects would chew their way out of their cocoons. However, that process would damage the silk. So growers don't allow it to happen.

Silk is a multibillion-dollar-a-year industry, with 80 percent of the world's silk production coming from China. Thousands of years of domestication has made silk moths blind and unable to fly.

The most common silkworms used for silk are *Bombyx mori*. These mulberry leaf-eating larvae are used for 90 percent of silk production. It takes about 2,500 silkworms to make a single silk robe. These tiny creatures have a brain and central nervous system, and can experience pain.

If you've never seen a silkworm that was allowed to become a moth, do a Google image search for "silk moth" or "Bombyx mori." They look like a Jim Henson character or something out of Pokémon. They have adorable furry bodies, antennae that look like hair clips, and wings that almost look felted.

Environmentally speaking, silk is bad news. Silk has the worst environmental impact of any textile, according to the Higg Index (an environmental-impact assessment by the fashion industry). A massive amount of fertilizers and irrigation is needed to turn the tons of mulberry leaves that silkworms eat into pounds of raw silk. The dyes used on silk are also highly carcinogenic, and can leach into water supplies.

Finally, the silk industry is associated with human rights violations like *bonded labor* (a form of modern-day slavery) and child labor.

Silk alternatives

TIP

Instead of buying silk, choose clothing or fabrics made with materials like nylon, cotton, bamboo, modal, or rayon.

Pearls

Naturally occurring pearls are rare, so pearl farmers expedite the process by inserting irritants like beads into oysters to produce what are known as *cultured pearls.* (All bivalves can create pearls, but oysters are the most commonly used in the pearl industry.) Some oysters die during this process.

The oysters respond to the irritant by coating it in crystalline *nacre,* which builds up and creates a pearl. This process takes 2 to 5 years. Then the pearls are harvested by opening the shells and removing the pearls.

After the pearls are removed, young oysters that produced quality pearls are put through the process again. Oysters that aren't producing the same quality pearls are sold to be eaten, or used for the mother-of-pearl on the inside of their shells.

Pearl alternatives

TIP

You can easily avoid pearls by choosing other types of jewelry. Seek out ethically sourced gemstones, synthetic or conflict-free diamonds, or jewelry made with recyclable materials.

While fake pearls exist, they're sometimes coated in animal-derived materials like mother-of-pearl powder, fish scales, or oyster scales. To be on the safe side, it's best to skip them or buy imitation pearls that are specifically labeled vegan.

Down or feathers

When you're buying pillows, cushions, comforters, or winter jackets and coats, you may see tags showing they're made with feathers or down. To acquire the feathers used inside these products, geese and ducks are plucked either after slaughter or while they are still alive.

During *live plucking*, the birds' feathers are painfully ripped out of their bodies without anesthetic while they are held down. Even more disturbing is that some ducks and geese are plucked repeatedly during their lives, all without any pain relief. Live plucking is illegal in the U.S. and the European Union. However, according to a 2016 article from cbsnews.com, 80 percent of feathers and down are produced in China, where live plucking is legal.

A 2020 article from Audobon.org states, "The vast majority of the 270,000 metric tons of commercial down produced each year is a by-product of goose and duck meat industries in Asia and Europe, where the birds might be live-plucked or force-fed for foie gras before heading to the slaughterhouse."

As for geese in the U.S., birds aren't protected by the Humane Methods of Slaughter Act (see the sidebar in Chapter 16 for more information). And they're often kept in terrible conditions before they're killed for food.

Like leather and wool, feathers and down are a lucrative business in their own right. According to Future Market Insights, the down and feather market is estimated at 7,567.3 million in 2023 and is projected to reach roughly 16,175.3 million by 2033. In addition to ducks and geese, other birds used for their feathers include swans, ostriches, and peacocks.

Down or feather alternatives

You can find animal-free, synthetic down pillows, comforters, and coats. Some of these products are even made from recycled plastic bottles. Fleece jackets and blankets are excellent at holding warmth and wicking away moisture.

TIP

When looking at coats, cushions, comforters, or pillows, stay away from those stuffed with down, and avoid accessories with feathers. Look for labels featuring words like cotton, synthetic, polyester fiberfill, or down alternative instead.

Bone china

As the name implies, *bone china* is made from the ash of burned animal bones (usually cows) from slaughterhouses. Bone china cups, plates, and bowls generally range from 25 to 50 percent bone ash.

TIP

You can sometimes tell that an item is made of bone china just from the way it looks. It's usually bright, milky white with a translucent quality. An even easier (and more accurate) way to know if a piece is bone china is by turning it over and looking at the label on the bottom. It will have a "bone china" stamp or signature.

As with leather, some people imply that bone china products are acceptable because they make sure no part of the animal goes to waste. However, bone china is a luxury business. More cows are killed so that their bones can be used as material in cups and saucers.

Bone china alternatives

Instead of bone china, choose tableware made of porcelain, stoneware, earthenware, metal like stainless steel, or glass.

TIP

In recent years, brands like Mikasa and other dinnerware makers have started selling vegan bone china. It is made without ash, but has a similar look, color, and translucence, thanks to mineralized calcium oxide. If you're in doubt, ask the company if their bone china contains bone ash.

Figuring Out What to Do with Your Non-vegan Clothing

Before I went vegan, I regularly purchased leather boots, shoes, and skirts. I associated leather with quality. But after I went vegan and found out more about leather and other animal-based materials, I didn't feel comfortable wearing those items anymore. Even touching or seeing them made me feel sad and uneasy. They didn't accurately represent my new convictions or what I wanted to present to the world.

So I tucked my leather and other non-vegan clothing items into bags for charity. Luckily, I already had plenty of other clothing options in my closet that happened to be vegan, so it wasn't a hardship choosing those cruelty-free items instead.

That may or may not be the case for you, however. You may not be able or willing to cut out the non-vegan products you already own. If you have a leather purse, wool sweater, or silk shirt in your closet, the items you own aren't creating further suffering. The damage has already been done. (Of course, I wouldn't advocate buying more of them.)

TIP

Depending on your comfort level, you can continue using the non-vegan items you already have. Then replace them as they wear out with non-animal versions. However, if the items make you feel unhappy or regretful, or if you don't like normalizing the use of animals for clothing, consider donating these items to charity. Then replace your non-vegan clothing with vegan alternatives when you are able, or use any vegan items you already have.

TIP

If you're looking to get rid of old fur coats, some charities distribute them to people in need who can't afford warm winter coats. Also, some wildlife rehabilitation centers take old fur coats to be used as warm bedding for injured and orphaned wildlife.

Finding Animal-Free Fashion

Nowadays it's easy to find animal-free fashion in almost any store. If it's summer or you live somewhere that's warm all year round, you'll have no problem finding clothing that features cotton, bamboo, modal, hemp, linen, or other vegan fabrics.

If it's winter or you live somewhere that's usually cold, you'll likely have to do more label reading. Animal hair like wool and cashmere pops up in a lot of sweaters. Many winter coats contain feathers or down, and gloves often include leather. Before you take an item to the dressing room, check the clothing label. By doing a brief scan, you'll know if you need to bother trying it on.

TIP

If you're doing your clothes shopping online, look under product details, features, or fabric and care to find the materials.

You'll also want to find a winter coat that will keep you warm all season long. Almost any store has vegan options. Just read the tag, and stay away from down. Choose puffer coats with sustainable filler or synthetic insulation.

For dress or casual shoes, including running shoes, search your favorite shoe sites with the word "vegan." From there, you'll get a bunch of non-leather options. You can also visit MooShoes online at https://mooshoes.myshopify.com (or in person if you live in or visit New York City). Everything on their site is vegan, including shoes, bags, wallets, and belts.

For purses and other accessories, check out Matt & Nat at https://us.mattandnat.com. Everything in their line is vegan, including bags, briefcases, shoes, and coats.

Choosing Cruelty-Free Cosmetics and Body Products

You likely already have favorite cosmetics and body products. See if those products happen to be vegan and cruelty-free. If they are, you're one step ahead of the game. If they aren't, start researching vegan products to buy in the future. As you finish a tube of lipstick, container of blush, or bottle of shampoo, swap it out with a vegan counterpart.

TIP

You can save yourself time reading labels by seeking out beauty products from 100 percent vegan companies. EcoTools makes vegan cosmetic brushes that are free from animal hair. For vegan makeup, check out Beauty Without Cruelty, e.l.f, Pacifica, Gabriel Cosmetics, and Zuzu Luxe. You can find loads of other fully vegan brands. A quick Google search will lead you to more options.

For shampoo and conditioner, you can choose from all-vegan brands like Avalon Organics (my choice), Aveda, Pacifica, and many more. I make my own deodorant with coconut oil, baking soda, and cornstarch. (You can find the recipe at https://cadryskitchen.com/diy-coconut-oil-deodorant/.) Or you can buy deodorant from brands like Booda Organics, Lavanila, Schmidt's, and more.

TIP

If you aren't buying from brands that are 100 percent vegan, you'll want to consider two things:

» Do these products contain animal by-products or ingredients derived from an animal source?

» Were they tested on animals?

Some companies label their vegan products. If a product is labeled as vegan, that means it doesn't include any animal products, like shellac or carmine (made from crushed beetles), and it wasn't tested on animals.

You can also look for symbols on the packaging noting that the product is vegan. Various organizations like People for the Ethical Treatment of Animals, Vegan Action, and The Vegan Society have vegan certifications.

If a product is labeled as cruelty-free, that means it wasn't tested on animals. However, it may still contain animal-based ingredients.

If you see a Leaping Bunny Logo on a package, it's the international symbol that means the company didn't use any new animal testing in developing their products, either by the company, their suppliers, or their laboratories. However, it may or may not be vegan. You still need to check the ingredients for any animal by-products.

Here are some ingredients to avoid:

>> **Animal hair:** Hair from horses, goats, raccoons, squirrels, badgers, and mink or sable are used in makeup brushes and hairbrushes. Boar bristle hair brushes are literally made with the hairs of boars.

   Hair for brushes can be retrieved in a variety of ways. Horse and boar hair is commonly obtained from slaughtered animals, mink and sable are kept in fur farms, and animals like squirrels are hunted and trapped.

>> **Beeswax** (also known as *cera alba*): It's made by bees to construct their honeycombs, protect their young, and store their honey and pollen for winter or a drought. It's used in mascara, lotions, and lip balms.

>> **Carmine or cochineal:** This red dye is made by boiling and crushing beetles. It's often in makeup and nail polishes.

>> **Casein:** Made from cow's milk, it's used in moisturizing products for the hair and face.

>> **Collagen:** It's made from animal ligaments, tissue, bones, and skin, and used in anti-aging products and lip-plumping products.

>> **Glycerin:** It's made from animal fats, ground-up hooves and horns, feathers, and animal hair. It's found in soaps, hair products, makeup, and moisturizers. Look for vegetable glycerin instead, which is made from soy or coconut oil.

>> **Guanine:** It's made from fish scales and used in nail polishes, eyeshadows, blushes, bronzers, and highlighters.

>> **Keratin:** It's made from animal hair and horns, and used in nail and hair products.

>> **Lanolin:** It's a wax made from sheep's wool found in lip balms and hair products.

>> **Oleic acid:** It's made from animal fat or tallow. It's used in nail polishes, soaps, moisturizers, and makeup.

>> **Shellac:** It's the resinous secretion made by female lac bugs and added to nail products and hair lacquers.

>> **Silk powder:** Made from the cocoons of silkworms, it's used in facial powders and soaps.

>> **Squalene:** Formulated from sharks' liver oil, it's used in lip balms, deodorants, and moisturizers. (Vegan versions can be made with olives. Look for vegetable squalene.)

>> **Stearic acid:** It's made from fat taken from the stomachs of pigs, cows, and sheep. It's used in deodorants, soaps, moisturizers, and hair products.

Chapter **18**

Dining Out

f you're new to dining out as a vegan, going to restaurants can feel like a challenge. Fully vegan restaurants may not be prevalent in your area. Non-vegan restaurant menus may look like a sea of animal products.

Don't worry! Dining out with friends doesn't have to end because of your compassionate lifestyle. In this chapter, you get useful tips for finding vegan restaurants and dining out at non-vegan restaurants.

Finding Vegan and Vegan-Friendly Restaurants

Before I stopped eating meat, I'd never visited a vegetarian restaurant, let alone a vegan one. I may not have even known that they existed! They weren't in the usual lineup of restaurants I patronized, and I didn't think about seeking them out.

So when I stopped eating animal products and started looking into vegan offerings, it was a wonderful surprise to unearth options I didn't know were out there. It's one of those cases where until you go looking for it, you don't know what you'll find.

Looking for vegan and vegan-friendly restaurants in your town? Here are some easy ways to find them:

>> **Do a Google search:** Start with a simple Google search. Put your city (or the city you're planning to visit) into the search bar along with the word *vegan*. After you hit enter, you'll see the top listings, including a map of your options.

Also included in the search results: reviews, travel sites, and blogs. Check out the listed restaurants, menus, and pictures of their offerings to see what looks appealing.

>> **Visit HappyCow:** Another terrific resource is www.happycow.net. This user-generated website and app compiles vegan options, firsthand reviews, and pictures. Type in your city to see if any vegan or vegan-friendly restaurants are listed.

TIP

The HappyCow app is incredibly useful when you're traveling. It's often the first thing I check when I arrive in a new city.

>> **Check out other review sites:** Search Yelp or Tripadvisor for vegan-friendly restaurants in your area. Users leave reviews and often include favorite dishes, photos, or tips on what to avoid.

WARNING

Be aware that any references to the keyword *vegan* will pop up in your search. So you may get some options that are notably not vegan-friendly if a reviewer writes something like "A vegan would hate this place."

Ordering a Vegan Meal at a Non-vegan Restaurant

If you have an abundance of vegan restaurants in your town, obviously that's an amazing option and a quality first choice when dining out. At vegan restaurants, it's a wonderful treat being able to order anything off the menu. Plus, you don't have to quiz your server about unexpected animal products sneaking in. However, vegan restaurants aren't available everywhere, and sometimes you want to branch out and try other things.

Before you visit a non-vegan restaurant, look at their online menu or social media pages. See if anything looks promising, and if they label their vegan options. While many restaurants can accommodate vegan diners, some places are going to have more satisfying offerings than others.

TIP

If a restaurant doesn't immediately look vegan-friendly, consider reaching out to them via phone or direct message to ask if they can accommodate vegan diners.

Some restaurants that don't immediately appear to be vegan-friendly may be able to prepare something plant-based using ingredients they already have on hand.

Table for two, please

The night has arrived, and you're out to dinner with friends. The server drops off menus at the table, and now is the time to choose your dinner. Here are some easy steps to follow on your way to getting a vegan meal:

1. **When you arrive, glance over the menu.** Make a note of menu items that look vegan-friendly or are "veganizable." Some restaurants put an asterisk, letter V, leaf, or other symbol next to menu items to show that they're vegan. That is super helpful and makes ordering easy. (If there is a designation, be sure to check that it means vegan and not vegetarian, and if it's vegan as listed or needs some adjustments.)

2. **Ask your server about those items, as well as suggestions for other vegan options.** If your server doesn't know what vegan means, clarify by saying that you don't eat meat, dairy, or eggs.

3. **See if any dishes can be made vegan by changing their preparation or omitting ingredients.** Sometimes it's as simple as cooking in oil instead of butter or leaving off cheese.

4. **Look at the side dishes for possible options.** If necessary, make a hodge-podge meal of sides. (Think french fries, a salad with balsamic vinaigrette, and steamed broccoli.)

5. **If there aren't any vegan options listed, ask if the chef is willing to make something off-menu.** Some chefs are happy to put together a plant-based option using ingredients they have on hand. I've gotten some wonderful meals this way!

Online ordering and apps

Many restaurants and fast-food places have online ordering available through their websites or apps. This option often makes it even easier for vegan diners to note which ingredients they'd like omitted, or how they'd like to customize their meal.

This is a great choice for tricky orders, because you can enter all the correct information yourself, without having to explain your order over the phone or to a server. It improves the likelihood that the person making your food will get all your requests right. On the website or app:

>> Check the box for your preferred protein, like tofu or beans.

>> Check any boxes that denote ingredients you want omitted, like eggs, dairy, or meat.

>> List your specific needs or requests in the special-instructions section. That's where I add the note "Vegan, please." If you'd prefer, you can say, "No meat, dairy, eggs, or honey, please."

Choosing Where to Eat and What to Request

When I was a brand-new vegan, my husband and I were getting together with extended family for brunch. We were coming in from out of town, so plans were made without our input. The restaurant they picked was a popular buffet known for their omelet bar, carving station, biscuits and gravy, fried chicken, and a place to make your own waffles. People often think buffets are a good choice because "anyone can eat there." And while that may be true, not everyone can eat *well* there.

Knowing the vegan options would be slim, I smuggled in a container of hummus and a small box of nondairy milk from a natural foods store. From the buffet line, I got some fruit, a few raw veggies, and a bagel. Then I slathered on my hummus, added the sliced vegetables to make a sandwich, and poured my nondairy milk into the unlimited cups of coffee.

Of course, I was happy to spend time with family I don't get to see often. But when the time came to pay our bill, it stung a bit to spend the same price as everyone who'd gotten full plates and hadn't brought in half of their meal in their purse. (By the way, if you're ever tempted to smuggle in your own food to a restaurant, be aware most establishments frown on that.)

That's why these days when I'm making dinner plans with friends or family, I advocate for myself and recommend a restaurant that offers satisfying and delicious vegan options. Dining out can be expensive, and if I'm going to splurge on a meal out, I want to feel like the money I spent was worth it. If a restaurant isn't interested in offering a quality vegan option, I'll take my business to one that is.

In this section, I offer restaurant options where you're going to have the highest likelihood of getting a hearty vegan meal, no smuggled hummus necessary.

Vegan-friendly cuisines

When you're making dinner plans with family and friends, steer them toward any of these vegan–friendly options: Ethiopian, Indian, Mediterranean, Middle Eastern, Mexican, Thai, or pizza places. Typically, it's easier to find dishes that are already vegan or that can easily be made vegan in those restaurants.

At any food establishment, when in doubt about the menu, just ask. Here are some special requests to keep in mind for easy ordering:

>> **Ethiopian restaurants:** Some of my favorite Ethiopian restaurants are exclusively vegan, but even non-vegan Ethiopian restaurants usually have loads of plant-based options.

Turn to the vegetarian section of the menu, where you'll find vegetable, lentil, and bean-based *wots* (stews). Ask your server if they use spice-infused butter (*niter kibbeh*) to cook their dishes. Many Ethiopian restaurants use vegan-friendly flavored oil instead.

Some of my favorite dishes are *gomen* (collard greens), *misir wot* (spicy red lentils), *kik alicha* (split pea stew), *shiro wot* (chickpea stew), *fasolia* (stewed green beans), and *atakilt wot* (potato, cabbage, and carrot stew). Scoop it all up with *injera,* a tangy flatbread.

>> **Indian restaurants:** Many Indian restaurants are exclusively vegetarian. Even in non-vegetarian Indian restaurants, you'll find lots of veg-friendly dishes like *chana masala* (chickpea curry) and *aloo gobi* (potato and cauliflower stew).

TIP

If vegan dishes aren't labeled on the menu, ask your server which of the dishes are made without *ghee* (clarified butter). For bread, look for roti, poori, or paratha without ghee.

Here are other words to look for on an Indian restaurant's menu:

- Aloo — potato

- Chana — chickpea

- Gobi — cauliflower

- Matar — pea

- Palak — spinach

- Saag — leafy green vegetable like spinach and mustard greens

Here are words on the menu to avoid:

- Paneer — cheese
- Ghee — clarified butter
- Korma — yogurt-based curry
- Makhani — dish with butter sauce

» **Mediterranean or Middle Eastern restaurants:** These cuisines are a vegan paradise with loads of plant-based options. Ask if the dishes contain any dairy like yogurt or feta and request that those ingredients be omitted.

Choose any of the following:

- Hummus — chickpea dip
- Baba ghanoush — smoky eggplant dip
- Falafel — fried chickpea balls
- Tabbouleh — parsley and bulgur salad
- Vegetable kebabs — grilled vegetables on a skewer
- Mujaddara — lentils and rice with sautéed onions
- Cucumber, tomato, or chickpea salads
- Dolmas — stuffed grape leaves (Make sure the dolmas aren't stuffed with meat.)

» **Mexican restaurants:** Scan the menu for veggie fajitas, bean or mushroom tacos, and bean burritos. Ask if they use lard in the beans or chicken stock in the rice. (You'll want to avoid both of those animal ingredients, obviously.) Ask them to leave off dairy-based cheese or sour cream.

» **Thai restaurants:** Scan the menu for tofu and vegetable dishes. Ask them to omit fish sauce, oyster sauce, shrimp paste, and egg from any dishes that look like they can be made vegan. If you're ordering a noodle dish, opt for one with rice noodles instead of egg noodles.

» **Pizzerias:** Look at all the vegetable toppings on offer and build a pizza around them. If they have vegan specialty toppings like veggie sausage or pepperoni, that's a big win. Ask if the crust and sauce are vegan. If they don't have vegan cheese available, ask for a pizza with no cheese.

» **Natural grocery stores:** If you're open to a very laid-back meal, many natural food stores have delis that offer sandwiches, salads, soups, and more. They tend to have vegan-friendly options that are clearly labeled.

Vegan options at chain restaurants

If your group visits a chain restaurant, you may be pleasantly surprised by the vegan options available. Some chains have made it easier by labeling and promoting their vegan options online or in the restaurant.

WARNING

Be aware that menus, ingredients, and food sourcing can change. What's listed below may be different or unavailable by the time you go. Ask about current vegan offerings and discuss your needs with the staff at the restaurant before ordering.

The following is a list of popular restaurant chains and a few vegan options you can try:

>> **Applebee's:** Start with brew pub pretzels, and replace the cheese dip and honey mustard with marinara. For your main course, order an Impossible Burger without cheese. Impossible Burger can also replace meat in certain bowls and salads. On the side, have french fries or waffle fries, or steamed broccoli with no butter.

>> **California Pizza Kitchen:** Begin your meal with chips and guacamole, lettuce wraps with Chinese vegetables, or a cup of smashed pea and barley soup. While they don't currently offer vegan cheese, you can order a California veggie or wild mushroom pizza, and request no cheese. They also have tomato basil spaghetti that's vegan as is.

>> **Cheesecake Factory:** Start with the Thai lettuce wraps with grilled avocado. Dip them in peanut or sweet red chili sauce. For your entree, the vegan Cobb salad and Impossible Burger are plant-based by default. On the side, enjoy french fries or sweet potato fries, or ask about getting one of their vegetable side dishes without butter.

>> **Mellow Mushroom:** This veg-friendly pizza chain has a separate vegan menu for in-person and online ordering. Start with a salted vegan pretzel with mustard for dipping. For pizza options, get the Vegan Veg Out, or build your own with either red sauce or an oil and garlic base. Then load it up with your favorite vegetable toppings, tempeh, and/or nondairy cheese. If you prefer, grab an avocado or tempeh hoagie, or a salad.

>> **Olive Garden:** Begin your meal with breadsticks and minestrone soup. (The garlic topping on the breadsticks is soy-based and contains no butter or other animal products.) For your main course, have spaghetti, angel hair, fettucine, rigatoni, or small shells with marinara. Enjoy it with a side of seasoned broccoli.

>> **P.F. Chang's:** For an appetizer, have vegetarian lettuce wraps, steamed edamame, or chili garlic green beans. Then for your main course, nosh on Buddha's Feast, mapo tofu, or stir-fried eggplant. On the side, enjoy white or brown rice.

>> **Red Robin:** Get the Impossible Burger without cheese or the veggie burger without cheese or aioli. On the side, enjoy steak fries or sweet potato fries, potato chips, steamed broccoli, or carrot sticks.

Vegan fast-food options

When you're on the road or short on time, fast food can be a convenient option. More and more fast-food places are adding vegan items to the menu.

Keep in mind that fast-food restaurants change their menus. Also, what's available in one part of the country or world may not be on offer in another region. Double-check with the restaurant about their current vegan-friendly options.

>> **Auntie Anne's Pretzels:** Order any of the following warm, fresh pretzels without butter: original, cinnamon sugar, sweet almond, jalapeño, or raisin. Be aware there will be a 5-minute wait to freshly make pretzels. For a dipping sauce, choose marinara or sweet glaze dip.

>> **Baskin-Robbins:** Try their Non-Dairy Mint Chocochunk, Lemon Sorbet, or Daiquiri Ice in a cake cone. They also have a variety of non-dairy fruit smoothies.

>> **Blaze Pizza:** Create your own pizza with your preferred vegetable toppings, vegan chorizo, and vegan cheese. For sauces, choose classic red, spicy red, barbecue, or olive oil. Both the traditional and gluten-free crusts are vegan. On the side, get cheesy bread made with vegan cheese.

>> **Burger King:** Order an Impossible Whopper with no mayonnaise or an Impossible King with no cheese. Other plant-based options include french fries, hash browns, applesauce, and French toast sticks.

>> **Carl's Jr.:** Pick up a Beyond Famous Star burger. Order it without mayo and cheese for a vegan option. Finish out your meal with french fries, waffle fries, or hash rounds.

>> **CAVA:** Put together your own bowl with lots of options like hummus, roasted eggplant dip, and roasted vegetables on brown rice. If you prefer a curated option, go with the lentil avocado bowl or crispy falafel pita, which are plant-based by default.

>> **Chipotle:** Get a burrito, bowl, salad, or tacos with *sofritas* (crumbled tofu simmered in a smoky sauce), black and pinto beans, fajita vegetables, rice, salsa, and/or guacamole.

>> **Dairy Queen:** Pick up a Non-Dairy Dilly Bar made with coconut milk ice cream and covered in a crunchy chocolate coating.

>> **Insomnia Cookies:** This bakery chain has several vegan cookie options, including vegan birthday cake, vegan chocolate chunk, and vegan double chocolate chunk.

>> **Jamba Juice:** Quench your thirst with one of their plant-based smoothies, like Apple 'n Greens, Vanilla Blue Sky, Greens 'n Ginger, Mega Mango, Peach Perfection, Pomegranate Paradise, Strawberry Whirl, and more.

>> **Moe's Southwest Grill:** Get tacos, salads, burritos, or bowls with black or pinto beans, rice, and/or tofu.

>> **Noodles & Company:** This fast-casual chain has one option on the menu that's vegan by default — Japanese pan noodles. They also have several menu items that can be prepared vegan with a few substitutions, like removing meat and dairy ingredients. For an extra bump of protein, add tofu or Impossible Panko Chicken to any dish.

>> **Panda Express:** They have a number of plant-based options, including chow mein, vegetable spring rolls, super greens, and white or brown rice. Some locations also have eggplant tofu.

>> **Peet's:** For breakfast, grab their Everything Plant-Based Sandwich or a Mediterranean flatbread with JUST Egg and Violife vegan cheese. Complete the meal with a soy latte.

>> **Taco Bell:** The menu at Taco Bell was made for personalized ordering. Swap out meat for beans or potatoes, and order your food "Fresco Style" to replace cheese, sour cream, and ranch sauce with pico de gallo. Use their website or app to make special ordering easy.

>> **White Castle:** Grab Impossible Burger sliders or veggie sliders. Request no cheese — unless you live in select locations where dairy-free cheddar is available. Fill out your meal with french fries or applesauce.

Dealing with Cross-Contamination

When you're dining out at a non-vegan restaurant, cross-contamination with animal-based ingredients is always a possibility. The staff may use the same preparation surfaces, food prep gloves, spatulas, grills, pans, or fryers for vegan items and non-vegan items.

If you have an allergy to any animal proteins, obviously this is a big issue. You should absolutely tell the staff about it, and avoid restaurants that don't take cross-contamination seriously.

However, if you don't have an allergy, it's up to you to decide whether you feel comfortable dining in a restaurant where cross-contamination is a possibility.

For some vegans, cross-contamination isn't an issue. To them, the point of being vegan is to reduce harm. No additional harm is created by cooking their vegan french fries in the same fryer as a meat eater's chicken nuggets.

However, others can't stand the thought of their vegan dish commingling with the remnants of non-vegan ingredients. If you don't feel comfortable with the possibility of cross-contamination, stick with exclusively vegan restaurants or restaurants that can guarantee strict adherence to keeping vegan items away from animal products.

IN THIS CHAPTER

» Identifying your dining options before traveling

» Finding vegan meals on the road

» Eating well at hotels, bed-and-breakfasts, or vacation rentals

» Flying the vegan-friendly skies

» Dining in style on a cruise

» Planning a plant-based campout

Chapter **19**

Vegan on the Road and in the Air

One of life's best pleasures is travel. It's such a treat to see another part of the world, have unique experiences, and, of course, try some new foods!

Like they always say, getting there is half the fun. In this chapter, you find tips for packing your car with vegan nibbles for a road trip, keeping a fully stocked hotel fridge, staying well fed at sea level or 35,000 feet, and even making the most of a plant-based camping trip.

Doing Your Research

Before you set out on your journey, research vegan and vegan-friendly restaurants in your final destination. Google the city you're visiting with the word *vegan* to see what kind of options are available. Check out travel websites, blogs, and reviews. Then make some notes on places you don't want to miss. (Plus, dinner reservations, if necessary!)

If you're planning a road trip, look at any major cities you'll pass through. See which interesting plant-based restaurants may be worthy of a pit stop.

TIP

Some of the U.S. cities that are best known for their vegan options include Los Angeles, New York City, Portland, Seattle, Chicago, Austin, Orlando, and San Francisco. Outside the U.S., great vegan options abound in Berlin, London, Toronto, Chiang Mai, Melbourne, Singapore, Bangkok, Amsterdam, Tel Aviv, and more.

Even if your travels take you to smaller locales, you may be pleasantly surprised at how veganism is growing in unlikely places.

Choosing Road-Trip Food

What's more fun than a good road trip? Whether it's a long weekend in a neighboring state or a cross-country excursion, setting off on the open road always fuels a spirit of adventure.

Of course, some places are more vegan-friendly than others. So packing meals and snacks is a good way to avoid "hangry" feelings and save some cash. With that in mind, this section provides road-trip ideas for breakfast, lunch, dinner, and snack time too.

REMEMBER

Think "picnic in a car" when planning your travel menu. Your meals can be as fancy or low-key as you want. Keep anything perishable in a cooler using frozen gel packs or ice. Shelf-stable items can be placed in a tote bag in the backseat to make them easy to grab.

Breakfast

Here are some simple breakfast ideas that are easy to throw together:

>> Baked donuts

>> Nondairy yogurt

>> Dry cereal with single-serving packs of nondairy milk

>> Bagels with vegan cream cheese

>> Single-serving oatmeal cups (Just add hot water from a thermos or gas station.)

Lunch or dinner

Sandwiches and wraps are super convenient for car lunches or dinners. You can either make them ahead of time or keep the fillings and bread separate in the cooler. Here are some simple meal ideas:

>> Peanut butter and jelly sandwiches

>> Vegan lunchmeat sandwiches with mustard, onions, and pickles

>> Eggless Egg Salad Wraps (Grab the recipe in Chapter 13.)

>> Raw vegetable sandwiches or wraps with hummus

>> Individual instant soup containers (Just add hot water.)

Before you go, pack several substantive salads for the trip. They can work as a side or a main course, depending on the dish.

>> Kale salad (Kale is so hardy, it holds up well in the cooler.)

>> Corn and bean salad

>> Mediterranean Couscous Salad (Grab the recipe in Chapter 14.)

>> Cold Peanut Noodle (Get the recipe in Chapter 12.)

>> Old School Chef Salad (The recipe for this meal-sized salad is in Chapter 13.)

Snacks

If you get peckish on your drive, it's nice to have some snacks to nosh on between meals.

>> Ready-to-eat veggies like baby carrots, celery sticks, sliced cucumbers, and bell pepper slices

>> Fruit like bananas, apples, oranges, and berries

>> Seeds, nuts, or trail mix

>> Vegan cheese and crackers

>> Vegan snack bars

>> Chips and salsa

>> Hummus and pita chips

>> Roasted Chickpeas (Get the recipe in Chapter 14.)

Gas station snack options

If your cooler rations are running low, pick up some vegan-friendly fast food, or grab a snack at a convenience store.

Consider these easy gas station options:

» Nuts and seeds

» Tortilla chips and jarred salsa

» Popcorn

» Energy bars

» Bananas, oranges, and apples

Vegan-friendly pit stops

Of course, some of the fun of getting away is trying new restaurants! If you'll be passing an excellent vegan or vegan-friendly establishment on the way to your final destination, consider stocking up on takeout orders that can be stored in the cooler for later.

TIP

I recommend picking items that hold up well and can be enjoyed cold. Salads, grain bowls, or sandwiches are all good options.

One time when I was driving across the U.S., I made a point of stopping every day at a different vegan restaurant in a new state. I'd enjoy one hot meal while I was there. Then I'd order another to eat at the hotel that night. It extended the fun, and allowed me to try more of each restaurant's menu.

At a stop in Denver, I hit up vegan restaurant Watercourse Foods. For lunch, I had a portobello reuben sandwich. Then for the road, I got a salad with grilled tofu. After several more hours of driving, it was such a relief to check into the hotel, put my feet up, and tuck into my delicious ready-to-eat dinner.

Keeping Yourself Well-Fed during Your Hotel Stay

When I was a kid, our vacations always involved a camper. So on those rare circumstances when I spent the night in a hotel, it was bliss. Watching cable television and ordering pizza to the room after swimming in the hotel pool was the ultimate luxury.

As an adult, the novelty of hotel stays can wear off — especially if you're there on business for days on end. You may not have the time, energy, or inclination to run to a restaurant for every meal. By staying in, you can put together meals that are a lot healthier than delivery pizza, and they're often a lot less expensive too.

In this section, I help you to fill your hotel fridge with satiating staples, take advantage of the complementary continental breakfast, and even order room service.

Stocking the hotel fridge

When possible, choose a room that has a mini fridge and microwave. With a well-stocked fridge and a way to warm food, you're on your way to a relaxing stay. Consider having a few things at the ready for quick lunches, dinners, snacks, and especially breakfasts. It's a great time and money saver.

Whenever I reach my final destination on a trip, my first stop is usually the local grocery store. If they have a natural grocery store like a co-op, Trader Joe's, or Whole Foods, I know they're going to have lots of options. However, even Target,

Walmart, and mainstream grocery store chains are really stepping up their game in terms of plant-based alternatives. It's amazing to see how many vegan specialty items are available. You can pick up sandwich fixings, oatmeal, dips and spreads, and other staples for your stay. (In the next section, I offer meal ideas you can make in your hotel room. Use that as a guide for ingredients you might want to procure.)

TIP

Natural grocery stores often have a wealth of vegan options at the deli and salad bar. Look for substantive salads like wheat berry–based salads, bean salads, or tofu salads, as well as prepared tofu. At the salad bar, you can make a hearty salad, or use the individual ingredients for meals in the room later. For example, a pile of raw vegetables can be a snack on their own, a dipping implement with your favorite dairy-free dip, or a sandwich topping. While you're there, see if any of the daily soups in the deli are vegan.

Finish your grocery store visit by picking up any drinks you want for the room, like sparkling water, coffee, or wine. (Much cheaper than paying later for something from the mini bar or a gourmet coffee drink!)

Preparing meals in the room

Here are some meals you can put together in your hotel room:

» **Chia pudding:** Put 2 tablespoons of chia seeds into a container with ½ cup of nondairy milk. If you like, add a squeeze of liquid sweetener like agave or maple syrup. Stir well. Let it sit for a couple of minutes, and stir again. Then pop it in the refrigerator overnight. The seeds will absorb the liquid, and become plump and pudding-like. In the morning, top it with sliced fruit, nuts, or granola.

» **Oatmeal:** Add hot water to an individual oatmeal cup or packet. Or make overnight oats by putting ½ cup of rolled oats into a container. Cover the oats with an equal amount of nondairy milk and stir. Pop it in the fridge overnight. In the morning, enjoy your oats cold or warmed in the microwave. Top with candied pecans, sliced bananas, or berries.

» **Breakfast sandwich:** Make a bagel breakfast sandwich with vegan cream cheese and a JUST Egg Folded, which is a vegan egg patty made from mung beans. You can find them in the freezer section of the grocery store, and they're ready to heat in the microwave and eat. For the bagel, many hotels offer a toaster oven in the breakfast area.

» **Toast with nut butter:** Top toasted bread with individual packets of nut butter. If you don't see nut butter packets at the grocery store, consider getting fresh nut butter, which you purchase by weight. (It's usually near the bulk bins.) That way you can buy the amount you need for the trip and not have to commit to a whole jar.

>> **Tofu sandwich or wrap:** Add baked marinated tofu slabs to bread or a tortilla with the condiments of your choice and lots of veggies.

>> **Yogurt parfait:** Nondairy yogurt is a delicious and easy option that has a bump of protein. Top it with granola and berries.

>> **Cereal:** Pick up your favorite dry cereal and some nondairy milk. (Don't want to commit to a large container of nondairy milk? Buy an individual-sized bottle or carton.)

>> **Soup:** Look for canned vegan soups with pull tabs, so you won't need a can opener. Pour into a bowl and heat in the microwave. Grocery stores also sell dried soups that just require hot water.

>> **Nachos:** Top tortilla chips with jarred vegan queso or vegan cheese shreds. Add spoonfuls of vegetarian refried beans or black beans. (Look for beans in pouches, which makes for easier opening.) Warm your nachos in the microwave. Finish with dollops of guacamole, salsa, and jalapeños.

>> **Premade or frozen meals:** Take a tour of the prepared and frozen foods area of the grocery store. Pick up one of these easy meals that you just have to heat and eat.

Having a bed picnic

One of my favorite meals at a hotel is a bed picnic. That's when you pull together a bunch of snacks for a meal of nibbles. Then you eat it all in bed, like the hotel version of a grazing board. (Worried about getting kicked out of bed for eating crackers? Dine at the in-room desk instead!)

Pick any or all of the following:

>> Fruit

>> Hummus

>> Nuts

>> Tofu slabs

>> Vegetable slices from the grocery store salad bar

>> Premade deli salads

>> Vegan deli slices

- » Vegan cheese
- » Crackers or crusty bread
- » Pickled veggies
- » Olives (jarred or from the grocery store olive bar)
- » *Dolmas,* or stuffed grape leaves (canned or from the grocery store deli)

Making the most of continental breakfasts and hotel buffets

While some all-vegan hotels and resorts do exist, many mainstream hotel breakfasts are on the underwhelming side for vegans. The usual fare includes buttery pastries, bacon, eggs, and non-vegan waffles. Outside of fresh fruit or dry cereal, plant-based options tend to be few and far between.

TIP

Some chains offer roasted potatoes, which can be pretty substantive on their own. If you have anything in your hotel room to eat with them, that's even better. For example, if you add the roasted potatoes to a tortilla with beans and nondairy cheese, you suddenly have a breakfast burrito.

Many hotels also offer oatmeal. Finish it with sliced banana, dried fruit, and nuts. Occasionally chains have nondairy milk available for coffee and cereal. Request it if you don't see it on offer.

Enjoying hotel room service and restaurants

If you're traveling to a city that's known for its vegan-friendliness like Los Angeles or New York City, you may be pleasantly surprised at the vegan options available from your hotel's in-room and on-site dining. In other locales, the offerings may be less than inspiring.

On occasions when choices were slim, I have cobbled together meals from room service like an omelet without the eggs. The omelet on the menu came with potatoes, onions, garlic, spinach, and bell peppers. I simply asked for all those fillings sautéed in oil. I completed the meal with a fruit bowl, toast, and jelly. It wasn't the best breakfast of my life, but I've had worse.

TIP

If you stay at a hotel that has a Starbucks location in the lobby, you're assured to have nondairy milk and a vegan breakfast option as well. When I'm traveling, I like to start my day with a soy latte and oatmeal with blueberries.

Some hotels promote that they make their coffee using Starbucks beans, but that isn't the same thing. Only actual Starbucks locations will have food options and consistently offer nondairy milk.

Many hotel restaurants have salad or pizza as a menu option. If they do, order salad with balsamic dressing, or pizza without cheese and with plenty of vegetables.

TIP

If you truly want to pamper yourself, seek out an all-vegan hotel or resort like Stanford Inn in Northern California, MOD Santorini in Greece, or Mother Earth Vegan Hotel in Costa Rica. At an exclusively vegan property you're guaranteed to have a wealth of options for room service and on-site dining.

Requesting Meals at Bed-and-Breakfasts

For a non-hotel option, bed-and-breakfasts (B&Bs) can be a good choice. It's awfully nice to wake up and have a hot breakfast waiting for you. To find a vegan-friendly B&B, simply google the area you're going plus "vegan bed and breakfast." If you're lucky, you'll discover a vegan gem like The White Pig B&B in Schuyler, Virginia, Pebble Cove Farm in Eastsound, Washington, or Black Sheep Inn and Spa in Hammondsport, New York.

Even if a B&B isn't strictly vegan, they can often prepare a plant-based meal. I've had great luck emailing B&B managers ahead of time (before booking) to see if it's an option. If the owner is unfamiliar with how to make vegan breakfasts, it doesn't hurt to email some ideas or links to recipes.

Early in our marriage, my husband and I traveled to the Cotswolds in England. We stayed at a B&B inside a renovated schoolhouse. Although it wasn't a vegan establishment, the proprietor took so much care making delicious plant-based meals for us every morning. While everyone else was having standard breakfast fare, we were dining on stuffed tomatoes, blueberry-laden porridge, and indulgent grain bowls. The other guests were getting jealous and asking for vegan meals too! The proprietor even made vegan cake to go with our afternoon tea. It was wonderfully cozy, and we felt truly pampered.

Another time we stayed at a B&B in St. Paul, Minnesota. Unbeknownst to me, the proprietor looked up recipes from my own website to serve me! I thought our breakfasts looked awfully familiar, and exactly like things I'd enjoy eating. So if it's not too much work, maybe start a vegan blog before you travel? Ha ha!

Eating Well While Staying at Vacation Rentals

These days a lot of people are opting for short-term vacation rentals like Airbnb. One major plus is that you have access to a kitchen and can stock it with vegan essentials. Some hosts are even willing to grab a few items for you before you arrive.

TIP

Before I reserve a place, I like to check Google Maps or www.happycow.net to see which locations are closest to vegan restaurants and natural grocery stores. I know I'll save on gas or rideshare costs if I can easily walk to the places I want to visit.

After you've made a reservation on Airbnb, you can fill out a form to tell your host why you're visiting. I like to let them know that I'm excited to check out the area's vegan restaurant scene. The reason I tell them that is twofold:

>> Hosts sometimes leave little treats in the rental like freshly made cookies or local snacks. I don't want them to go to the trouble of getting non-vegan things I won't eat.

>> Once the hosts know I'm vegan, they occasionally leave vegan snacks instead, like one host who stocked a snack bowl with a variety of vegan muffins. Sometimes they also give me great recommendations for vegan restaurants I need to try.

The hosts of an Airbnb where I stayed in Milwaukee, Wisconsin, also happened to be vegan. We messaged back and forth, and they basically wrote up a full itinerary of all the places I needed to go in the city, plus what to order while I was there. I love getting that kind of insight from locals who really know the scene.

Navigating Meals in Airports

If you're planning to travel by air to get from point A to point B, you've got to contend with the airport first. While some large airports offer a wealth of vegan riches, at others the vegan options include such highlights as potato chips and a banana. (Shout-out to Iowa's Cedar Rapids airport! Womp, womp.)

Even if you're going through a vegan-friendly airport, you never know when a delay will cause a tight connection that doesn't allow for grabbing a bean burrito or veggie burger. Plus, a missed flight can mean you're spending a whole lot more time at the airport than you'd planned — sometimes after hours when the restaurants have closed.

So I always like to pack for flights as if I'm going on a long adventure, even if it's supposed to be a quick jaunt. I'd rather be overprepared with snacks I can eat at my destination than ravenous and stuck in a middle seat with a grumbling stomach.

Here are some things to consider when you're preparing airplane meals yourself:

>> **Remember the Transportation Security Administration's (TSA) 3-1-1 liquids rule.** One passenger is allowed one quart-sized bag of liquids, gels, creams, or pastes in their carry-on. The containers cannot exceed 3.4 ounces (100 milliliters). The 3-1-1 rule includes any foods that qualify as liquids.

Note that while you *can't* pack a jar of vegan mayo in your carry-on, you *can* spread some on your packed sandwich without a problem.

>> **Be wary of pastes.** Other foods to be careful about are ones that resemble pastes, like guacamole, hummus, peanut butter, or vegan cream cheese. They're a no go in a carry-on, unless they're slathered on a sandwich.

>> **Pack an empty reusable water bottle in your carry-on.** While you can't take a filled water bottle through security, once you've been screened, you can fill it at a water fountain on the other side.

Carrying on your own food

Here are some easy meal ideas to make at home and take on the plane:

>> Deli sandwich with store-bought vegan deli slices, vegan mayo, lettuce, and tomato

>> Pasta salad tossed in balsamic vinaigrette

>> Kale salad with roasted chickpeas (Because of the liquid rule, don't pack the dressing separately. Toss it with the kale before you go.)

>> Veggie wrap

>> Slabs of marinated baked tofu (Great for snacking or adding to a sandwich.)

>> Instant noodle cups and oatmeal cups (Most airplanes have hot water available.)

>> Hard vegan cheese slices, crackers, and pickles (Soft cheeses would be confiscated because they're a paste.)

Here are a few snack ideas for the plane:

>> Popcorn

>> Fresh or dried fruit

>> Chips

>> Vegan jerky

>> Crackers

>> Nuts other than peanuts (in case someone on the plane is allergic)

>> Sunflower or pumpkin seeds

>> Pretzels

REMEMBER

Don't forget a fork or spoon! Unless an airline has dinner service on their plane, they usually won't have extra sets of flatware around.

TIP

Return flights can be a little trickier for meal and snack packing if you don't have access to a kitchen at your destination. In those instances, I like to grab an extra meal at my final restaurant stop, or visit a natural grocery store to get a vegan to-go item.

HOW TO KEEP FOOD COLD ON THE PLANE

Just like packing a lunch for work or school, you'll want to use common sense for keeping foods cold and within safety standards. Using an insulated lunch bag is an obvious first step.

According to the TSA guidelines, an ice pack can go through the security checkpoint as long as it's frozen solid during screening. If the pack has started to melt, is slushy, or has left behind liquid at the bottom of the container, it will have to meet the 3-1-1 liquid requirements, or it won't be permitted.

To keep things cold, freeze your ice packs well ahead of time, and don't put them into your insulated container until you're heading out the door. Adding a frozen food, like frozen grapes, can also help keep things cool.

Finding airport food options

Depending on how large the airport is, your choices will vary greatly. Smaller, out-of-the-way airports may only have a newsstand. Huge regional hubs have large food courts with fast-food places, lounges, and restaurants. (At the Denver airport, you can even get vegan donuts at VooDoo Doughnuts!)

If you have time when you land, do a quick Google search for vegan options at your airport. You'd be surprised at the number of up-to-date online guides, which can help pare down your options.

Here are some ideas about where to look for vegan food to tide you over until you reach your destination:

> » **Newsstands:** At these stands you often can find trail mix, fruit, nuts, chips, pretzels, and crackers.

> » **Fast-food chains:** More and more fast-food places are offering vegan options. Grab an Impossible Whopper from Burger King, nondairy ice cream from Ben & Jerry's, bean tacos at Qdoba, a pretzel without butter at Wetzel's, a falafel rice bowl at Garbanzo, a bagel with hummus at Einstein Bros., or a fruit smoothie at Jamba. (Check out Chapter 18 for a lot more vegan fast-food ideas.)

> » **Restaurants:** It's rare to find airport restaurants with clearly labeled vegan options, but it does happen occasionally. When in doubt, ask the staff for help. Look for dishes like stir-fried vegetables with rice, vegetarian burritos and tacos (hold the cheese and sour cream), hummus plates, falafel pita wraps, cheeseless vegetable pizza, veggie burgers, or pasta with marinara.

> » **Lounges, airline clubs, and bars:** These types of places usually offer crackers, bread with oil and vinegar, pretzels, nuts, olives, wine, and hot beverages.

TIP

At some airports, different gates are easy to access through a belowground tram. If you have plenty of time on your hands, consider venturing to another gate for better food options. Just don't miss your flight!

Ordering a vegan meal for your flight

Some domestic flights offer snacks for purchase onboard. Vegan options often include chips, popcorn, or hummus. In place of the peanuts or pretzels of yore, flight attendants often hand out complimentary Biscoff cookies, which are vegan.

Going on an international flight? When making your reservation, request a vegan meal. Most airlines require that vegan meals be booked at least 24 hours before takeoff. Look for the meal code VGML (Vegetarian Vegan Meal).

TIP

When you get to the airport check-in counter, confirm with the agent that your special meal request has been noted on the flight plan. You may not be able to get a vegan meal onboard if the request didn't go through, but at least you'll know to pick something up in the airport before getting on the plane.

Also try to alert the flight attendants of your special request when you're sitting down before takeoff. Doing so helps them keep you in mind and note where you are so your meal doesn't end up on someone else's tray table. (One bonus of getting a special meal is that you're usually served first, before the passengers with standard meals.)

The offerings and quality of meals vary from one airline to the next. In the best-case scenario, you'll be treated to a spicy lentil stew, bean chili, or spaghetti marinara. In the worst case, they'll forget to load your meal onto the plane, and you'll be rationing out potato chips for your long-haul flight.

TIP

If, for some reason, your special meal didn't make it on the plane, ask if any suitable first- or business-class meals are left. The attendants may be able to remedy the situation with extra fruit, bread, or appropriate snacks if your meal was mislaid.

"Seasing" the Day: Vegan Dining on Cruises

Ready to trade dry land for a floating city? Get on board a vegan-friendly cruise. Most ships offer a huge variety of food around the clock. Certain cruise lines like Oceania, Virgin, Princess, Regent Seven Seas, and Holland America are more vegan-friendly than others. So if you have the opportunity, do your research and find a boat that caters more specifically to you and your vacation dreams.

Do a Google search of the cruise line you're considering plus the word *vegan*. Lots of bloggers like to share pictures of the meals they ate on their trips. It gives you a chance to see an unedited version of what to expect.

Disney cruises, especially aboard the *Disney Wish*, are known to be vegan-friendly. There's usually a vegan appetizer and entree on each menu that's labeled as plant-based. Plus, chefs are happy to veganize meaty dishes. You can also order off-menu with options like avocado toast, vegan chicken tenders, vegan Mickey waffles, or a vegan omelet.

Royal Caribbean offers a full vegan dinner menu in their main cabin with different options available every night.

You can even book all-vegan cruises like Vegan Culinary Cruises and Holistic Holiday at Sea. Along with a 100 percent plant-based menu, Holistic Holiday at Sea offers presentations with health experts and leaders in the vegan community. In the past, they've also had themed parties like nondairy ice cream socials, vegan pizza parties, and nacho nights.

Even if it's not an entirely vegan cruise, any cruise ship will be familiar with and offer many vegetarian options. When you book your trip, fill out any of the necessary online forms regarding your dietary needs. If you're booking through a travel agent or over the phone, let them know that you're vegan. If in doubt, send a message through the special needs email address or call the cruise line's customer service department with any questions or concerns.

TIP

Consider getting a room with a mini fridge, so you can store nondairy milk for coffee and cereal, any snacks you like, plus future food finds from your ports of call. You can also bring along shelf-stable foods like instant soup mixes, energy bars, or nuts.

REMEMBER

On the first night of your cruise, let the head waiter know about your dietary needs at the beginning of dinner service. The chef will most likely veganize something from their regular or vegetarian menu. If you're really lucky, they'll bring out a menu of vegan options. Once dinner is nearing its end, you'll be given the option to order future meals in advance, along with any alterations you prefer.

While you're on the ship, here are a few more to-do's:

>> Check out the menus of any restaurants onboard. Ask the staff to confirm with the chef what can be prepared vegan.

>> Visit the buffet to load up on roasted veggies, rice, pasta, and fruit. If the ingredients aren't labeled, ask a staff member for guidance.

>> Some cruise lines have apps that show vegan options or allow you to make special requests. If your cruise line has one, download it before you go.

WARNING

It's worth noting that some vegans take issue with cruising because of environmental concerns like air pollution, sewage treatment, the effect on fragile habitats, marine life, and coastal communities, worker treatment, and food waste. Before booking a cruise, you may want to do more research into these issues if they are a concern for you.

Chowing Down on Camping Trips

Camping getaways have only gotten more popular in recent years. They're a great way to escape from it all, enjoy the beautiful outdoors, and avoid crowds.

With so many vegan camping meal options to explore, you can cook while you're at the campsite, prepare sandwiches and salads in advance, or do a combination of both.

Packing prepared foods

When you're camping, you may not want to start a fire every time hunger strikes. So it's nice to have some premade options that you can enjoy right away. Pack any of these foods ahead of time, and then savor them in nature:

>> Homemade vegan muffins or banana bread

>> Store-bought or homemade bean dip, *baba ghanoush* (smoky eggplant dip), *muhammara* (walnut and roasted red pepper dip), salsa, or olive tapenade (They can all be used on sandwiches, in wraps, or as dips.)

>> Tortilla Pinwheels (For a complete recipe, see Chapter 13.)

>> Potato salad (Make it with vegan mayo. Consider adding lots of crunchy pickles, minced onion, and shredded carrots for more veggie goodness.)

>> Pasta Salad with Creamy Dressing (Get the recipe in Chapter 14.)

>> Coleslaw (Make it with vegan mayo for a tasty side dish or sandwich topping.)

>> Vegan chicken salad (Enjoy it on a sandwich, scoop it onto crackers, pile it into hollowed-out tomatoes, or roll it into a tortilla. Use the Chicken-Free Salad Sandwich recipe in Chapter 13.)

Cooking at the campsite

Hiking, boating, and biking really get your stomach grumbling! Here are some food ideas for the grill or campfire:

>> **Cast-iron breakfast skillet:** Add veggie sausage patties and crumbled super-firm tofu to an oiled cast-iron skillet. Top the tofu with seasonings like cumin, chili powder, paprika, granulated onion, and salt. Add any veggies you enjoy, like onions, bell peppers, mushrooms, or dark leafy greens. Close the

grill cover, and allow it all to warm. Once it's brown and toasty on one side, flip with a long spoon or spatula, and continue cooking until everything is beautifully browned.

» **Refried bean quesadillas:** Slather a tortilla with homemade or store-bought refried beans. Then sandwich it with another tortilla. Cook it in a grill basket or cast-iron skillet over a fire until browned on one side. Then flip it to brown the other. Serve with sliced avocado or guacamole.

» **Toasted peanut butter and banana tortillas:** Follow the directions for refried bean quesadillas, but use peanut butter and slices of banana for the filling.

» **Veggie burgers or dogs:** Grab store-bought veggie burgers or dogs for quick grilled meals. (Keep in mind that burgers and dogs made from seitan or pea protein hold up better on the grill than burgers made from beans or veggies alone.) Put the grilled burgers or dogs in toasted buns, and finish with your choice of condiments and veggie toppings.

» **Veggie fajitas:** Toss sliced vegetables with seasonings, oil, and a squeeze of lime juice. Pop them in a grill basket, and cook until they're fire-licked and caramelized. Warm corn tortillas on the grill to go with them. Then pile on guacamole or sliced avocado to finish.

» **Marinated tofu:** Before you head to the campsite, throw slabs of super-firm tofu in a sealed freezer bag with a lemon and garlic marinade. Then when you get to the campsite, start the fire, and grill the marinated tofu for about 10 minutes on each side (until dark grill marks form).

» **Grilled vegetables:** Toss thickly sliced vegetables in an herb vinaigrette, and marinate for about 30 minutes. Think zucchini, bell peppers, button mushrooms, grape tomatoes, red onions, and steamed baby potatoes. Spear the vegetables with long metal skewers, and grill for 8 to 10 minutes. Remember to rotate often for even cooking. (Grab the complete recipe for Grilled Vegetable Skewers in Chapter 14.)

» **Grilled portobello mushrooms:** Marinate portobello mushroom caps in an herb vinaigrette for about 30 minutes. Then grill for about 4 minutes on each side. Enjoy them as a main course, side dish, or burger alternative.

» **Corn on the cob:** Remove the silks and husks, oil the corn, and grill for about 10 minutes, turning as needed with tongs. The corn picks up the smokiest flavor this way. If you'd prefer, you can grill the corn in the husk. Just remove the silks, and pull the husks back up to cover the corn. Grill for 15 to 20 minutes, turning often to char the husks evenly.

>> **Chili or stew:** Place a cast-iron Dutch oven over your fire to make a hearty chili or stew. Use your choice of veggies, beans, plant meat, fire-roasted tomatoes, and spices for a satisfying meal.

>> **Campfire nachos:** Put a layer of tortilla chips into a lightly oiled cast-iron Dutch oven. Top with salsa, shredded vegan cheese, and pinto or black beans. Add another layer of chips and toppings. Then cover the Dutch oven and place it on the metal grill over your campfire. Cook for about 15 minutes or until the cheese has melted. Serve with any other toppings you enjoy, like guacamole, cilantro, olives, jalapeños, or vegan sour cream.

Chapter **20**

Navigating Tricky Social Situations

Here's a secret you should know about veganism: The food is the easy part.

People often assume that figuring out meals or getting enough protein are what's complicated. Nope, that stuff works itself out. Once you've made a few simple swaps and created new habits, you can just coast. And although it may seem impossible to believe in our protein-obsessed culture, getting enough protein while on a plant-based diet is a cinch.

However, no matter how long you're vegan, you always have to interact with other people. You make friends, get hired at new jobs, become acquainted with the neighbors, or stumble into awkward conversations with people you've known for a long time.

Whether you've been vegan for a day or a decade, there will be times when you have to navigate a tricky conversation or situation.

On *Sesame Street* they sang, "One of these kids is doing his own thing . . . Come on, can you tell which one?" They'd show three kids happily jumping rope while the fourth kid was doing something different — like jumping jacks. The kids seemed entirely content, but outside of public television, a person may feel self-conscious when breaking away from what's expected.

Living vegan in a non-vegan world means that sometimes you're the only one in a group doing something different. Because of that, you have to advocate for yourself, and give words to your needs. Depending on your personality, it may take time, patience, and energy to get acclimated.

In this chapter, I empower you to be proactive about your dietary requirements and offer ways to handle sticky conversations with grace. I also lay out the reasons why feeding the trolls isn't worth the effort.

Following Party Etiquette as a Vegan Guest

I have a non-vegan friend who is an amazing host and cook. I know if I go to her home for dinner, she's going to serve elaborate cocktails, homemade focaccia with dill cashew dip, tempeh satay, and almond cheese–stuffed figs for dessert. If you have a similar friend, lucky you! Bring along a bottle of wine to share, and call it a day.

However, most of the time when you're a vegan guest at the home of non-vegans, you need to be a little more hands-on with your preparation. Whether you're invited to a party for a birthday, graduation, or retirement, go in with a plan. A prepared vegan is a happy vegan.

Eat before you go

If it's an informal gathering like someone's retirement party or a backyard graduation party, there's a good chance that the vegan offerings will be slim (unless the person who is being honored is vegan too).

TIP

I recommend going with the assumption that nothing will be vegan, and don't arrive famished. Then if you're greeted by some accidentally vegan food like a fruit tray, carrot sticks and hummus, potato chips, or tortilla chips and salsa, it's a nice surprise.

Sometimes people go out of their way to include something plant-based, but better safe than sorry!

Ask about the menu

You've been invited to a large dinner party with some kind of food theme like a sandwich bar, taco bar, or pizza party? Talk to the host ahead of time.

Ask questions about the type of food they're planning. If they need suggestions for a vegan option to include, recommend things that fit with what they're already making.

>> If it's a sandwich bar, hummus, or vegan deli meats are an easy choice. They can just pick up prepared items if they don't want to make their own.

>> If it's a taco bar, warmed black beans and soy chorizo are simple options.

>> If it's a pizza party, suggest a cheeseless pizza with lots of vegetables.

TIP

Always offer to bring something to help ease the load. It's best to ask first, so the host doesn't go to a lot of work and then feel like your dish is "competing" with what they've made. If the host takes you up on it, choose something that's sub-stantive enough to be your main course but is also a complementary side dish for others.

Make a vegan version of the menu

Another option is to find out what's being served and bring along a vegan version of the menu. This trick is often suggested for the parents of vegan children.

For example, say a vegan child is going to a birthday party where deli sandwiches and potato chips will be served for lunch. Then for dessert, they'll have chocolate cake. Pick up vegan deli slices to make a sandwich, and of course, potato chips are already vegan. Then bring along a slice of vegan cake for the vegan child to eat.

TIP

You can make a whole cake and send the child with a slice. Or you can stop by a natural grocery store to pick up vegan cake sold by the slice. (I recommend telling the birthday girl or boy's parents you're sending along lunch and dessert, in case they already have a vegan option in mind.)

The vegan child's 7-year-old peers won't know the difference if they're eating turkey or Tofurky. It's important to some kids that they "fit in" and not feel like they stand out for eating differently.

Even though kids are the ones who often have that reputation, I don't think adults are so far off sometimes. When you're having dinner, you don't always want the conversation to turn to you and what you're eating or not eating.

A while back my husband and I were invited to my niece's birthday party for dinner and cake. On her birthday, she always requests her favorite lasagna. A different year, my sister-in-law threw some noodles in for us along with jarred pasta sauce. It totally worked. But this time I decided to do something different, especially since I knew my brother and sister-in-law had their hands full getting the house ready for guests and preparing for the party. I assured them that we could handle our dinner for the evening.

The night before the party, I made a small tray of vegan lasagna. My husband and I had it for dinner. Then I cut out two large pieces and put them in a glass storage container for the next day.

When the time came for dinner, I heated our lasagna. Since we were eating lasagna like everyone else, we avoided the sometimes awkward discussions that start with, "Now, what are YOU having?"

It takes a little more planning, but in the right circumstances, making a vegan version of the planned menu can be a fun alternative.

Remember what's important

I'm always thankful when people invite me into their homes, often going out of their way to make me feel included and considered. But at the end of the day, what we remember about celebrations has very little to do with the food.

It's about celebrating the birthday boy or girl, spending time with family and friends, and just enjoying being together. Although many celebrations seem to revolve around food, the ultimate goal is connecting.

If your dinner one night is an odd menagerie of side dishes, it's just one meal. There will be others. Stay in the present moment, enjoy yourself, and remember that what makes events special are the memories you're creating.

Attending Gatherings at Meat-Heavy Restaurants

Recently a chef made headlines because he banned vegans from his restaurant. Apparently, someone who is vegan had called to ask about plant-based options for an upcoming dinner gathering. The chef said he would accommodate her. But when she arrived for dinner, he had forgotten about it. It was a busy night, and the only option he had was lacking and expensive. She gave the restaurant a negative review, and the chef took it to heart and put out a blanket ban on vegans.

Many people who commented on the online article were confused about why a vegan would go to a meat-heavy restaurant in the first place. One reason is that sometimes vegans aren't the ones choosing. Vegans have non-vegan friends who have celebrations at steakhouses. Vegans have jobs and sometimes have to attend organized business lunches.

In Chapter 18, there's a full section on how to order vegan meals at restaurants, and which restaurants have the highest likelihood of offering satisfying vegan options. However, if you end up at a meat-heavy restaurant, here are some suggestions:

» **Look at the menu ahead of time.** See if there's anything vegan or "veganizable" on the menu.

» **Call the restaurant or direct message them on Facebook or Instagram, if necessary.** Ask about their vegan options, or see if the chef is willing to prepare an off-menu vegan option.

   It's a lot more comfortable to ask these questions ahead of time than with an audience of 12 other dinner guests staring at you. Plus, on a busy night, the server and chef are juggling a lot. Preplanning helps everyone involved.

   If it's a work dinner that someone else is organizing, I still recommend that you call and speak to the restaurant yourself. It's like that game of telephone. What you tell your coworker may not be what the chef hears. Perhaps your coworker doesn't know the difference between vegetarian, vegan, and gluten-free. Or maybe your coworker thinks that a small side salad with oil and vinegar qualifies as a vegan dinner option. Talk to the restaurant yourself for a higher chance of success.

» **Eat ahead of time if the restaurant doesn't appear to have many vegan options.** Then when you go, order a drink, side salad, or french fries. Or plan on having a nice dinner on your own afterward at some place more vegan-friendly.

   Depending on where you live, breakfast and brunch places are often the trickiest for finding vegan options. Outside of oatmeal and potato side dishes like hash browns or country potatoes, there's usually not a whole lot on the menu that's vegan. I recommend pregaming with a light breakfast at home, and then getting a small second breakfast at the restaurant.

Arranging Vegan Meals at Conferences

My husband loves to tell a story about a work trip he took a few years back. The conference was in a hotel, and they'd provided a form to note special dietary requests. He had high hopes because of that. Maybe they would pull through with a good vegan option — especially since it was in a larger city?

However, that dream was dashed at the first dinner. He was sitting with a lot of people he didn't know well, and multiple servers kept trying to give him the standard main course of salmon.

He kept telling the servers that he'd ordered the vegan option. Finally, one of them told him, "Oh, this is the vegan option. The salmon is prepared vegan."

My husband sent it away and was offered leftovers of the grilled vegetables that had been on the buffet line earlier in the day. He became very familiar with those grilled vegetables, as they were lunch and dinner the next day too. (Not a huge surprise, he ordered Thai food to his room later.)

When you're going to a conference for business or leisure, use these handy pointers:

>> **Ask the planners about vegan options.** When you're signing up for the conference, make a note of your needs on the appropriate form.

>> **Bring plenty of snacks in your checked luggage.** Or make a stop at the grocery store to stock your hotel room fridge. (Chapter 19 includes lots of ideas for hotel room meals.)

>> **Do a quick online search for nearby vegan options.** You can also check out the HappyCow app for possibilities. Then make a dash for a quick lunch or dinner if the conference's vegan options are lacking.

>> **Place a late-night order to your hotel room for a more substantive dinner, if needed.** A delivery order from a local Thai, Ethiopian, Indian, or Mediterranean restaurant will almost make you forget about the conference's meager options.

Understanding That Some People Have a Bias Against Vegan Food

In Chapter 1, I emphasize that vegan food is just food. And it is. It's vegetables and fruits. It's nuts, seeds, mushrooms, and grains. It's ordinary, everyday stuff. You know that, and I know that. But not everyone does.

Some people have really unfortunate ideas about what *vegan food* entails. The only thing they know about it is that it's the butt of many jokes. They assume it has to be terrible, flavorless, or really weird.

Research backs this up. A 2023 study from Massachusetts Institute of Technology (MIT) looked at the bias against vegan and vegetarian food labels. For one part of the study, researchers had people choose between two lunch options — a veggie hummus wrap or a Greek salad wrap. They found that when the hummus wrap was labeled "vegan," people were significantly less likely to order it. When the label was removed, people ordered it more often.

The study's lead author, Alex Berke, who is vegan, wasn't surprised by the results. She said, "Anyone who has been vegan or vegetarian for a while would not be surprised. They see the bias against these foods."

So it's not surprising that when a vegan walks into the room with cookies to share, some people are wary. They think, "No, thanks. I don't need any broccoli-flavored cookies." (Never mind that they probably already have vegan cookies in their pantry that go by the name of Oreo.)

In the time that I've been vegan, I've had people ignore my platters and bowls at gatherings. Some folks were suddenly "not hungry" once they realized the restaurant we popped into was vegan, and the fries they ordered were, gasp, also vegan. I've brought salsa to get-togethers and had other people eye it speculatively.

"Now what is that exactly?" they said cautiously.

"Tomato salsa."

It was vegan, just like every other salsa they'd ever eaten.

Another time I was disappointed that the vegan label was removed from the amazing cinnamon rolls at my local natural grocery store. When I asked the store about it, they said not to worry. The cinnamon rolls were still 100 percent vegan. It was just that shoppers wanted their baked goods to feel indulgent, and the vegan label worked against that. The store kept the same plant-based ingredients, but removed the label. Then they sold like hotcakes, or you know, cinnamon rolls.

One time my cousin jokingly told me I should stand far away from my "pariah cookies" so people would eat them. I did, and sure enough, people loved them.

For reference, vegan chocolate chip cookies are made with the following ingredients:

>> All-purpose flour

>> Baking powder

>> Baking soda

>> Sugar

>> Salt

>> Maple syrup

>> Oil

>> Vanilla

>> Semi-sweet chocolate chips

That's all ordinary stuff that most people eat. But once people hear it's vegan, watch out. Some folks suddenly recoil. Depending on your mood, it can be amusing or disappointing.

Now, some people will say, "Oh, well. More for me then!" And if that's how you feel, wonderful. But it can also be a little disheartening when you know something is delicious, but people reject it because of its branding. Plus, if you've spent time, money, and energy making dessert for 15, you may not feel great if you go home with enough leftovers for 14.

Here's some advice for making food for non-vegans at potlucks and holidays:

>> **Prepare your dish with positivity.** Remember that whatever dish you bring to share, many people will be receptive, delighted, and surprised by the delicious food the vegan at the potluck made.

>> **Make a dish because you like it.** Make something that you enjoy preparing and eating. If it's something involved or arduous, do it for you.

>> **Avoid announcing that it's vegan ahead of time.** People will likely figure it out if the vegan in the group brought it, of course. But in general, wait until they've enjoyed it to let them know. Just say, "I brought chocolate chip cookies!" Not "I brought *vegan* chocolate chip cookies!"

When people with negative preconceptions eat something vegan, they often go in looking for what's missing instead of just enjoying what's there.

REMEMBER

>> **Brace yourself that some people may not even try it.** If this happens to you, try to detach. Though it can be disappointing, it's not about you, what you brought, or your cooking. Try not to take it as a rejection.

>> **Consider how open your friends and family are to eating vegan dishes.** Once you've cooked for specific people a time or two, consider how receptive they are to plant-based dishes. Then weigh that against the amount of time you spend on cooking.

If it will make you happy to spend hours in the kitchen cooking, do it. But if spending a lot of time preparing food only to have it ignored will hurt your feelings or ruin your day, make something that's less involved — for your own happiness.

>> **Pick up takeout or store-bought items instead.** It can be a lot easier to not take things personally if you weren't involved in making the dish. Plus, sometimes people are more receptive to branded foods they recognize. And who knows? Maybe you'll turn them on to a great vegan product they can pick up at the store next time.

Responding to Jokes about Vegans

When you first go vegan, you may be surprised at the jokes aimed your way. You may get some timeless classics like, "Yeah, I love animals too . . . Next to the mashed potatoes."

Here are three reasons for the onslaught of jokes:

>> **They heard the joke, and they've been itching for an opportunity to tell it.** Here you are — a vegan right in front of them. This is their chance.

>> **Jokes are often used to defuse uncomfortable situations.** When people are suddenly aware of themselves or their habits in a way that makes them

feel defensive or uncomfortable, jokes are an easy release valve. They're a way of voicing that discomfort in a socially accepted way.

That's understandable and something we all do in one way or another at times. However, when veganism is totally new to you, and you're suddenly being teased regularly at mealtimes, it can get . . . tiresome.

>> **Jokes highlight beliefs that separate us or unite us.** Sometimes when you're a new vegan or the only one in the group, jokes create an interesting us-versus-them power dynamic, which can be very startling when you're suddenly in the minority. It can feel like you're getting piled on.

As a new vegan, what do you do? Become grumpy and let people think you're a spoilsport? Or laugh even when that tired joke is at your expense? (I mean, to the bald guy, is the tenth Mr. Clean joke funny? Probably not.)

Plus, when you are vegan for the animals, it can feel like the joker-in-question is not only laughing at you, but also making light of the very personal reasons you chose to go vegan in the first place.

TIP

Remember that misplaced jokes don't really have anything to do with you, even though they can feel personal. These wisecracks say more about the joker's views than they do about you.

Here's some good news:

>> **It gets easier.** After a while, the jokes slow way down. People run out of them, or they've already said their "best" ones so it's not an interesting topic anymore. It's old news.

>> **People become more comfortable with you being vegan.** They don't need to defuse an uncomfortable situation because they aren't uncomfortable.

>> **They realize you're still the same person you always were, and you're going to keep being vegan.** Why would they continue commenting on something that's not going to change?

Nowadays when I hear jokes, it's in one of two circumstances. It's either when I'm meeting new people and my veganism randomly comes up. Or it's when I'm with people I know very well who are comfortable with me being vegan.

In the first case, it's easier now to give people some slack. I get it. There was a time that veganism seemed very unfamiliar to me too. The only way I can communicate that vegans are warm, open, and have a sense of humor is if I give the same compassion I want to receive.

In the second situation, when my close family and friends joke with me about veganism these days, it's good-natured. They know I care very deeply about animals. They get it. And it feels entirely different when a joke is born out of long conversations and shared history. It's the kind of joke that recognizes our commonality.

Handling Awkward Conversations

Sometimes when people hear you're vegan, they can't help but steer the conversation toward meat. It's like a compulsion. All these words start falling out of their mouths, and you're there to witness it.

It's kind of fascinating really. They meet the person who wants to hear about it the least, and then they must tell you every last detail. Suddenly you're having a Forrest Gump–style conversation about the various meats they've enjoyed and the most obscure meats they've ever eaten.

I can't tell you how many times I've been at a vegan restaurant, and I've overheard people who thought they were hilariously unique by ordering steak. Or they talk at length about the most off-the-wall meats they've ever eaten. (At a vegan restaurant in Chicago, I overheard a guy at the next table telling his Tinder date about all the ways he'd eaten cicadas, including on pizza. Even she seemed perplexed.)

My husband and I stayed at an Airbnb a few months back. The owner was there to show us to the apartment. I had mentioned that I'm vegan and we were looking forward to trying the city's vibrant vegan scene.

She said, "So . . . vegan? You don't eat cheese or eggs?"

"Nope."

"Never?" she said, unable to believe her ears.

"No, never."

"No fish?" she asked.

"No, no fish."

Then she said, "Oh, I could be vegetarian. I don't eat much meat. I don't even really like it . . . except for bacon. I love bacon."

I tried to change the subject, but she just kept bringing it back to bacon . . . over and over again.

"Yes, a lot of people say that," I told her.

I don't know if she even realized she was doing it. That kind of thing happens often.

Or you go out to dinner with someone, and they apologize to you for ordering meat. Mind you, that didn't stop them from ordering it. But while it's there in front of them, they feel uncomfortable, like they've committed a faux pas.

In that kind of situation, I really don't like being apologized to. If a person wants to abstain from meat around me of their own volition, that's lovely, and I appreciate the consideration. But when someone apologizes once the meat is on the table, what's the expectation? It puts me in a position where I'm supposed to make them feel okay about it.

Most people in the world aren't vegan, and 99.9 percent of the people in my day-to-day life eat meat. But I really don't want to be the one who's expected to make other people feel all right about it. Plenty of people are out there doing that work. It doesn't have to be me.

If someone apologizes for eating fried chicken in front of you, try saying, "Why are you apologizing to me? I'm not a chicken."

Dealing with Bullies Online and in Real Life

Veganism is something that many people have opinions about — whether they're vegan or not. Because of that, it's a topic that people just love to argue about.

A folksy, country-themed restaurant offered plant-based sausage on their menu a while back. When they posted about it online, meat-eating commenters were furious. The post generated more than 22,000 comments, many from people who were irate about the plant-based addition. They accused the restaurant of being "woke," simply for having a meatless option. Mind you, the restaurant hadn't taken away any of their meat options. They were just offering something new for those who wanted it.

Whether it's a Facebook post by a restaurant announcing their new vegan options or your uncle who loves playing devil's advocate, when some folks hear the word *vegan*, they have an immediate and obvious knee-jerk reaction: They're ready to argue about it.

If you happen to be in the firing line, please remember this: Just because you're invited to an argument, that doesn't mean you have to accept the invitation.

Consider that the stakes may be higher for you. Most people who are vegan have researched the many reasons behind it and given it a lot of careful thought. It's usually not something a person does lightly. You may have deep, personal reasons why you chose this lifestyle. However, that may or may not be true of the people who would like to argue with you about it.

People who argue for the sake of arguing are rarely looking to understand someone else's viewpoint. They just want to win the argument. When there's an imbalance of skin in the game, there's really no way to come out the other side feeling good about it. It often just leads to frustration. You can usually tell when a person is asking a question because they're sincerely interested in knowing something, or when they just want to debate.

Remember that Google exists. You're not required to be someone else's search engine. If you feel like it, you can suggest some websites or books like this one, where they can get more information. If they seem disingenuous, just let it go, and save yourself some work.

TIP

If it's a public social media post, I recommend staying away altogether. Like they say, don't read the comments. Responding to someone who is strongly anti-vegan only means they'll direct their ire toward you. Save yourself. It's not worth it.

Something else that's important to remember about trolls online is that the argument is public. Think about when you were in high school, and a fight broke out in the hallway. Onlookers would chant, "Fight! Fight!" People would gather around as if a professional wrestling match was going to take place. With that kind of attention, it would have been very hard for one of the angry high schoolers to say, "Hey, I think this has gone too far. We should talk it out." Instead, the fight didn't end until a teacher broke it up.

Although the internet isn't your high school hallway, it is a public forum. When people see an argument brewing, they start piling on with comments, adding emojis, and fanning the flames of conflict. In that setting, it's difficult to have a productive conversation. It's hard to hear someone else's viewpoint or have a changed perspective when an ego is on the line.

Those types of debates are rarely useful. Be assured that information about veganism is out there and easily accessible. If someone truly wants to know more, there are plenty of places to find it. You don't have to be the one doing unpaid labor decoding veganism for someone else.

6

Veganism in All Walks of Life

Meet your nutritional needs while pregnant and nursing.

Help your children blossom — from infancy through their teenage years — with nutritious and filling meals.

Dive into the vegan lifestyle on your college campus.

Flourish as a vegan athlete with a plant-powered diet.

Get a boost by embracing veganism in middle age and beyond.

IN THIS CHAPTER

» **Planning for a healthy vegan pregnancy**

» **Understanding daily nutrition requirements when eating for two**

» **Preparing meals during pregnancy**

» **Dealing with common issues that pop up in pregnancy**

» **Providing yourself with great nutrition and self-care after giving birth**

Chapter **21**

Healthy Vegan Pregnancy and Postpartum Period

C ountless people have brought healthy babies into the world while eating a vegan diet. So don't feel like you're venturing into unknown territory. A well-planned, healthy, and diverse vegan diet can meet your needs for pregnancy, breastfeeding, and beyond.

Plus, a diet that's rich in fruits and veggies may protect against certain pregnancy complications like gestational diabetes and *preeclampsia* (high blood pressure). Additionally, it may reduce your baby's risk of developing diseases like diabetes, eczema, asthma, and even certain cancers.

Here is the position from the American Dietetic Association:

"It is the position of the American Dietetic Association that appropriately planned vegetarian diets, including total vegetarian or vegan diets, are healthful, nutritionally adequate, and may provide health benefits in the prevention and treatment of certain diseases. Well-planned vegetarian diets are appropriate for individuals during all stages of the life cycle, including pregnancy, lactation, infancy, childhood, and adolescence, and for athletes."

Proper nutrition is important before and during pregnancy, as well as while breastfeeding. This chapter covers the basics that any vegan who is planning on getting pregnant needs to know.

Focusing on Nutrition and Preparation

Preparedness is a must for parents-to-be. After all, once the baby arrives, just leaving the house will require packed bags full of extra clothes, sunscreen, toys, plenty of baby wipes, food, beverages, and so on. You and every other person who is expecting — vegan or not — need to plan ahead for your nutritional and health needs.

If you want to get pregnant in the next few years, or if you're actively trying to conceive, start eating the proper quality of foods now. That way when the test comes back positive, you're already on the right path.

Vegan foods are naturally high in many of the nutrients pregnant folks need. Get familiar with the U.S. Recommended Dietary Allowance (RDA) for iron, calcium, and other nutrients for the average person who isn't pregnant. (You can find all the details in Chapter 6.) Eat a varied diet of whole, fresh, and nutrient-dense foods to prepare your body for optimal health.

Consider prenatal vitamins

When you're pregnant, the extra nutrient demands for yourself and a growing fetus may feel like a stretch. A prenatal vitamin isn't a replacement for a healthy and varied diet, of course. But when you're struggling with morning sickness or random food aversions, prenatal vitamins can help fill any nutrition gaps, support your body, and help with your future child's development.

There are many vegan prenatal vitamins on the market. You'll have no problem finding one that suits your needs.

Here are a few options:

>> Garden of Life mykind Organics Vegan Prenatal Multi

>> Naturelo Prenatal Multivitamin

>> Deva Vegan Prenatal Multivitamin & Mineral

>> Freeda Prenatal One Daily

>> Ritual Essential Prenatal Multivitamins

Talk to your healthcare provider about which prenatal vitamin is best for you.

Involve healthcare professionals

As with all pregnancies, having a medical team behind you for support is paramount. Going to all your regular doctor visits, and getting their expertise is imperative.

If your doctor isn't well versed in vegan nutrition, consider finding a physician who can appropriately support you throughout your pregnancy. Or seek out a registered dietitian who fully understands the ins and outs of a vegan diet as it pertains to pregnancy and beyond. Even if there isn't a vegan dietitian in your area, you can connect with one online. (Just do a simple Google search to find one you like.) They can go over your current diet and future needs via video calls.

Knowing What to Include in a Well-Planned Diet

Throughout your pregnancy, you'll want to make sure you're meeting your calorie goals, as well as getting all the nutrients you need.

Caloric needs don't increase during the first trimester of pregnancy. However, they do increase in the second and third trimesters. In the second trimester, you need an extra 340 calories a day. In the third trimester, that amount goes up to an extra 450 calories a day. Depending on your weight, you may need more or fewer calories. Weight gain during pregnancy helps determine the calories needed.

Plant-based foods that are high in fiber may naturally fill you up quickly. So it's important to be aware of increased calorie needs and to monitor weight gain throughout pregnancy.

Become familiar with the recommendations in the following sections for folate and folic acid, protein, calcium, vitamin D, iron, vitamin B12, zinc, iodine, choline, and omega-3 fatty acids.

Protein

When you're pregnant, most protein recommendations hover around an extra 25 grams a day, especially during the second and third trimesters.

>> **For the first trimester:** You want to get about the same 45 to 50 grams of protein a day that you aim for when you aren't pregnant (or calculate 0.8 grams per kilogram of your prepregnancy body weight to get your individual protein needs).

>> **For the second and third trimesters:** Add 25 grams of protein for a total of between 70 and 75 grams (or 1.1 grams of protein per kilogram of your prepregnancy body weight). This level of protein is easily attainable — even on a plant-based diet. You can either eat larger portions of the protein you're already eating. Or you can add other protein-rich foods that may also help amp up your other nutrient needs, like calcium and iron.

Focus on eating a wide variety of plant foods like lentils, beans, tofu, whole grains, and vegetables. Table 21-1 shows you some easy ways to get extra protein along with some other great nutrients in one fell swoop.

TABLE 21-1 **Options for Extra Vegan Protein (and Other Important Nutrients)**

Protein Source	Serving Size	Protein (g)	Calcium (mg)	Iron (mg)	Zinc (mg)
Lentils, boiled	1 cup	17.9	37.6	6.59	2.52
Chickpeas, cooked	1 cup	14.5	80.4	4.74	2.51
Black beans, cooked	1 cup	15.2	46.4	3.61	1.93
Enriched pasta	1 cup	6.21	7.49	1.37	0.54
Silk unsweetened soy milk	1 cup	7	299	1.07	0.60
Hemp protein powder	4 tablespoons	12	44	6.01	Unlisted

Source: U.S. Department of Agriculture's FoodData Central

Vitamin B12

Vitamin B12 helps you maintain a healthy nervous system and produce blood cells. This vitamin crosses the placenta into the fetus. It's needed to help make DNA and other cell material.

Because many vitamins and minerals are needed in higher quantities during pregnancy, it's no surprise that B12 requirements are higher too. If you are pregnant or nursing, aim for between 2.6 and 2.8 micrograms (mcg) per day.

Vitamin B12 may be found in standard multivitamins, as well as prenatal vitamins. Or you can take a separate B12 supplement to make sure you're getting enough. Additionally, B12 can be found in foods like fortified nutritional yeast, enriched nondairy milks, vegan meats, and fortified cereals.

REMEMBER

Breastfed babies get their B12 through breast milk. They can store enough B12 from what they get in the womb to last 6 months to 1 year. So optimal intake during pregnancy and nursing is key. For more information on vitamin B12, refer to Chapter 6.

Omega-3 fatty acids

Omega-3's are essential fatty acids that build and protect your brain, organs, and eyes. They're necessary in greater amounts when you're pregnant.

There are three types of omega-3 fatty acids:

>> *Docosahexaenoic acid* (DHA)

>> *Eicosapentaenoic acid* (EPA)

>> *Alpha-linolenic acid* (ALA)

DHA and EPA are found in cold-water fish, algae, and krill, but you don't need fish or fish oil supplements for omega-3s. Plant-derived ALA is found in flaxseed, hemp seeds, edamame, seaweed, algae, and walnuts. Your body can convert ALA into EPA and DHA, which is important for proper fetal and infant development.

The National Academy of Medicine has set an Adequate Intake of 1.4 grams a day for ALA during pregnancy. To get your dose of omega-3 riches, grind flaxseed for smoothies, snack on walnuts, sprinkle hemp seeds on your salads, or make chia pudding. Or take a microalgae-based DHA and EPA supplement. The Academy of Nutrition and Dietetics and the World Health Organization (WHO) have issued various recommendations for DHA, ranging from 200 to 500 milligrams a day.

TIP

An easy way to integrate certain omega-3–rich oils, like flax oil, into your diet is to drizzle your daily serving on salad, steamed vegetables, or pasta. Or use it as a dip for warm bread along with balsamic vinegar. Heat damages the health benefits of these oils, so don't cook them. At 7 grams of ALA per tablespoon for flax oil, you're just a drizzle away from reaching your ALA needs for the day!

Calcium

Getting enough calcium while pregnant or breastfeeding shouldn't pose any problems while maintaining a vegan diet. The amount you need while pregnant is the same as before you were pregnant because the efficiency of calcium absorption from foods increases during pregnancy.

If you are 19 or older, the RDA for calcium during pregnancy and breastfeeding is 1,000 milligrams per day. For those who are 14 to 18 years old, the RDA is 1,300 milligrams per day during pregnancy. The WHO recommends similar calcium intake levels to prevent complications during pregnancy and early labor, and to promote proper fetal development.

Focus on healthy sources of calcium. Think dark leafy greens, tofu, enriched non-dairy milk, nuts, grains, figs, tahini, enriched cereal, sunflower seeds, and beans. Calcium-rich foods like these can help you reach your daily goal. (Flip to Chapter 6 for a list of vegan foods that supply calcium.)

TIP

Your body absorbs calcium and iron best when they're taken separately, so plan your vitamin intake accordingly. Calcium citrate is easier to absorb than calcium carbonate, so supplement with this form if supplementation is required to meet your needs. Take no more than 500 milligrams of calcium at a time for best absorption.

Vitamin D

Calcium doesn't work alone. It also needs vitamin D. Our bodies turn sunlight into vitamin D through the conversion of UVB rays. Get regular, short doses of sun exposure.

TIP

Getting 15 to 30 minutes of sunlight around noon each day has been shown to be most effective. Your body then uses the vitamin D to properly absorb calcium. Be aware that people with darker skin or who live far from the equator may need a longer time in the sun to produce enough vitamin D.

See Chapter 6 for more information about vitamin D.

Iron

Getting enough iron is important to ensure a healthy rate of development for your baby. It also helps with a strong and energized pregnancy for you. Your body is making extra blood for the baby now. You need more iron than ever, about 27 milligrams a day.

Focus on including iron-rich foods in your diet. Squeeze in dark leafy greens, beans, dried fruits, nuts, seeds, whole grain breads, and cereals.

Of course, a prenatal supplement that contains iron also helps make blood production go smoothly. Most vegan prenatal vitamins provide 100 percent of the iron you need. Talk with your healthcare provider about which supplement to take. And be sure to include lots of vitamin C–rich foods to help your body absorb the extra iron you're consuming.

REMEMBER

Note that the extra iron is important, but it may also cause constipation. Lucky for you, a plant-based diet offers lots of fiber to prevent constipation. Make sure you're getting a variety of whole plant foods to ensure adequate fiber intake. And drink plenty of water to keep the fiber moving through your digestive system.

To read more about iron, including a list of great vegan food sources, check out Chapter 6.

Folate and folic acid

One of the first nutrients that comes up in pregnancy discussions is folate, which is also known as folic acid. *Folate* is a B vitamin that's found naturally in many vegan foods. *Folic acid* is the synthetic form that people take in supplements.

This nutrient gets a lot of press because it helps the body produce new cells, especially during the rapid cell division and growth of pregnancy. A lack of folate can lead to birth defects. Luckily, deficiency is easily avoidable with proper nutrition and a well-chosen prenatal vitamin.

Table 21-2 lists some of the best natural vegan sources of folate to help you reach the recommended minimum of 600 micrograms per day during pregnancy and 500 micrograms per day while lactating.

Zinc

Zinc is especially important during pregnancy because it's needed for energy production, cell growth, and brain development in your growing fetus.

TABLE 21-2 ## Natural Vegan Sources of Folate

Food Source	Serving Size	Folate (mcg)
Blackeyed peas, canned	1 cup	252
Spinach, cooked	1 cup	179
Asparagus, cooked	1 cup	85.1
Green peas, cooked	1 cup	101
Vegetarian baked beans, canned	1 cup	30.5
Broccoli, frozen, cooked	1 cup	103
Broccoli, raw	1 cup	58.5
Avocado, raw	1 fruit	122
Orange, raw	1 fruit	43.1
Banana, raw	1 fruit	18.9

Source: U.S. Department of Agriculture's FoodData Central

If you're pregnant and 19 or older, aim for 11 milligrams of zinc per day. For pregnant people 18 or younger, get 12 milligrams per day.

Choose foods like beans, nuts, fortified nutritional yeast, and fortified cereals. Table 21-3 lists some great sources of zinc.

TABLE 21-3 ## Vegan Sources of Zinc

Food Source	Serving Size	Zinc (mg)
Vegetarian baked beans, canned	1 cup	5.79
Cashews, dry roasted	½ cup	3.83
Brazil nuts, dried	½ cup	2.7
Lentils, boiled	1 cup	2.52
Chickpeas, cooked	1 cup	2.51
Peanuts, roasted	½ cup	2.39
Almonds, whole	½ cup	2.23
Black beans, cooked	1 cup	1.93
Kidney beans, cooked	1 cup	1.52
Tahini	2 tablespoons	1.38

Source: U.S. Department of Agriculture's FoodData Central

Note: Certain components in food can hinder your zinc absorption. Too much calcium in your diet, for example, can impede your body's ability to absorb zinc. Some calcium supplements now come with added zinc to offset this disparity.

Found in the outer layers of seeds, beans, grains, nuts, peas, and legumes, *phytic acid* can keep your body from absorbing zinc properly. Luckily, simply soaking these foods in water will remove much of the phytic acid. Similarly, soy milk contains large amounts of phytic acid. Make sure you're getting plenty of zinc from other healthy foods, and don't drink gallons of soy milk. Moderation is key.

Iodine

Iodine is an essential trace mineral, found in the ocean and in soil. It's called *essential* because it's not made in the body. To reach your RDA, you need to eat foods or supplements that contain it.

In order to support proper fetal growth and neurological development, the RDA for iodine is higher for people who are pregnant or breastfeeding.

Here is the RDA for iodine:

>> Before pregnancy: 150 micrograms

>> During pregnancy: 220 micrograms

>> Breastfeeding: 290 micrograms

Meet your RDA by using iodized salt or eating seaweed like kombu, wakame, and nori. (The iodine in sea vegetables varies. Check the label to be sure you're getting enough, but not too much.) You can also talk to your doctor about recommending a prenatal multivitamin that contains sufficient amounts of iodine.

REMEMBER

The amount of iodine in breast milk varies, depending on whether or not the pregnant or breastfeeding parent is deficient. If they are deficient then the fetus or infant may be at risk for iodine deficiency and associated risks, like cognitive impairments.

For more information about iodine, see Chapter 6.

A WORD ON SUPPLEMENTS

Adding well-chosen supplements to your well-rounded diet ensures that you and your growing fetus are getting everything you both need in the way of nutrients. Take a realistic look at your diet and talk with your healthcare provider about what you may be lacking. Safeguard your and your baby's health with a few vitamins and minerals or take an all-inclusive prenatal vitamin.

For example, if you're concerned about your iron intake, discuss it with your midwife or doctor. Many people, vegan and non-vegan alike, experience anemia during their 40 weeks of pregnancy. You can choose from various types of iron supplements: iron sulfate, chelated iron bisglycinate, and ferrous fumarate. *Iron sulfate* (also known as *ferrous sulfate*) can cause upset stomach, black stools, and constipation. The easier types of iron to digest are called *chelated iron bisglycinate, ferrous succinate,* and *ferrous fumarate*. If you take separate calcium and iron supplements, take them a few hours apart, because calcium and iron can interfere with each other's absorption.

Similarly, if you aren't getting sufficient sunlight on a daily basis, talk with your healthcare provider about taking a vegan vitamin D supplement. While some foods are fortified with vitamin D, it may not be enough to reach the levels required during pregnancy to ensure proper calcium absorption.

In general, vitamin and supplement tablets and oils should be kept away from heat and sunlight and be stored in opaque containers to prevent oxidation and breakdown. Liquid supplements are usually easier to digest and absorb during pregnancy, but chewables seem to be second best. Chapter 6 provides more detail on choosing vegan supplements.

Choline

Choline is necessary during pregnancy for developing healthy cell membranes, nerve cells, and brain and tissue cells. The Adequate Intake recommendation for choline during pregnancy is 450 milligrams per day.

Choline can be found in tofu, navy or kidney beans, some vegetables, nuts, and grains. Some prenatal vitamins also contain choline in amounts ranging from 10 to 55 milligrams. Consult with your healthcare provider to see if a supplement is needed based on your current diet.

Making Meal Prep Easy

Navigating pregnancy and your hectic day-to-day life can be a lot to manage. You may need to work until a few days before your due date. You may be scrambling to get your house ready for a new baby. You may already be caring for other children. Whatever your situation, it can be difficult to maintain a healthy diet when there's so much to do.

Use the following tips to keep healthy foods at the ready, and to make cooking well-rounded vegan meals more manageable:

>> **Cook once and eat twice.** When preparing meals like homemade soups, pasta dishes, casseroles, stir-fries, or curries, make a double or triple batch. When you're already chopping vegetables, it's not that much harder to chop a few more. Eat the leftovers for lunch, or save individual servings in the freezer for easy reheating later. (This can be an especially good way to prep for post-birth meals.)

>> **Start a cooking co-op with vegan friends.** Ask friends to cook extra servings of their favorite meals, and trade once or twice a week. This gives you a variety of vegan meals from which to choose.

>> **Rely on your grocery freezer section occasionally.** Freshly prepared foods are ideal. However, some great vegan frozen meals are available for those times when you're just too tired to cook. Choose hearty frozen dishes like whole grains with vegetables and tofu, bean burritos, and lasagna. These easy meals are super convenient.

>> **Ask a friend to be prep chef for you.** After a big shopping trip, ask a family member or friend to come over and do some of the prep work for you, such as washing, drying, and chopping vegetables. Bagging prepped veggies, lettuce, and chopped fruit cuts down on cooking time later in the week. Plus, it provides grab-and-go snacks. Of course, this is also a fine time to choose pre-chopped veggies from the market for an even easier setup!

Managing "Morning" Sickness

Nausea or morning sickness varies a lot from one pregnant person to the next. For some people, it's minimal. Others may have endless queasy feelings no matter the time of day. Your upset stomach may be accompanied by a slight headache, a sour taste in your mouth, and vomiting.

REMEMBER

These symptoms are all normal during the first trimester. However, if you can't eat at all or have excessive vomiting, talk with your midwife or doctor. Ask them for advice if you seem dehydrated, lose weight, or feel lightheaded. These symptoms can all lead to complications if not addressed quickly.

During this time, you may not be able to tolerate some foods that used to be regular favorites. And certain times of day may be better or worse for you.

Here are some tips that can help you get through pregnancy nausea:

» **Eat small snacks and meals throughout the day.** Eating small amounts more often instead of big meals will help your sensitive stomach.

» **Keep a sleeve of plain saltine crackers next to your bed.** Eat a few if you wake up nauseated in the middle of the night and immediately upon waking in the morning.

» **Avoid strong smells.** Gasoline fumes, cooking food, perfumes, and heavily scented home products may aggravate your symptoms.

» **Stay cool during the day and avoid overheating.** Suck on store-bought or homemade popsicles.

» **Relieve your nausea by eating watermelon and drinking naturally sweetened ginger lemonade.** Peppermint tea is also known to calm an upset stomach. Another stomach smoother, ginger tea can be made by steeping freshly cut pieces of ginger in water. Enjoy it iced or hot.

» **Exercise moderately and regularly.** You may not feel like it, but some light movement can help.

» **Open windows to get fresh air in your home, when possible.** A nice breeze keeps the house from smelling stale, improves indoor air quality, and helps to get rid of smells that may cause nausea.

» **Avoid skipping meals.** If at all possible, try to eat regular meals even if you have only a few bites at a time.

» **Eat mild foods.** Make sure your foods are free of excessive spices and flavorings and eat plain whole grains, tofu, avocado, crackers, or toast.

» **Avoid lying down for at least 30 minutes after eating.** If you must lie down, use a pillow to elevate your head and shoulders.

» **Find your acupressure points on your wrist.** To help stave off nausea, use acupressure wrist bands or apply pressure with your index finger and thumb.

Caring for Yourself Postpartum

After your bundle of joy has finally made their debut into the world, much of the attention will likely shift from you to the baby. However, it's important to remember that you have just been through a major physical, emotional, and hormonal shift.

REMEMBER

Plan ahead and think about how to make your entrance into parenthood as smooth and supported as possible. Talk with your friends and family beforehand to line up assistants to help take care of your older children, cook and clean, or even hold the new baby while you take a shower.

Will your family and friends be helping with meal prep? If yes, go over vegan menus and ingredients to help them cook for you and satisfy your needs.

Here are some freezer-friendly vegan dishes to suggest:

>> Baked oatmeal

>> Bean burritos

>> Black bean or jackfruit taquitos

>> Breakfast burritos with tofu and potatoes

>> Pancakes or waffles

>> Three bean chili

>> Vegetable, bean, or lentil soups

>> Vegetable lasagna with tofu ricotta

TIP

If your loved ones prefer to give gift cards for postpartum meals, suggest ones to your favorite grocery stores, meal delivery services, or vegan and vegan-friendly restaurants in your area.

There are many ways to ensure that you feel supported and cared for as you begin to provide for your new baby and growing family. The following sections offer some details.

Choose certain vegan foods for strength

Recovering from childbirth and labor can be a slow process. Having meals planned in advance offers an easier transition.

>> Plan to make a few meals that can be frozen in the weeks before your due date.

>> Stock your cupboards and refrigerator by going on a big shopping trip shortly before your due date as well.

>> Be sure anyone cooking for you, like a spouse or partner, knows how to prepare healthy vegan meals that support your energy needs. The meal-planning chart included in Chapter 8 can help them prepare for the days after your labor.

REMEMBER

High-energy foods like whole grains, avocados, nuts, and bean soups are filling and provide you (and your family) with excellent nutrition. If you lost a lot of blood during labor, plan to have more iron-rich foods to replenish your blood supply. (Chapter 6 includes a list of foods that can boost your iron intake.) Stay hydrated with plenty of water and enriched soy milk for your protein and nutrient intake.

Meet calorie and other nutrient requirements

REMEMBER

If you plan to breastfeed, be aware that it requires an extra 500 calories a day for the first six months. After six months, it drops to 400 calories. (That's when children begin eating some solid foods, such as baby food, infant cereals, and soft fruits and veggies.)

Your protein needs are also still high during breastfeeding. Experts recommend 1.05 grams of protein per kilogram of body weight per day. However, research published in 2020 in the peer-reviewed journal, *Current Developments in Nutrition*, shows protein needs may be even higher.

Just like when you were pregnant, it's important to choose a variety of foods that offer good sources of protein, calcium, iron, B vitamins, zinc, and other nutrients. That way both you and your baby will get everything you need.

Chapter **22**

Bouncing Baby Vegans

Congratulations on your new little one!

If you're planning on raising your child vegan, rest assured that babies and toddlers can receive complete nutrition from a plant-based diet. A little planning and creativity can make the job of vegan parenting easier and more successful. Plus, starting kids on a plant-based diet from the very beginning offers them a lifetime of healthy habits and benefits.

What children eat in their first few years can set their eating habits for life. Offering children a colorful diet of whole plant–based foods will ensure that they grow up healthy and loving their veggies.

This chapter discusses infant and toddler nutritional needs. I cover various ways to feed babies and toddlers with nutritious plant-based menus. Keep in mind that these are general guidelines. Of course, you should keep your doctor or qualified healthcare professional involved every step of the way with regular visits for your baby or toddler. Talk to them about any concerns you may have and to get specific advice for your situation.

Nourishing Your Newborn

Because a baby's digestive system is still quite immature and sensitive, for the first six months or so, nutrition is pretty straightforward. It's best to provide either breast milk or formula.

Those who are able to breastfeed can ensure that their milk is rich, ample, and filled with the necessary nutrients by consuming a wide variety of plant-based foods and supplementing with additional nutrients as needed. (See Chapter 21 on postpartum nutrition for specifics.) However, breastfeeding isn't always possible for a variety of reasons. Luckily, plant-based formula exists for those who prefer to use it.

Breastfeeding: So perfectly vegan!

People are sometimes confused about whether or not vegans support breastfeeding. They assume that since vegans don't drink cow's milk, all types of milk are off the menu. That couldn't be more wrong!

As surprising as it may be to some, vegans are pro milk. They think that a mother's milk is the perfect food — for her baby. Human's milk is the perfect food for human babies. Goat's milk is the perfect food for baby goats (also known as kids). Sheep's milk is the perfect food for lambs. When you want to raise a strong, full-grown cow, cow's milk is the way to go.

People hear the words "dairy cow" and wrongfully assume cows are lactating constantly throughout their entire lives. Like humans, cows lactate only after giving birth. In the dairy industry, cows (as well as goats and sheep) are impregnated so that they will lactate. Their offspring are taken from them (either to be sold for meat or to become dairy cows themselves), and the animals' milk is given to humans instead. That's what vegans are against.

But a parent feeding their child the food that's perfectly designed for them is 100 percent vegan.

The benefits of breastfeeding

Breastfeeding has many benefits — for both parent and child.

>> **It's free, while formula can get expensive.** You don't have to worry about keeping your pantry fully-stocked with formula or running out.

>> **It's good for the baby.** Babies who are breastfed tend to have better neurodevelopmental and dental health. Plus, they have lower risks of diarrhea, Crohn's disease and ulcerative colitis, celiac disease, sudden infant death syndrome (commonly known as SIDS), asthma, diabetes (types 1 and 2), leukemia, and more.

>> **Parents who breastfeed also reap some benefits.** They have less risk of hypertension, type 2 diabetes, and rheumatoid arthritis. They also have a lower risk of developing breast, ovarian, endometrial, and thyroid cancers.

Amazingly, breast milk changes over the course of a baby's life to provide the child what they need to thrive and grow at that particular time. As their nutrition needs change, so does the milk. Mothers also pass on their *antibodies* (protective proteins that defend against infection), which helps babies develop a strong immune system, and improves their ability to fight off illness.

The first milk that's produced is immunity-building *colostrum*. It's easy to digest, high in carbohydrates and protein, and low in fat. That makes it the perfect first food for a baby. This rich milk is full of antibodies, which provide nutrients that aid in proper growth and development in addition to boosting immunity.

REMEMBER

Because breastfed babies receive vitamin B12 through breast milk, lactating parents should remember to supplement appropriately. The Centers for Disease Control and Prevention (CDC) recommends vitamin D supplementation of 400 international units (IU) for breastfed children under 12 months old. For children 12 to 24 months old, the CDC recommendation increases to 600 IU.

Breastfeeding timeline

The longer you're able to breastfeed your baby, the better. The American Academy of Pediatrics (AAP), World Health Organization, and UNICEF all recommend that babies should be breastfed within the first hour after birth. From there, babies should be breastfed exclusively for the first six months of their lives. After that time, breastfeeding can be combined with complementary foods for two years and beyond. Iron-rich sources are recommended as the baby's first food.

REMEMBER

Breastfeeding is optimum because of the many compounds contained in breast milk that can protect babies from infections and disease. Breastfed babies have fewer hospitalizations and incidence of ear infections, allergies, diarrhea, and asthma than formula-fed babies.

TIP

Breastfeeding can come with challenges like difficulty latching on and low milk supply. Ask your pediatrician, obstetrician, or midwife for recommendations for a certified lactation consultant if you need expert help.

Formula feeding

If breastfeeding isn't possible for some reason, infant formula is a healthy alternative that will give your baby the nutrients they need. You can find plant-based formulas that will do the job, whether your baby is exclusively or supplementally formula fed.

Be aware that some plant-based formulas, especially for infants, include vitamin D3, which may or may not be vegan. D3 typically comes from sheep's wool, also known as *lanolin*. But some formula makers like Else Nutrition use algae-derived D3, a vegan source.

Vitamin D3 is added to formula to meet U.S. Food and Drug Administration regulations. If you're unsure of the vitamin D3 source and want to make sure it's vegan, check the formula manufacturer's website or reach out to the them and ask. Once children are older than 12 months, more options become available.

If you're unable to find a plant-based formula with vegan D3, don't let perfect be the enemy of good. Just do your best with the options you have available.

Here are some plant-based formula options:

>> Earth's Best Non-GMO Plant Based Infant Formula

>> Enfamil ProSobee Simply Plant-Based Infant Formula Powder

>> Similac Soy Isomil Infant Formula

>> Gerber Good Start Gentle Soy Powder

>> Baby's Only Organic Plant Based Pea Protein Formula

>> Else Nutrition Plant-Based Complete Nutrition for Toddlers

WARNING

Soy milk isn't the same as soy formula. The nondairy milk you use on your cereal doesn't contain the proper nutrition for babies to thrive. *Do not give infants nondairy milk in place of formula.* It's also not advisable to make your own formula. Homemade formula doesn't support adequate nutrition or contain the required fats, protein, and calories for infants.

Starting Older Babies on Solid Foods

When your baby is 4 to 6 months old, you may decide to start offering them solid food in addition to breast milk or formula. Not only must a baby's digestive system evolve slightly to allow for some solid food, but their mouth muscles also need to develop enough to move food around and swallow.

Around the age of 4 to 6 months, your little one will begin to hold up their head. They will develop stronger neck muscles for swallowing, as well as begin sitting up with some help. According to the CDC, these milestones are all important markers on the way to eating solid foods. Other signs that show your child may be ready for solids include:

>> Trying to grasp for small objects, food, and toys

>> Bringing objects to their mouth

>> Opening their mouth when food is offered

>> Moving food from the front of the tongue to the back, as opposed to pushing food out onto their chin

The CDC recommendations state that the main source of calories should be breast milk or formula until a child is at least 6 months old. After that point, they advise that "continuing to breastfeed while introducing solid foods through 12 months or older is recommended."

WARNING

Even though your baby may be ready to begin trying some solid foods, hold off on introducing any type of milk — dairy or nondairy. The AAP recommends that cow's milk not be fed to children under the age of 1 because it can cause digestive problems and allergies.

As a vegan, you likely aren't buying cow's milk anyway. However, you still need to wait to give your baby soy milk until after they're 1 year old. Stick to breast milk, formula, or a bit of water to wash down solids for now. (Water is not suitable for babies under 6 months old, unless recommended by a doctor.)

Slow and steady wins the race

If your little vegan has reached those pivotal milestones of development and starts grabbing for your dinner, you can start experimenting with different foods. Take it slow and introduce foods one at a time. According to the AAP, most children don't have to receive foods in a certain order. Go with what makes the most sense for your little one.

REMEMBER

Choose only one food at a time, giving each a trial of three to five days. For instance, feed your baby a few spoonfuls of mashed avocado a couple times a day for up to a week. If your baby has no noticeable reactions, try mashed banana the next week, on its own. If they still have no reactions, you can move forward in this manner with a different food every few days.

If your baby has a reaction to a certain food, you know not to try it again for a while. Keep in mind that if you were to make a mash of several foods at once and your baby reacted, you wouldn't know which food was the culprit. Always introduce one food at a time.

Deciding what and how to feed your growing baby

What should you choose for your baby's first solid foods?

TIP

Iron-fortified infant cereal is a popular first food for vegan and non-vegan babies alike. Choose a variety of fortified infant cereals like barley, multigrain, and oat. (It's not advisable to give babies rice cereal exclusively because it can increase their exposure to arsenic.) Cereal can be mixed with a little breast milk or formula to thin it.

Experts used to recommend that vegetables come before fruit in a baby's first forays into solids. The concern was that by starting with sweet foods, babies would develop a lifelong preference for them. However, research hasn't borne that out. Nowadays parents are free to start with whatever foods they choose, in whatever order they prefer.

Mashed ripe avocados or bananas are easy on the digestive system for most kids. They have a soft, creamy texture and a mild flavor. Bananas are also lauded for their potassium and vitamin C. Fully cooked and mashed potatoes or sweet potatoes, green beans, peas, carrots, and natural unsweetened applesauce are other options. Remember to include good sources of iron like lentils, tofu, and chickpeas.

Buying premade baby food is an option, but it isn't a requirement. It wasn't until the 1920s that store-bought baby food became a thing. Infants just ate a mashed-up form of whatever their parents were eating. Most babies around the world are still fed like this today. It's cheaper and generally easier than buying hundreds of little containers of premashed food. Plus, the baby gets a head start on trying family favorite ingredients, which may expand their palate and influence their preferences for years to come.

Many people assume that baby food has to be bland, but that's not backed up by science. In fact, breastfed babies are already used to seasoned food, because a mother's milk takes on the flavors of what she eats. If she has a delicious plate of *chana masala* (chickpea curry), her breast milk is going to take on some of that flavor. So don't be afraid to incorporate herbs and spices with your baby's food too. Just skip any that are overly hot and avoid adding sugar. The USDA and the Department of Health and Human Services recommend that children younger than 24 months not consume any added sugars.

TIP

You can puree foods with a blender or food processor. Low-cost baby food mills that grind your adult food into a consistent paste are available online and at big-box stores. These mills are easy to clean and transport.

Once your baby is able, you can transition them away from pureed food and toward soft chopped, mashed, or ground foods that they can eat with their hands or a spoon. (This generally happens when they're 10 to 12 months old.)

Watching Them Grow: Food for Toddlers

Toddlers develop their personality quicker than you may expect. They express their likes and dislikes for foods with no reservations. After the explosive growth that most babies experience, the slowing weight gain of toddlerhood can cause a decrease in appetite.

When your child's decrease in appetite is coupled with their innate pickiness, you can easily become frustrated. Don't allow it to upset you. Most parents experience a similar situation. Just keep offering healthy choices and nutritious snacks.

TIP

Don't give up on the greens! Most kids need a new food introduced many times before they accept it. Keep cooking wholesome foods, show your child you enjoy them, and don't force them to eat something.

REMEMBER

After your baby's first birthday, you can begin to wean them off formula, and switch to fortified soy milk or toddler formula. If you opt for fortified soy milk for your toddler, be sure that the type you choose has appropriate levels of fat, calcium, protein, and vitamins D, B2, and B12.

QUIETING THE NAYSAYERS

Your loved ones may be concerned about the healthfulness of raising a vegan child. You can reassure well-intentioned family and friends with some insights from experts.

The position of the Academy of Nutrition and Dietetics states that "appropriately planned vegetarian diets, including total vegetarian or vegan diets, are healthful, nutritionally adequate, and may provide health benefits for the prevention and treatment of certain diseases. Well-planned vegetarian diets are appropriate for individuals during all stages of the life cycle, including pregnancy, lactation, infancy, childhood, and adolescence, and for athletes."

(continued)

(continued)

A 2021 article on the Academy of Nutrition and Dietetics website states that, "For infants, children, and adolescents, a well-planned vegetarian diet can promote normal growth."

Loved ones may mention their concerns about the alarming headlines they've read over the years. *(Trigger warning: child abuse and infanticide.)* Sadly, some well-publicized but misleading headlines have implied that parents whose children were malnourished died because of a vegan diet. Take a look at some of these cases:

- In one case, an 18-month-old hadn't been fed for a full week before passing. Before he was starved, his diet was inadequate and inappropriate, consisting of nothing but raw produce and breast milk. The baby died of starvation, malnutrition, and dehydration. Obviously, that has nothing to do with veganism. That's abuse and neglect, of which the parents were convicted. (They had older children who were also abused and neglected.)

- In another case, the parents had been feeding their baby only tomato juice and water.

- In yet another case, an 11-month-old was given only small amounts of berries and nuts.

- Finally, one case involved parents who fed their 6-month-old only wheatgrass, coconut water, and almond milk.

These incidents are positively horrifying. Blaming these tragedies on veganism grabs headlines, but it's sensationalism and an inaccurate portrayal of abuse. Starvation and neglect were to blame in each case. No reasonable person would look at the diets these children were fed and think they're adequate for anyone. You can point this out to any concerned family members, and assure them that you will be feeding your child appropriately and regularly, as well as following your doctor's advice if any issues arise.

Choosing nutrient-dense foods over fiber

The nutritional needs of toddlers are similar to your own, but they're scaled to children's smaller body size. They need a good variety of healthy fats, protein, calcium, iron, vitamin B12, vitamin D, and all the other minerals and nutrients that adults require.

REMEMBER

Vegans tend to eat more fiber than the average person, which is great for adults. The problem with vegan toddler food is that kids can fill up on fiber and then not want to eat other valuable nutrient-rich foods. Because kids have smaller stomachs, it's easy for them to fill up with fruit and whole grains.

Ensure that your child is getting enough nutrition by focusing on nutrient-dense foods like avocado, nut and seed butters, enriched whole grain products, and enriched nondairy milk.

WARNING

To safeguard against strong reactions to nuts or seeds, including food sensitivities and allergies, avoid giving your child these foods until after the age of 2 if similar allergies run in your family. If that's the case for you, and you would like to introduce nut and seed butters before the age of 2, talk with your pediatrician about testing a single seed or nut butter for any reaction before making it part of your child's diet.

Keep track of your child's growth and weight gain to make sure they're getting enough calories and nutrition. Choosing healthy fats is also important to guarantee proper growth and development. The Academy of Nutrition and Dietetics recommends aiming for 0.7 grams of omega-3 fatty acids a day. You can get there by adding flaxseed, chia seeds, hemp, walnuts, soybeans, or vegan omega-3 oils to your child's food.

Outsmarting finicky eaters

The most frustrating thing about kids' tastes is that they change — often. What they like for lunch one day is a no go the next.

Here are some tips for presenting healthy foods in a way that entices your little one:

>> **Let your child help in the kitchen.** Kids can dump premeasured items into a bowl, stir ingredients, or put napkins on the table. When they help prepare a meal, children get excited to eat the finished dish.

>> **Offer several small bowls of different foods.** Studies have shown that when given lots of healthy choices, kids will most likely make a well-rounded meal for themselves.

>> **Make food fun.** Create faces out of veggies on your child's plate, use fruit as decoration, cut sandwiches into shapes with cookie cutters, or set steamed broccoli in mashed potatoes as trees. Get creative!

>> **Avoid forcing them to eat.** If your child won't eat one meal, don't make a fuss over it. As long as they have access to wholesome snacks throughout the day and consume a variety of foods over the course of several days, they're likely going to get what they need. Just keep offering healthy foods.

>> **Set a good example.** Prepare and eat fruits, vegetables, whole grains, and beans to demonstrate that nourishing food is good for the whole family — yourself included.

>> **Incorporate antioxidant-packed greens.** Pureeing cooked kale, broccoli, or spinach and mixing it into pasta sauce, soups, or even smoothies is a healthy trick.

>> **Remember: Don't become a short-order cook.** Make a variety of foods that kids can choose from and let them decide how much of which foods they will eat.

Satisfying your little snacker

Snacks tend to make up a hefty portion of a toddler's diet. A small stomach and constant play makes little ones hungry for frequent small meals. Offer nourishing and safe snacks. They can be an important part of proper nutrition, even if meal-times are less than perfect.

REMEMBER

Develop your child's love for healthy foods by offering them fresh fruits and vegetables every day. Even if they don't eat them every time, they'll become accustomed to seeing fruits and veggies on the table, and will choose them more often in the future.

Here are some excellent nutrient-dense foods that toddlers and preschool-age kids will love:

>> Bagels spread with nut or seed butter, or mashed avocado and hummus

>> Blueberry Banana Oatmeal (Get the recipe in Chapter 11.)

>> Chicken-Free Salad Sandwich (Grab the recipe in Chapter 13.)

>> Happy Pigs in a Blanket (Find the recipe in Chapter 13.)

>> Mashed potatoes and vegan gravy

>> Nondairy yogurt with fruit

>> Oven-baked sweet potato fries

>> Pancakes topped with sunflower seed or nut butter

>> Peanut butter and jelly sandwich

>> Peanut Butter Banana Smoothie (Find the recipe in Chapter 11.)

>> Pizza Bagels (See Chapter 13.)

>> Quesadilla with nondairy cheese and avocado

>> Tomato soup with a vegan grilled cheese sandwich

>> Tortilla Pinwheels (Find the recipe in Chapter 13.)

>> Vegan Chicken Noodle Soup (Get the recipe in Chapter 12.)

>> Whole grain or enriched pasta with marinara sauce

WARNING

To avoid choking hazards when providing snacks to your toddler, be sure to do the following:

>> Finely grind nuts in a spice grinder or blender instead of offering whole or coarsely chopped nuts.

>> Spoon out half teaspoonfuls of nut butter rather than large globs.

>> Chop vegan hot dogs into pea-sized bits.

>> Quarter or halve cherry tomatoes, olives, grapes, pitted cherries, and any other large, round foods.

>> Grate raw carrots into shreds rather than offering small chunks.

>> Avoid popcorn and gum until your child is older.

>>

IN THIS CHAPTER

» **Ensuring children get proper nutrition**

» **Setting a solid foundation for healthy eating for life**

» **Discovering kid-friendly vegan food choices**

» **Preparing meals as a family**

» **Making sure kids eat well away from home**

Chapter **23**

Vegan Diets for Kids and Teens

There comes a time in a child's life when they realize that the chicken out in the field is the same as the chicken on their plate. For many kids, this is a rude awakening. Suddenly, they may no longer want to eat old favorites like chicken nuggets. Some parents scramble for a response, not knowing what to do.

» Do they assume it's a phase and cross their fingers that their child will forget by dinnertime?

» Do they go along with it and just hope their kid won't ask what's up with turkey and fish next?

» Do they lie to their child and sneak animal-based foods onto their plate?

Since you're reading this book, you may be one of those parents who decided to embrace your child's innate compassion and start making animal-friendly meals for them. Or you may be a vegan adult who's interested in transitioning your whole family to a vegan lifestyle.

Meat eating is seen as "neutral" in many cultures because that's what the majority does. But whether a parent tells their kid that eating meat is good and natural or that it's cruel and unnecessary, both viewpoints are an expression of the parent's values.

If you're ready to raise a vegan child, there's never been a better time for it. You're in good company as more and more families discover the benefits of a plant-based way of life.

The key to raising a child vegan is doing it in a kid-friendly way while avoiding common pitfalls. This chapter guides you through the process with dietary recommendations, shopping and cooking tips, and meal ideas. Plus, I offer helpful suggestions for when your kids are eating away from home.

Defining the Four Vegan Food Groups

As with any diet, you can follow it in an optimal or a suboptimal way. Hypothetically speaking, a kid could go vegan and eat a diet of french fries, Oreo cookies, and Sour Patch Kids. It wouldn't be the healthiest diet by any stretch, but it would be vegan. On the other hand, a kid could go vegan and eat a balanced plant-based diet with beans, tofu, whole grains, lots of dark leafy greens and other vegetables, and fruit. The second child would almost certainly see a much better health outcome than the first.

To have healthy, happy vegan kids, make sure they're eating a wide variety of nutritious whole foods. They'll be way ahead of the game, because that's something most kids aren't achieving.

>> According to a 2023 study from the Centers for Disease Control and Prevention, many children aren't eating fruits and vegetables daily. Their findings showed that nearly one-third (32.1 percent) of pre-school aged kids didn't eat a daily fruit, and nearly one half (49.1 percent) didn't eat a daily vegetable.

>> A 2020 study published in *Health Equity* noted that 63 percent of American children don't consume the nationally recommended amounts of fruits per day, and 90 percent don't eat the recommended amounts of vegetables per day.

By putting plants at the front and center of meals, vegan kids are at an advantage.

The following list provides an overview of the plant-based food groups that should be incorporated into every vegan's diet — both young and old. Take note of the serving sizes listed here and in Table 23-1 for a clearer idea of how much of each food your child needs.

>> **Whole grains:** Kids reap the rewards of fiber, protein, magnesium, iron, and B vitamins when they eat whole grains. Good sources include brown rice, barley, breads, pasta, quinoa (technically a seed), and cereals (both hot and cold).

One serving is equal to a slice of bread, 1 cup of cold cereal, ½ cup of cooked rice or pasta, or a 6-inch tortilla.

>> **Vegetables:** Veggies are the way to go for children to get ample amounts of folate, potassium, vitamin C, fiber, and beta-carotene. Offer everything from dark leafy greens like kale and collards, to orange vegetables like sweet potatoes and carrots, and red veggies like tomatoes and beets. Continue with starchy vegetables like potatoes and corn, as well as wholesome veggies like green beans, celery, and onions.

For the most part, one serving is ½ cup of cooked or raw vegetables. The only exception is raw leafy greens (like spinach or romaine), which need 1 cup to make a serving.

>> **Protein-rich foods like legumes, nuts, seeds, and soy:** Children have much to gain from these protein-rich foods — like zinc, iron, fiber, and B vitamins. Plus, by eating walnuts, flaxseed, chia seeds, hemp seeds, and soy products like tofu, kids get heart-healthy omega-3s. (If they fall short on those foods, algae-derived omega-3 supplements are available.)

Offer up black beans, pinto beans, chickpeas, lentils, tofu, and split peas. For nuts and seeds, consider almonds, cashews, pumpkin seeds, sunflower seeds, and natural nut butters.

One serving of cooked beans, lentils, or tofu is ½ cup. A serving of mixed nuts is an ounce, and a serving of nut butter is 2 tablespoons.

>> **Fruits:** Kids gain the benefits of fiber, vitamin C, potassium, and folate when they nosh on fruit. Have them reach for fruits like bananas, mangoes, strawberries, blueberries, apples, oranges, or pineapple.

One serving is a small whole fruit like an apple, or ½ cup of chopped fresh fruit like mango or banana.

TABLE 23-1   **Serving Recommendations for Kids and Teens**

Age Group	Whole Grains	Vegetables	Proteins (Legumes, Nuts, Seeds, and Soy)	Fruits
Females 3–6 Males 3–5	4–5 servings	1 serving dark green, orange, and red vegetables 1 serving starchy vegetables 1 serving other vegetables	1 serving beans and lentils 1–1½ servings nuts, seeds, and soy	2–3 servings
Females 7–18 Males 6–11	5–6 servings	1–2 servings dark green, orange, and red vegetables 1 to 2 servings starchy vegetables 1 serving other vegetables	1–1½ servings beans and lentils 1½–2 servings nuts, seeds, and soy	3–4 servings
Males 12–18	7–10 servings	2–3 servings dark green, orange, and red vegetables 2 servings starchy vegetables 2 servings other vegetables	1½–2 servings beans and lentils 2–2½ servings nuts, seeds, and soy	4–5 servings

Source: Physicians Committee for Responsible Medicine (www.pcrm.org/good-nutrition/nutrition-for-kids)

Examining Nutritional Requirements for Children

Children and adults alike need the same macronutrients, minerals, and vitamins. The only difference is in amounts. That's why children's needs change as they grow.

In this section, I highlight the purpose of macronutrients like protein, minerals like calcium and iron, and a variety of vitamins. While you read, check out the various tables, where you can find your child's daily requirements by age.

Calcium

Kids need calcium for growing bones and healthy teeth. While many people think calcium is synonymous with cow's milk, plenty of plant foods are rich in this mineral. Plus, the human body absorbs calcium more efficiently from many vegetables than it does from cow's milk products.

Beans, grains, greens, vegetables, seeds, and nuts can supply everything your child needs for optimum nutrition and proper growth. Table 23-2 lists the calcium requirements in milligrams (mg) for children. (Amounts are the same for girls and boys.)

Daily Calcium Requirements for Children

Age	Amount (mg)
1–3 years	700
4–8 years	1,000
9–18 years	1,300

Source: The National Institutes of Health

Chapter 6 provides a list of vegan foods that are great sources of calcium. Be sure to give your child a variety of these foods so they can meet the proper calcium requirements for their age group.

Iron

Growing kids need iron-rich foods to ensure consistent energy levels and healthy blood production. Table 23-3 provides recommendations for how much iron in milligrams (mg) kids need at various stages. Fill your child's diet with items from the list of iron-rich vegan foods in Chapter 6.

REMEMBER

Children who have begun their menstrual cycle require more iron to compensate for the blood loss.

Daily Iron Requirements for Kids and Teens

Age	Males (mg)	Females (mg)
1–3 years	7	7
4–8 years	10	10
9–13 years	8	8
14–18 years	11	15

Source: The National Institutes of Health

Iron-rich foods that also contain vitamin C are especially good, because vitamin C enhances the body's ability to absorb iron. Broccoli, kale, and unpeeled potatoes are some of these nutritious foods.

You can also pair foods to gain the same effect. Here are a few ways to pair iron-rich foods with foods that contain vitamin C:

>> **Breakfast:** Make your child oatmeal with blueberries.

>> **Lunch:** Serve tacos with black beans and tomato salsa.

>> **Dinner:** Make vegan lasagna with shredded zucchini, tofu ricotta, and marinara.

Protein

Growing bodies need protein to create muscle, build blood, and repair tissues. Many folks are obsessed with getting enough protein, but the fact is, true protein deficiency is rare in the developed world. In fact, most people are getting way too much of it. As long as you and your family are getting enough calories from a wide variety of plant-based foods, you're likely getting the protein your body needs.

Use Table 23-4 to create kid-friendly menus based on your family's changing protein needs.

TABLE 23-4

Daily Protein Requirements for Kids and Teens

Age	Males (g)	Females (g)
1–3 years	16	16
4–6 years	24	24
7–10 years	28	28
11–14 years	45	46
15–18 years	59	44

Source: The National Institutes of Health

TIP

Focus on offering a variety of protein-rich foods throughout the day. Your child's body will accumulate all the amino acids it needs to create complete proteins.

Daily doses of whole grain products, different kinds of beans or legumes, and a variety of nuts, seeds, and soy foods all ensure that your child meets their protein needs. Flip to Chapter 5 to see a list of vegan sources of protein.

Essential vitamins

Vegan kids need the same vitamins that adults need. They may need a bit more or less at certain ages and stages. Rest assured, eating a well-balanced vegan diet will provide your child all the essential vitamins they need.

The following vitamins are required on a regular basis for proper development:

>> **Vitamin A:** Colorful vegetables like carrots, sweet potatoes, kale, and spinach are great sources of vitamin A. The body uses this vitamin for eye and bone health, growth, and reproductive functions, just to name a few.

>> **Vitamin B12:** Fortified nutritional yeast, fortified nondairy milk, B12 supplements, and vegan multivitamins are all good sources of B12. (See Chapter 6 for more info on vitamin B12.)

TIP

Check the label on your vegan multivitamin to see if it includes vitamin B12. If it doesn't, a separate B12 supplement is recommended.

>> **Vitamin C:** Fruits and veggies are the best sources of vitamin C, which aids the body in absorbing iron, increasing immune function, and repairing tissue. Papaya, red bell peppers, broccoli, Brussels sprouts, and countless other fresh plant foods provide this useful vitamin.

>> **Vitamin D:** You can find this vitamin in fortified vegan foods. Getting regular doses of sunlight or supplements can help keep your child's vitamin D levels adequate. (Check out Chapter 6 to understand why vitamin D is important.)

>> **Vitamin E:** Known for its importance in blood, brain, eye, and skin health, this nutrient also strengthens the body's natural defenses against illness and infection. Almonds, avocados, hazelnuts, olive oil, sunflower seeds, and sunflower seed butter all supply good quantities of this antioxidant-rich vitamin.

>> **Vitamin K:** This vitamin, which is crucial for blood clotting and healthy bones, is found in green leafy vegetables, parsley, avocados, and kiwifruit. Because it's a fat-soluble vitamin, sautéing greens with olive oil or pairing them with another fat (like seeds or avocado) helps the body use vitamin K better.

TIP

Because some kids may not adhere to the best eating habits every day, offering a daily vegan multivitamin is good health insurance. Chewable vitamins, liquid vitamins, or vegan gummies ensure that a child's intake is sufficient. Talk to your doctor about which one is the best choice for your child. Here are a few options:

>> Garden of Life mykind Organics Kids Multi Gummies

>> Nutracelle Nutramin Kids Multivitamin Gummies

>> Mama Bear Organic Kids Multivitamin Gummies

>> Llama Naturals Plant-Based Multivitamin Gummies

>> VegLife Vegan Kids Multiple Chewables

Making Fruits and Veggies More Enticing

Eating a diet that's rich in fruits and vegetables affects your child's health now. It may even inform their eating habits for the rest of their lives.

When you're trying to entice your kid to eat more fruits and vegetables, think about what appeals to you. Empathize with them, and build on what works.

>> **Add more veggies to the dishes your child already likes.**

- When you have spaghetti, add vegetables like zucchini, broccoli, kale, spinach, onions, garlic, fresh basil, or eggplant to the pasta sauce.

- Throw a handful of greens like spinach or kale into their fruit smoothies.

- Add sautéed red bell peppers, onions, or zucchini to their tacos.

- Top pizza with flavorful produce like bell peppers, onions, mushrooms, spinach, fresh basil, olives, pineapple, or artichoke hearts.

- Put lots of fresh vegetables, including lettuce, onion, and tomato, on their sandwiches or veggie burgers.

>> **Cut veggies into bite-sized pieces.** If you were going to try a new food, would you prefer a great big bite or a small taste? Depending on the food, most of us would rather commit to a small sample than a heaping mouthful. When you add veggies to a dish, cut them into small, manageable pieces. This works especially nicely in chopped salads, stir-fries, pasta salads, and rice dishes.

>> **Let kids serve themselves the amount they want.** Depending on their age, let kids dish out the amount of food they'd like to eat and decide how much of each dish they want to try. They can always go back for seconds if it's something they really love.

This is a good way for children to take ownership of their meals and to listen to their own hunger cues. If they spoon out too large a serving (more than they can comfortably eat), simply wrap it up and refrigerate it for later when they're hungry again.

>> **Keep introducing new foods.** Encourage your kids to try at least one bite. You may be surprised at how they come around after enough exposure.

>> **Talk about the benefits of good nutrition.** Instead of forcing kids to eat their peas, share with them what makes these legumes good for growing kids as well as adults. Eating healthy food shouldn't be seen as a chore or a punishment. When you serve a new fruit or vegetable, tell them about the nutritional benefits. You can even pull out your phone and research together what makes a specific fruit, vegetable, bean, or grain good for you. Get curious with them!

>> **Extend your family dinner time.** There's a lot of go, go, go in today's world. But slowing down to appreciate your dinner has the potential to make a big difference. A small 2023 study published in the *Journal of the American Medical Association* suggested that children ate significantly more fruits and vegetables when family dinners lasted 10 minutes longer than usual.

For example, if a family's average dinner lasted 20 minutes, stretching it to 30 minutes meant kids ate more produce. (It's worth noting that the intake of other foods, like bread or dessert, didn't increase with the added time.)

>> **Add a dip.** Don't underestimate the power of a delicious dip to make veggies more palatable. Hummus, vegan ranch dressing, barbecue sauce, vegan honey mustard, guacamole, or ketchup can go a long way toward making cauliflower florets, broccoli, carrots, celery, sugar snap peas, oven-baked fries, or sweet potato fries more inviting.

>> **Try different preparation methods.** If your kids haven't liked certain vegetables one way, try a different cooking method. Boiling is rarely the most delicious way to prepare veggies. Try serving them raw or use a variety of cooking methods, such as air frying, baking, roasting, sautéing, or steaming.

TIP

Make a game of it! Try cauliflower (or another vegetable) multiple ways — make cauliflower rice, cauliflower "wings," steamed florets with nondairy butter, roasted florets, and mashed cauliflower. Also enjoy the florets raw with a dip or in a salad. You may end up with a cauliflower lover after all!

>> **Add a sauce.** By coating vegetables in a sauce, you're able to enhance some flavors and mute others. Make sauces like vegan pesto or vegan alfredo from scratch, or use a jarred marinara, barbecue, or curry sauce.

>> **Cover veggies in crispy breading.** When vegetables are coated in crispy breading, they're downright addictive! While you may assume you have to fry them in oil, that often isn't the case. Air frying is my favorite way to make breaded vegetables. Baking them in the oven on parchment paper usually works too.

Start with any of these veggies:

- Broccoli florets
- Cauliflower florets
- Artichoke hearts, jarred (blotted dry)
- Mushrooms
- Onions, sliced into rings
- Zucchini slices

Pour some panko breadcrumbs into a shallow bowl. (If you like, add seasoning salt for extra flavor.) Next, make a simple batter (the consistency of pancake batter) with flour, water, baking powder, and salt. Dip the vegetables in the batter and tap off any excess. Then dredge the veggies in panko breadcrumbs and place them in a single layer in the air fryer basket.

Spritz the breaded veggies with oil and air fry at 360 degrees for 8 to 12 minutes or until browned, stopping once to flip. Serve with a dipping sauce like marinara, cocktail sauce, ketchup, or vegan ranch dressing.

TIP

If you're the kind of cook who prefers specific measurements and instructions, you can find recipes for air fried zucchini, artichoke hearts, onion rings, eggplant, green tomatoes, vegan jalapeño poppers, and more at https://cadryskitchen. com/. (Use the search bar to find what you want.)

Keeping a Well-Stocked Fridge and Pantry

Offering nutritious snacks and meals at home is the first step in creating a lifetime of good eating habits for kids and teens. By providing constant access to fresh, wholesome treats, you're offering a valuable lesson in how to plan and succeed in being a healthy vegan.

Use these guidelines to help stock your kitchen:

>> Stock whole grains like brown rice, polenta or grits, and oats. They make filling bases for meals.

>> Keep nuts and seeds like almonds, cashews, pecans, walnuts, sunflower seeds, sesame seeds, and pumpkin seeds on hand. They're protein-filled snacks that kids can reach for any time they need a pick-me-up. Nut butters make healthy snacks even tastier.

>> Fill your pantry with several types of canned or dried beans and lentils, including black beans, chickpeas, pinto beans, red lentils, brown lentils, and cannellini beans. Always have a block of vacuum-packed tofu in the fridge. These inexpensive and protein-rich ingredients give dishes some staying power.

>> Make sure you have plenty of fresh fruit on hand. To encourage kids to eat it, place clean fruit in a bowl on the counter. Or put cut fruit in a sealed container in the fridge — and make sure it's always accessible for snacking.

>> Buy both frozen and fresh vegetables. Cut a variety of raw veggies for snacking: cherry tomatoes, jicama, bell peppers, carrot sticks, celery, and cucumbers.

TIP

If you're short on time, buy precut vegetables and fruits in your grocery store's produce section. Broccoli and cauliflower florets, pineapple chunks, baby carrots, sugar snap peas, and apple slices are all handy shortcuts.

Turning Meal Planning into a Family Affair

Every member of the family can help plan menus and make shopping lists. Here are some ideas to get them involved:

>> Encourage them to look through cookbooks for meal ideas or talk about which dinners sound good this week. Let every family member pick at least one meal for the week.

>> Put a weekly menu chart on the table, and have each family member participate in filling it. (Weekly menu charts can be found in Chapter 8.)

>> After you figure out which ingredients you need, kids and adults in the household can go through the cupboards and refrigerator to see what should be added to the shopping list.

>> Kids can tag along to the grocery store and farmers market to help pick out the week's ingredients.

By training your kids early on how to plan, shop for, and prepare wholesome meals, you're imparting invaluable life skills that they'll use for years to come. Plus, kids who are active participants in meal planning and preparation are often more willing and excited to eat those dinners.

Cooking with your kids

Start cooking with your kids when they're young to ensure they're comfortable preparing meals. Kids as young as about 2 years old can help with meals by picking out fruit at the grocery store, pouring premeasured ingredients into a bowl, and stirring ingredients with adult supervision.

As kids get older, they can take more responsibility in the kitchen by doing food prep (like grating or shredding carrots), and even preparing family or individual dinners on their own. If a new vegan food trend takes off on TikTok, encourage them to make it for the family. (Or maybe your vegan kid will start their own trend!)

When dinnertime arrives, you can make simple plant-based tweaks to meals your family already enjoys. (Get ideas for veganizing dishes in Chapter 9.)

Serving kid-friendly vegan meals

Here's a list of easy, kid-friendly vegan meals for breakfast through dinnertime:

» Cereal with nondairy milk

» Oatmeal with apples and cinnamon

» Pancakes topped with bananas, peanut butter, and maple syrup

» Waffles with fresh or frozen berries

» Baked potato fries smothered in vegan chili

» Veggie burgers, vegan hot dogs, and sandwiches with vegan deli meats

» Tomato soup with grilled cheese sandwiches made with nondairy cheese

» Peanut butter and jelly sandwiches

» Bean and rice burritos

» Tofu nuggets with corn and barbecued baked beans

» Taco salad with soy chorizo and beans in a crispy baked tortilla bowl

» Spaghetti with tomato sauce (Mix in some cooked lentils or vegan meatballs for extra protein.)

» Vegetarian refried bean tostadas topped with shredded lettuce and tomatoes

» Lentil sloppy joes

» Falafel in a whole grain pita with hummus, cucumbers, tomatoes, and olives

» Cold Peanut Noodles (Recipe in Chapter 12.)

» Chickpea tacos

» Vegan lasagna with shredded zucchini

» Veggie pizza with nondairy cheese

Offering healthy snacks

Running and playing can burn off a lot of calories. Keep your kids energized with these simple snacks:

» Applesauce sprinkled with ground cinnamon

» Tortilla chips with salsa, guacamole, or vegetarian refried beans

» Fresh berries and fruit cut into bite-sized pieces

» Fruit smoothies

» Ants on a log (nut butter inside celery sticks with raisins on top)

» Nondairy yogurt

» Fruit leather

» Homemade popsicles made from fruit juices or fruit smoothies

» Hummus with veggies and pita chips

» Baby carrots and cauliflower with vegan ranch dressing

» Apple or banana slices dipped in nut butter

» Roasted Chickpeas (Find the recipe in Chapter 14.)

» Dates stuffed with nut butter

» Pitted olives or pickled cucumbers

» *Edamame* (cooked green soybeans) in pods

» Vegan cheese sticks, spreadable cheese, or cheese wedges with whole grain crackers

>> Popcorn drizzled with melted vegan butter and nutritional yeast flakes

>> Trail mix

>> Pretzels dipped in mustard or barbecue sauce

Modeling good eating habits

Sometimes parents complain that their kids don't eat fruits and vegetables, and then it comes out that the parents don't eat those foods either! It's unrealistic to think kids are going to nosh on salads and crudités if their parents never let a leafy green pass their lips. It's important to lead by example and expose children to nutritious foods.

Show your kids with your actions that vegetables, fruits, whole grains, and beans are foods that all of us eat — from kids to adults alike.

>> Load up your plate with colorful produce, whether you're eating at home or dining out.

>> Offer a bite of your dish to curious kids and introduce them to things they may not have tried before.

>> Share your food story with them. Let them know what you ate growing up and which foods are your favorites. Tell family stories involving recipes. By sharing why certain foods and dishes are special, you give them even more reasons to try and enjoy different things.

Knowing Your Children Won't Go Hungry When They're Away from Home

When field trips and other school-related activities are on the calendar, you have to think ahead and make some strategic decisions about what your kids will eat. The tips in this section can help make mealtime away from home easier and more stress-free for your little vegan. Lunch periods, parties, away games, and other competitions can all be exciting adventures with a little preplanning.

TIP

Although this section focuses on school-related activities, you can also plan for events outside of school. If your child is going to party or sleepover at a friend's house, contact the child's parents ahead of time to let them know about your child's dietary needs. Since many children have specific dietary needs or allergies,

I'm sure they won't be the only one. You can offer to send your kid with a meal and a dessert, or you can offer suggestions. If the parent is ordering a cake, they may be able to get a vegan cupcake from the same location. (Vegan cupcakes are often more expensive than the nonvegan variety. Offering to pay for your child's treat is a nice gesture.)

Navigating the school cafeteria

Most school cafeterias offer foods like chicken nuggets, walking tacos, pizza, hot dogs, and cheeseburgers. While demand for vegan options in schools and beyond is growing, the offerings are still few and far between. Some school menus are more inspiring than others.

>> In 2022, California made a $700 million investment to help schools procure plant-based foods, becoming the first state to support plant-based school meals. Menu items include enticing dishes like mushroom street tacos with cilantro cream sauce.

>> New York City schools have vegan Fridays, where they offer meals like black bean bowls with plantains, bean tacos, pasta primavera, and Mediterranean chickpeas with rice.

>> As of August 2023, an Illinois law requires schools to provide a nutritious plant-based meal to any student who requests it.

>> In Washington D.C., vegetarian meals are available daily upon request.

Depending on where you live, you may be able to contact your child's school about their specific dietary requirements.

If you don't have time to make a packed lunch, your child may be able to cobble together a meal at the salad bar or make a meal of side dishes. But for the most part, sending your child to school with a homemade lunch is usually the best option.

Get kids involved with the planning for best results. Depending on their age and development, they can pack their own lunches. Some brown-bag lunch ideas for your child include:

>> Vegan deli meat sandwich

>> Pasta Salad with Creamy Dressing (Get the recipe in Chapter 14.)

>> Ultimate Homemade Chili (see the recipe in Chapter 12) or vegetable soup in a thermos

- » Hummus Bagel Sandwich (Get the recipe in Chapter 13.)

- » Vegan-style snackable or lunch kit with vegan deli meats, vegan cheese, grape tomatoes, pickles, and crackers

- » Eggless Egg Salad Wrap (Get the recipe in Chapter 13.)

- » Chicken-Free Salad Sandwich (Grab the recipe in Chapter 13.)

- » Burrito bowl or taco salad

- » Build-your-own pizza bites with crackers, vegan pepperoni, tomato sauce, and vegan cheese, plus a side of carrot sticks

- » Falafel wrap with fresh veggies and hummus

- » Old School Chef Salad (Get the recipe in Chapter 13.)

- » Tortilla Pinwheels (Get the recipe in Chapter 13.)

- » Cold pizza

TIP

Plan ahead and do a little research into what other kids are eating at school. For instance, is pizza being served as the hot lunch on Friday? If so, make a vegan pizza for dinner on Thursday. Then send a couple leftover slices for lunch the next day.

Vegan kids may feel pressured or bullied by classmates when it comes to eating differently. Help your child feel more at ease by asking them which vegan options they're most comfortable with for lunch.

Depending on their age, personality, and how long they've been vegan, they may prefer to have bagged lunch options that are inconspicuous, like a vegan deli meat sandwich, potato chips, and an apple. Or they may be happy to stand out in a crowd and choose breaded tofu with dipping sauce, sugar snap peas, and potato salad. Obviously, what seems "normal" will vary from one place to the next.

Preparing for away games or field trips

When your kid is going away without you on a school trip, remember to talk with their chaperones well in advance. Make sure the chaperones understand what a vegan diet is, and find out as much as you can about planned mealtimes and locations. Give them your phone number so they can contact you if any issues, questions, or concerns arise.

If they're stopping at a fast-food place during the trip, make sure your kid and the chaperones are aware of the vegan options. (You can read about fast-food options in Chapter 18.) If your child's group plans to stop at a specific dine-in restaurant while on a trip, check out their menu online to find vegan options.

Some kids love to try new foods on school trips. Others want the comforts of home while they're away. A lot of these feelings depend on age. An older teenager, for example, may feel confident going to dinner in another state with their soccer team. They can look at a restaurant menu and pick out vegan-friendly options, or ask the server to help.

However, because they aren't yet making their own decisions, younger kids may need prepared meals for the trip, depending on where they're going. Stock a cooler with snacks and sandwiches, if necessary. You can also send along shelf-stable treats like cookies, muffins, or homemade banana bread.

Sending treats for school parties

When you're a kid, parties and celebrations at school are a wonderful diversion. They break up the school day with a bit of color and fun. Vegan kids don't have to miss out on the joy of social events. However, they may require a little preplanning.

TIP

At the beginning of the school year (or throughout the year), give your child's teacher a box of shelf-stable vegan treats. That way the teacher can pull out a treat for your child when the class is having a celebration. Choose things like candy bars, lollipops, or vegan gummies. For ideas on vegan treats, check out the Halloween section in Chapter 10. (When in doubt, ask your kid for suggestions of things they'd like to have.)

If the school celebration is for a holiday, you'll obviously have more warning. When there's a school party on the schedule, plan ahead by making or buying a vegan cookie or cupcake. Take the fun up a notch by getting one that's decorated for the holiday, like a jack-o'-lantern cupcake or snowman cookie.

IN THIS CHAPTER

» Finding vegan options in the dining hall

» Stocking your dorm or apartment fridge

» Exploring restaurants in your community

» Bonding with new friends over shared beliefs

» Informing your parents about your new vegan lifestyle

Chapter **24**

Exploring Veganism as a Young Adult

here's nothing quite like getting dropped off at college your freshman year. Suddenly, your bedroom, living room, and kitchen are all in a single room that you share with a stranger. You're meeting new people, exploring a new community, and getting exposed to new ideas. For those reasons, college is a time when many people first consider veganism.

According to a 2019 study from College Pulse, 14 percent of college students follow a vegetarian or vegan diet. Students' biggest motivating factors are environmental concerns and animal rights, followed by health reasons.

If veganism is something you've been thinking about since high school, college is a good time to put your thoughts into motion. This is a period when you're discovering newfound independence and managing mealtimes on your own. When you're developing new patterns and habits, it's a great opportunity to reconsider what you eat for breakfast, lunch, and dinner.

In this chapter, you get acquainted with vegan options in the dining halls and outside your college campus. I offer suggestions for stocking your pantry and outfitting your apartment kitchen with all the necessary gadgets. I encourage you to connect with like-minded friends, and offer ways to help your parents understand your new lifestyle.

Living the Vegan Life on Campus

If you're still in the planning stages of picking a college, see how the ones you're considering fare for vegan options.

TIP

Check out a university's website or app to get more information about the vegan menus they offer. Many schools accommodate special diets, including vegan, vegetarian, gluten-free, and religious diets. Don't see a mention on their website? Send an email to the director of the dining halls for more information.

If you take an in-person campus tour, visit the dining hall, and check out the food options. Even better, order something and taste it for yourself. If the food is delicious, you're more likely to make use of cafeteria dining, and not order another pizza instead.

TIP

You can also take a peek at a school's vegan report card to see how they fare. Visit https://collegereportcard.peta.org/. Schools are given a letter grade, depending on whether they have at least one vegan entree every meal, label vegan dishes, offer nondairy milk, have an all-vegan food station, and more. The report card also indicates how happy students are with the offerings.

Eating vegan in the dining halls

Many students begin their college years by staying in the dorms. Getting on a meal plan is often mandatory or included in your housing costs. While dorm cafeterias used to have a pretty bad reputation, many have seriously upgraded their offerings. According to a 2017 study from peta2, 70 percent of colleges offer at least one vegan daily meal option and 19 percent have all-vegan dining stations.

TIP

Before hitting the dining hall, visit the school's website or app for the day's menu. That way you'll know where to go first.

At breakfast, look for things like oatmeal, hash browns, fruit, and bagels. Slather toasted bagels with peanut butter, hummus, or vegan cream cheese, if it's available. Depending on the school, they may offer more elaborate choices like a tofu scramble or vegan omelet bar. Stop by the soy milk dispenser to add a splash to your coffee or cereal.

For lunch or dinner, possible vegan options include veggie burgers and vegan hot dogs, vegetable curry, bean or lentil tacos, and tofu stir-fry. If your school has a sandwich station, make a panini-style sandwich with lots of veggies plus hummus to seal it together. Before you leave, grab a piece of fruit for later!

If your school has less than thrilling vegan options, get creative by pulling from various food stations to make a complete and satisfying meal. Check out the salad bar, hot bar, and other themed stations to see what the plant-based options are.

TIP

If you have any questions, talk to the cafeteria staff about what's available. If they know students want vegan options, they may start including more of them.

Some colleges allow students to use their dining allowance at other on-campus restaurants. If yours does, check out the menus to see if any are vegan-friendly. Some on-campus dining options include popular fast-food restaurants, which are increasing their vegan options every year. (See Chapter 18 for ideas.)

TIP

It may be worth downgrading your dining plan to just one meal per day if your school's vegan options are on the slim side. Then you can put that money toward meals you make yourself. (*Note:* In general, lunch and dinner menus tend to have more vegan-friendly offerings than breakfast.)

Filling your grocery cart with vegan foods

Of course, college students are always trying to stretch their dollars. Visit the grocery stores in your area to see who has the best prices and selection for produce and other plant-based foods.

If you have a hankering for well-loved college mainstays like frozen pizza, ramen, and mac and cheese, you're in luck. You can find loads of vegan versions. However, now is a great time to build healthy habits that will pay dividends for the rest of your life.

Plus, while vegan specialty foods and convenience items can get expensive, whole plant foods tend to be a lot cheaper. Save money by filling your shopping cart mostly with vegetables, fruits, grains, and beans.

Get some recipe ideas on vegan food blogs, Pinterest, YouTube, and TikTok, or visit your local library for cookbooks. If you're living in a dorm, you'll likely be limited to what you can cook in a microwave.

TIP

If your dorm room is large enough, consider getting a dorm fridge of your own, as opposed to sharing with your roommate. All that produce can take up a lot of space! (If your dorm has rooms with kitchenettes, that's another good option.)

Here are some grocery ideas for the dorm and on the go:

» Baked tofu slabs (Eat them right out of the package, or add them to salads, rice bowls, and ramen.)

» Beans, canned: black, pinto, and garbanzo (chickpeas)

» Bread, crackers, tortillas, and tortilla chips

» Cereal

» Condiments: ketchup, vegan mayonnaise, mustard, and salad dressing

» Energy bars

» Fresh vegetables like carrots, cucumbers, bell peppers, tomatoes, onions, celery, potatoes, and romaine lettuce

» Frozen brown rice (Great for rice bowls!)

» Frozen veggies like green beans, corn, broccoli, and peas

» Fruit like apples, bananas, and oranges

» Hummus

» Nondairy milk

» Nondairy yogurt

» Nuts, seeds, nut butters, and trail mix

» Oatmeal (Make overnight oats or buy microwaveable packets.)

» Olives

» Pickles

» Salsa

» Vegan cheese

» Vegan deli slices for sandwiches (Tofurky is inexpensive and readily available at Target.)

» Vegan jerky

TIP

Don't have a car? Use a grocery delivery service like Instacart to get your groceries brought to you. Or use a ride-sharing app to go pick up groceries yourself. You can also order groceries online through a variety of services, or get shelf-stable foods on websites like Amazon.

ESSENTIAL KITCHEN GADGETS FOR YOUR OFF-CAMPUS APARTMENT

If you're living in the dorms, your kitchen setup will likely be limited to a dorm-sized fridge and microwave. However, once you move into your own apartment, you can take your cooking game to the next level.

Fill your apartment kitchen with basics like a cutting board, knives, pots, and pans. Then if you have the budget for it, consider adding specialty items like an air fryer, which can be a terrific time-saver for quick-and-easy meals. (Multitask by throwing frozen items like vegan chicken strips or vegetable samosas into the air fryer. Then round out your meal with something fresh like a leafy green salad or veggie stir-fry.)

Use this handy list as a guide for filling your kitchen:

- Air fryer
- Blender
- Can opener
- Coffee maker
- Colander
- Cutting board
- Food processor
- Food storage containers
- Grater
- Knives
- Ladle
- Measuring spoons and cups
- Microwave
- Potholders, oven mitts, or oven gloves
- Plates, bowls, cups, and silverware
- Pots and pans
- Sheet pan(s)
- Spatula
- Toaster

TIP

Many residence halls have a community kitchen. While students often don't take advantage of it, you should! You can prep several meals or hearty side dishes and just reheat them in the microwave later. Access to a kitchen gives you a much wider variety of recipe options. Plus, it means you can make vegan cookies to share!

If this is your first time cooking regular meals, don't get overwhelmed! Remember that most people make the same five or six things week after week. Find a handful of recipes you like, and prepare them until you know them by heart. Then, as time goes on, you can tweak those recipes for variety, as well as add some new ones to your repertoire. (Be sure to check out Chapter 13 for college-friendly recipe ideas!)

Grabbing a Bite Off Campus

College towns are often wonderful havens for vegan food options, even in less vegan-friendly states. Restaurateurs know that students are more likely to want plant-based options, so they cater to the younger crowd with vegan menu items.

Oftentimes, college towns are home to a lot of vegan-friendly eateries, like Mediterranean, Indian, Thai, Middle Eastern, and Ethiopian restaurants. If you didn't grow up eating some of these cuisines, it's a perfect time to expand your palate and make some new favorites. (Before I went to college, I'd never had hummus or Indian food. My tastebuds didn't know what they were missing!)

Of course, you can also find ample vegan options at many fast-food places. Get tofu sofritas at Chipotle, build your own vegan chorizo pizza at Blaze, dive into Japanese pan noodles at Noodles & Company, or grab a bean burrito without cheese at Taco Bell. (See Chapter 18 for more vegan fast-food options.)

TIP

Do a search on Google, Yelp, or the HappyCow app to see what your vegan options are off campus. While you're doing a search online, see if anyone has written a vegan city guide to your town. Obviously, larger cities get a lot of focus on the bigger websites, but you may luck out with write-ups for smaller cities on niche sites.

Check out vegan hashtags for your city or university on Instagram. For example, if your school is in Nashville, look up #vegannashville. Then you can see at a glance what looks inviting. (Don't miss the fried chicken–style seitan with turnip greens and vegan mac and cheese at The Southern V!)

If you don't see much for your area, start sharing your own food pictures and videos on Instagram, TikTok, or YouTube. It can be fun to showcase what you're making and eating (or wearing if you're a cruelty-free fashionista).

Finding a Community of Like-Minded Individuals

When all your high school friends have scattered in different directions, making new friends at college can take a little bit of time. One way to step up your friend game is by joining a club with like-minded folks. Check out your university's website to see if they have any vegan clubs or groups. If they don't, consider starting one yourself!

Many groups have regular meetups. They often have potlucks, bake sales, movie nights, field trips to local animal sanctuaries or vegan events, and even a shared Thanksgiving meal. It can be a wonderful way to meet people with common interests, as well as discover vegan-friendly restaurants and events in your town.

Plus, it can really add a lot of fun and enjoyment to your new way of eating when you hang out with people who understand where you're coming from. Bond over delicious recipes and favorite restaurants. Then plan a weekend road trip to the nearest vegan-friendly city.

Telling the Folks Back Home about Your New Lifestyle

At some point you'll go back home for weekend visits, as well as winter and summer breaks. The reactions to your plant-based diet from your parents and siblings will, of course, vary from one person to the next. Maybe your parents are vegan too, so it's a no-brainer that they'll have plant-based options available in the fridge. Or maybe your parents aren't entirely sure what being vegan entails, or they have some negative preconceptions.

If you think your parents will react poorly, cushion the blow. Try this: "Hey, Mom. My boyfriend and I eloped in Vegas. Just kidding. I eat tofu now!" That should put it all in perspective. Ha ha!

But seriously, whatever your situation, consider letting your parents know ahead of time, so they can plan accordingly.

Parents are frequently surprised by the way their daughter or son changes during their time apart. A lot of growing up happens in just that first semester, and students form more fully into the adults they're becoming. Your parents may be used to the way you ate as a 10-year-old. They still know all your childhood favorites and remember you eating sandwiches without crusts. It may take some time for them to get on board with your new way of eating.

Share your "why" with your parents. Letting them know the reasons behind your dietary changes will help them understand you and your motivations better. It may also help with any pushback if they understand why veganism is important to you.

TIP

If your parents are amenable, suggest some things that would be nice to have in the fridge back home. Or plan on going shopping with them when you get back. Of course, if you do your own grocery shopping, you can just keep doing what you usually do.

Your parents may or may not be up for making fully vegan dinners for the family. So plan on getting involved at mealtimes or making your own meals.

Take the opportunity to make your parents dinner one night and share a favorite meal with them. Seeing you putting in the work goes a long way toward making them feel confident in your decisions.

Many college students subsist on a diet of burgers, buffalo wings, fries, and soda, and live to tell about it. And yet your parents may have questions or concerns about you getting enough nutrients on a vegan diet. They may need some assurances that you're eating healthfully.

TIP

If they have specific worries about you meeting nutrient markers, consider tracking your meals for a day or a week using a food tracking app. Show them how you're regularly getting enough protein, carbohydrates, fat, fiber, vitamins, and minerals. (And if you aren't meeting any of those markers, use this as an opportunity to fill in those gaps.)

If your parents have more questions than you feel equipped to answer, share this book with them, or point them in the direction of any documentaries or websites you've found helpful.

Chapter **25**

The Vegan Athlete

hen you're an athlete, the importance of what you eat cannot be overstated. It's up there with sleep in terms of performing your best. When you're not getting the right foods or enough of them, you feel it in your performance.

Did you know that plant-based foods offer 64 times more antioxidants than animal-based foods? When athletes engage in vigorous workouts, they break down muscle fibers. By chowing down on antioxidant-rich plant foods like ginger, garlic, turmeric, berries, greens, nuts, and soy, athletes reap the rewards of their anti-inflammatory effects. That helps fight inflammation and results in faster recovery.

It's no wonder that an increasing amount of professional and amateur athletes are turning to plant-based diets to fuel workouts and shorten recovery time. You can find vegan athletes in every sport — from ultramarathoners to professional soccer players, tennis greats, powerlifters, and even professional football players.

Carl Lewis, the nine-time Olympic gold medal track star, is often quoted as saying, "My best year of track competition was the first year I ate a vegan diet."

People who are committed to running at the top of their game, lifting more, and pushing their body to the ultimate edge of endurance are proving that a vegan diet isn't a hindrance. In fact, it's a help. In this chapter, I share how to maximize your vegan diet for greatness and soar over any nutritional hurdles with ease.

Boosting Strength and Stamina with Macronutrients

Because athletes burn more calories than the average person, they also require more calories to replenish their energy reserves. If you don't eat enough calories, good luck having enough energy to power through your workout.

Every athlete's training should include vibrant and energizing foods that help build muscle and stamina. To create this kind of energy, the body needs *macronutrients* — protein, fats, and carbohydrates — in proper amounts. Healthy snacking and quality foods will improve your energy levels, physical ability, and focus.

In the following sections, I give you the lowdown on each of the macronutrients that athletes need. Head to Part 2 in this book for more on the nutrient requirements for vegans who aren't athletes.

Increasing protein consumption for performance

Our bodies use protein to do all sorts of things like:

>> Making muscle

>> Repairing tissues damaged during training

>> Providing structure and connective framework

>> Creating hormones and enzymes

>> Maintaining proper pH

Athletes require extra protein to keep up with their active lifestyle. These increased protein needs can easily be met by adding more of the same protein-packed plant foods already found in the typical vegan diet.

According to the National Academy of Medicine, 10 to 35 percent of a person's calories should come from protein.

>> If you get moderate to light exercise, your daily Recommended Dietary Allowance (RDA) is 0.8 grams of protein per kilogram of your weight.

>> If you exercise regularly, your needs are 1.1 to 1.5 grams per kilogram.

>> If you are an athlete, you require 1.2 to 2.0 grams per kilogram.

By choosing larger portions of protein-rich foods, vegan athletes can meet their body's needs. Eating a protein-rich snack every few hours can help with recovery from regular strenuous workouts.

TIP

Plant-based foods that are rich in protein include the following:

>> Amaranth, quinoa, brown rice, and wild rice

>> Beans and lentils

>> Breads made from sprouted grains

>> Green peas

>> Nutritional yeast flakes

>> Nuts like peanuts (technically a legume), almonds, pistachios, and cashews (whole or processed into nut butter)

>> Oats and oatmeal

>> Seeds like pumpkin, sunflower, and hemp (whole or processed into seed butter)

>> Seitan

>> Tofu, tempeh, edamame, and soy milk

>> Vegan meats

Fueling your muscles with fat

Vegan athletes need to include high-quality plant sources of fat in their diet. The body uses fat to cushion organs and lubricate joint movement. Eating too little fat while training can lead to muscle fatigue. Plus, the body needs fat to utilize certain vitamins, minerals, and *phytochemicals* (beneficial compounds found in plant foods).

However, vegan athletes don't need any more fat in their diet than nonathletes. Vegan athletes should stick close to the normal RDA range, which means 20 to 35 percent of your daily calories should come from fat. For saturated fat, aim for 10 percent or less.

TIP

Select high-quality whole-food vegan sources of fat to ensure that your body gets what it needs. As a bonus, vegan sources of fat offer two-for-one benefits, such as protein from nuts and seeds, and anti-inflammatory properties from cold-pressed flax oil or extra-virgin olive oil.

Avocados deliver a powerhouse supply of good-quality fat while also providing nutrients and minerals like potassium, vitamins C and K, folic acid, copper, sodium, and fiber. You can also find healthy plant-based sources of fat in chia seeds, flaxseed, pumpkin seeds (and other seeds), walnuts (and other nuts), tahini, tofu, olives, and dark chocolate.

Loading up on carbs for endurance and brain power

A 2020 study was published by the *European Journal of Clinical Nutrition* titled "Is a vegan diet detrimental to endurance and muscle strength?" It followed 56 physically fit young women over two years. Some of the participants were vegan; others were not.

Researchers took a variety of measurements, including participants' body composition, estimated maximal oxygen consumption, submaximal endurance, muscle strength, and dietary factors. In the end, the vegans and non-vegans were comparable in activity levels, body fat, and muscle strength. Endurance was where vegans had a significant advantage, the results suggested.

Perhaps part of the vegan diet's secret sauce is that it's rich in carbohydrates, and carbohydrates fuel physical activity. They are the body's main source of energy. They play an important role in giving your body and brain the power they need to train and compete.

The body stores carbohydrates as *glycogen*, an easy-to-use form of *glucose* (or sugar), in the liver and muscles. During workouts the body taps the reserves of glycogen in the liver to maintain blood sugar levels, which keeps the brain and nervous system in working order.

TIP

If you're moderately active, about half of your calories should come from carbohydrates. If you're an endurance athlete, you require a little more — in the range of 55 to 65 percent.

Complex carbohydrates are digested more slowly, which helps you stay fuller longer and regulates blood sugar spikes. Eating enough complex carbohydrates helps ensure that you have a steady supply of fuel for endurance and repetitive strenuous training exercises.

Choose items from this list on a daily basis to ensure you can go the distance:

» Beans, lentils, and edamame

» Starchy vegetables like sweet potatoes, yams, winter squash, potatoes, corn, and peas

>> Whole fruits like bananas, apples, oranges, and berries

>> Whole grains like brown rice, oats, buckwheat, millet, quinoa (technically a seed), barley, and wheat

>> Whole grain flour products, including multigrain high-fiber breakfast cereals and whole wheat pastas

REMEMBER

Focus on eating complex carbohydrates as opposed to simple ones like white bread, pastries, or soda. While simple carbohydrates may supply a quick fix of energy, it doesn't last as long as the energy you get from complex carbohydrates and can lead to faster burnout.

Identifying Sources of Iron, Calcium, and Other Minerals

Those tiny trace minerals that the average person needs for daily living are even more important to an athlete. Having enough iron and calcium are paramount to doing your best on the road, field, track, and court.

Don't worry, though. Despite popular belief, you don't need meat and dairy products to get iron, calcium, and other minerals in your diet.

Finding vegan iron sources

Athletes of all stripes (both vegan and non-vegan) have a greater risk of being iron-deficient in comparison to the general public. According to a 2021 study in the peer-reviewed journal, *Life*, athletes are more prone to iron deficiency because of increased iron loss (through sweating and gastrointestinal bleeding), elevated iron demand, and decreased absorption.

To maintain consistent performance, healthy iron levels are key. Choose from this handy list of vegan sources of iron:

>> Beans and legumes like black beans, chickpeas, lima beans, lentils, and kidney beans

>> Blackstrap molasses

>> Dark chocolate

>> Dried fruits like prunes, raisins, and apricots

- ≫ Iron-enriched whole grain cereals

- ≫ Low oxalate leafy greens like kale, collards, and arugula

- ≫ Nuts and seeds like almonds, pumpkin seeds, hempseed, cashews, sesame seeds, and Brazil nuts

- ≫ Potatoes and sweet potatoes

- ≫ Quinoa, *teff* (an ancient grain native to Ethiopia), and amaranth

- ≫ Tofu, tempeh, and soybeans

- ≫ Vegetables like peas and broccoli

Don't forget the vitamin C! It helps the body absorb vegan sources of iron, the *nonheme*, or plant-based, variety. Boost the power of iron-rich foods by pairing them with any of these vitamin C superstars:

- ≫ Bell peppers, red or yellow

- ≫ Broccoli

- ≫ Brussels sprouts

- ≫ Grapefruit or grapefruit juice

- ≫ Kale

- ≫ Kiwi

- ≫ Lemons

- ≫ Mango

- ≫ Oranges or orange juice

- ≫ Papaya

- ≫ Pineapple

- ≫ Red cabbage

- ≫ Strawberries

- ≫ Tomatoes and tomato juice

In addition to vitamin C, you can pair iron-rich foods with allium vegetables (like garlic and onions) or foods high in carotenes (like carrots and sweet potatoes) to boost iron absorption.

Athletes who menstruate may need to pay special attention to their iron levels and ensure adequate daily intake.

Be aware that vegans aren't any more likely to develop anemia than non-vegans. However, if you start feeling lethargic or your performance starts to decline, consider having your iron levels checked out by a doctor.

Iron overdose is very serious. Always have a blood test before taking a supplement.

For more information about calculating and meeting your iron requirements, see Chapter 6.

Protecting your bones with calcium

Calcium supplies one of the building blocks for the strong bones athletes need for running, throwing, and jumping. Ensure that you're reaching the RDA by including naturally calcium-rich foods in your meals.

Don't worry about getting extra calcium as an athlete. Research has shown that the calcium needs for athletes aren't wildly different from the needs of nonathletes.

These simple vegan foods should be a part of your calcium strategy:

>> Almonds

>> Beans, peas, and lentils

>> Broccoli

>> Dried figs

>> Fortified nondairy milk and nondairy yogurt

>> Greens like kale, spring greens, and bok choy

>> Okra

>> Oranges

>> Seeds like poppy, pumpkin, flaxseed, and chia seeds

>> Soy products like tofu, edamame, miso, soy milk, and tempeh

>> Tahini

Female athletes especially need to stay on track with their calcium intake. Excessive training, which is defined as more than seven hours a week, can lead to a decline in hormone levels. These lower hormone levels can compromise bone health and lead to premature *osteoporosis,* a weakening of the bone matrix.

You can find more information about calculating and meeting your calcium needs in Chapter 6.

Meeting your other mineral markers

Because of their constant training and exercise, athletes need to consume more minerals and vitamins than their nonathletic counterparts. Keep in mind, however, that the human body absorbs nutrients better from fresh foods than from supplements. So vegans should mine their mineral needs from healthy whole foods on a daily basis. Here are a few more minerals to consider on your way to peak performance.

Making sure you get enough magnesium

Magnesium is a mineral athletes may want to focus on when designing their diet for optimum levels of performance. Magnesium helps the body regulate muscle contractions and is necessary for metabolizing carbohydrates and protein.

Fortunately, most of the foods that contain the highest amounts of magnesium are vegan.

Here are a few options:

>> Avocados

>> Black beans

>> Dark chocolate

>> Pumpkin seeds

>> Sesame seeds

>> Soybeans

>> Spinach

>> Sunflower seeds

>> Swiss chard

Boosting your chromium intake

Chromium is used by the body to regulate insulin, metabolism, and blood sugar levels.

You can find good vegan sources of chromium in the following foods:

>> Apples

>> Broccoli

>> Fortified nutritional yeast flakes

>> Grape juice and red wine

>> Onions

>> Potatoes

>> Romaine

>> Whole grains

Counting on copper

Copper is an athlete's ally because it creates cellular energy and strengthens connective tissue. Copper also acts like an antioxidant, helping to reduce inflammation.

Get copper into your diet by eating following foods:

>> Almonds

>> Cashews

>> Edamame

>> Hazelnuts

>> Lentils

>> Lima beans

>> Mushrooms

>> Dark chocolate

>> Oats

>> Quinoa

Zeroing in on zinc

Zinc levels may be lower in athletes, and it's needed for healthy skin and wound repair. You can easily meet the RDA of 8 to 11 milligrams a day with good food choices. Vegan sources of zinc include:

>> Beans and lentils

>> Fortified cereals

>> Fortified nutritional yeast flakes

>> Miso paste

>> Nuts and seeds

>> Quinoa

>> Tofu

>> Wheat germ

Planning Your Diet before an Athletic Event

Choose nutritious whole foods during athletic training to prepare for the main event. Eating well ensures a better outcome for your future athletic goals.

Because whole plant foods have more fiber than processed foods, be consistent with the foods you're consuming during training and competition. Avoid experimenting with new fiber-rich foods on the day of competition to avoid having to run to the bathroom.

REMEMBER

If you know you have a sensitive stomach (or a nervous stomach before competitions), reduce your fiber intake 24 to 48 hours before the big game or meet. Instead, try choosing other high-calorie foods, such as potatoes and whole grain pasta, to fuel your energy needs.

Many athletes eat a large meal of 800 to 1,000 calories about four or five hours before an event, and have a small high-quality snack of 150 to 200 calories, such as cereal with soy milk, an hour or two before. You want to give your digestive system time to absorb the nutrients and energy from the food while allowing the stomach time to digest.

IN THIS CHAPTER

» **Understanding nutritional needs and pitfalls in middle age and beyond**

» **Regaining your cardiovascular health with a plant-based diet**

» **Alleviating menopause symptoms**

» **Dealing with digestive issues**

» **Creating a lifestyle that promotes wellness**

Chapter **26**
Vegan after 40

The thing to remember about growing older is, the goal isn't just to extend the number of years you'll live. Rather, it's to lengthen the number of healthy years you'll enjoy. Prolonging the years you feel vibrant, full of life, and able to be an active participant in the lives of those you love is the ideal.

According to the World Health Organization, "Evidence suggests that the proportion of life in good health has remained broadly constant, implying that the additional years are in poor health. If people can experience these extra years of life in good health and if they live in a supportive environment, their ability to do the things they value will be little different from that of a younger person."

So as we think about ways to extend our lives, we can focus on what will help us continue living in a way that's pleasurable, energizing, and happy.

REMEMBER

Taking on the vegan ethos later in life has the potential to make you feel years younger. A well-planned vegan diet supports good health, and potentially lowers your likelihood of having heart disease, cancer, diabetes, and strokes.

According to the Academy of Nutrition and Dietetics, vegans have lower rates of heart disease, type 2 diabetes, and cancer overall. Vegans tend to have lower blood cholesterol levels, body mass index, and blood pressure.

If you're looking for more reasons to adopt a vegan diet later in life, here are a couple good ones:

>> A 2021 study published in the *American Journal of Lifestyle Medicine* indicated that older vegans had 58 percent fewer prescribed medications than non-vegans.

  The authors of the study said, "Our results show that eating healthy, especially a vegan diet, may be protective in leading to a reduced number of pills taken, either by preventing the development of risk factors and/or cardiovascular disease or by helping on the controlling of such conditions."

>> A 2022 study from the Rush Institute for Healthy Aging found that a plant-based diet slowed the rate of cognitive decline by almost 30 percent in older Black adults. This news is especially welcome because Black Americans are about twice as likely to develop dementia in comparison to non-Hispanic whites.

In this chapter, I discuss the nutritional needs of people over 40, as well as what you have to gain by transitioning to a vegan diet in middle age or beyond. After all, older age is often when many diet-related diseases come to a head. Think heart disease, cancer, diabetes, and hypertension. Making healthy choices now has the power to pay off in meaningful ways.

Examining Nutritional Needs after 40

A well-planned vegan diet that's based on whole foods, including whole grains, beans, nuts, seeds, vegetables, and fruit, provides a strong foundation for adults in middle age and beyond.

The nutritional needs for vegans over the age of 40 are similar to those for younger adults, but there are a few important differences. To ensure that your body has enough of every necessary nutrient, it's important to be educated about the sources and quantities of those nutrients.

Strengthening your bones

According to the Bone Health & Osteoporosis Foundation (BHOF), approximately 10 million people in the United States already have *osteoporosis* (decreased bone mass). Another 44 million Americans have low bone density, which puts them at an increased risk for developing the disease.

BHOF notes that half of all women and a quarter of all men will break a bone due to osteoporosis. For women, this is a more sizable risk than breast cancer, heart attack, and stroke combined. While men over age 50 are more likely to break a bone due to osteoporosis than get prostate cancer. Osteoporosis can have grave consequences. In the year following a hip fracture, 24 percent of patients age 50 and older die.

Many people in this demographic have lived their entire lives being marketed to by the dairy industry. They've been told time and again that dairy is the best source of calcium, and cow's milk is the ideal way to build strong bones and avoid osteoporosis. However, while Americans consume more dairy than most people living in other nations, we also have one of the highest osteoporosis rates.

>> A study published in 2023 in the scientific journal *Osteoporosis International* suggests that older adults who follow a healthy plant-based diet may be at a lower risk for osteoporosis.

   The study, which followed 9,613 participants, found that a healthy plant-based diet was associated with a significantly lower risk for osteoporosis than eating animal foods and unhealthy plant foods. Foods that were especially beneficial included whole grains, fresh produce, nuts, and legumes.

>> A 2022 study published in the *Journal of Cachexia, Sarcopenia, and Muscle* found that a higher intake of plant protein over animal protein resulted in a lower risk of frailty among older women. (The characteristics of frailty include fatigue, weak muscle strength, weight loss, and a slowed walking speed.)

   The study analyzed data from 85,000 women age 60 and older. It also suggested that replacing animal protein with plant protein could help people avoid developing frailty altogether.

Here are the calcium needs in milligrams (mg) for adults, according to the National Institutes of Health (NIH):

>> Women 19 to 50 years old — 1,000 mg

>> Women 51 to 70 — 1,200 mg

>> Men 19 to 70 — 1,000 mg

>> All adults over 71 years of age — 1,200 mg

To reach your calcium goals, eat a plant-based diet full of green leafy vegetables like collards, kale, turnip greens, and bok choy. For more calcium-rich plant foods, see Chapter 6.

Dark leafy greens like spinach, kale, and collard greens also contain the antioxidants *lutein* and *zeaxanthin*. They can help prevent *macular degeneration*, which is a common cause of visual impairment in older adults. Other sources of these antioxidants include broccoli, avocados, and peas.

TIP

Help your body use calcium properly by getting enough vitamin D from the sun. The top layers of your skin make vitamin D (which is actually a hormone) when exposed to sunlight. You can get this benefit with daily sun exposure of 10 to 30 minutes. Be aware that people with more *melanin* (dark pigment) in their skin require a longer amount of time in the sun to produce ample amounts of vitamin D.

If it's winter and you live in a Northern climate, or if you want to limit your sun exposure, consider taking a vegan vitamin D supplement.

Getting your vitamin B12

Despite occasional food recalls and outbreaks of foodborne illnesses, we live in an age of unparalleled food safety when it comes to cleanliness. Proper sanitation is necessary when one factory or processing plant is manufacturing thousands of pounds of food from hundreds of sources every day.

The flip side of this widespread disinfection and sanitation is that our fruits and vegetables are virtually free of bacteria. This seems like a win, and in many ways, it's for the best. However, some bacteria are good for humans.

Vitamin B12 is produced by bacteria. Because livestock animals have these bacteria in their diet (which is often supplemented with B12), people who eat meat consume B12 from the animals they eat. Vitamin B12 is necessary in sufficient quantities for every human. The Recommended Dietary Amount (RDA) for adults is 2.4 micrograms per day.

WARNING

Older adults are at a higher risk of vitamin B12 deficiency, because they make less stomach acid, which separates B12 from proteins. Plus, many are on prescription drugs that interfere with B12 absorption.

As people age, sufficient amounts of vitamin B12 can help protect the nerve fibers in the brain, as well as safeguard the body against anemia and dementia. Muscle coordination, balance, memory, and depression are all helped with adequate B12 intake.

TIP

Vegans can ensure they're getting enough vitamin B12 by taking a supplement. Fortified nondairy milk and nutritional yeast are also vegan sources of B12. Don't count on food alone for your vitamin B12 needs, however.

Consuming enough protein

As people get older, they progressively lose (and struggle to build) muscle. Around the age of 50, *sarcopenia* (muscle loss) can range from .5 to 2 percent of total muscle mass each year. While it used to be the conventional wisdom that increased protein intake in older adults would lead to bone loss and kidney issues, experts now believe that consuming more protein can help with bone health and the maintenance of muscle mass.

Research shows that regular resistance exercise in tandem with adequate protein intake can help older people to overcome the body's struggle with muscle growth. Experts say that consuming up to 35 percent of daily calories as protein is safe for older people, unless there's a medical reason against it. In order to gain and maintain muscle mass and function, current studies suggest that most people over age 65 should consume about 1 to 1.2 grams of protein a day per kilogram of body weight.

You can boost your protein intake by consuming lentils, beans, seitan, vegan meats, nuts, seeds, and soy products like tofu. And don't forget about breakfast! While many folks eat lightly in the morning, getting by on toast and coffee, you can easily increase your protein intake for the day by adding something protein-dense at breakfast. Consider slathering nut or seed butter on toast, or adding a side of Eggy Tofu. (Get the recipe in Chapter 11.)

For more information on meeting your protein needs, turn to Chapter 5.

Eating the right fats

Fat makes food taste good. It's also necessary for optimum health. The right kinds of dietary fat aid in healthy skin, lubricated joints, and proper brain function. Wholesome plant-based fats help your body utilize several vitamins and many phytonutrients, which contributes to better overall health.

The fatty acids *linoleic*, or omega-6, and *alpha-linolenic*, or omega-3, are good for you. These fatty acids are converted in the body to form the long-chain fatty acids your body needs to perform various physiological functions. Most people consume plenty of omega-6, so the key is focusing on adding omega-3s to your diet.

According to Harvard Health Publishing (HHP), most Americans eat 10 times more omega-6s than omega-3s. On their website, HHP notes, "A low intake of omega-3 fats is not good for cardiovascular health, so bringing the two into better balance is a good idea. But don't do this by cutting back on healthy omega-6 fats. Instead, add some extra omega-3s."

TIP

Plant-based sources of omega-3 fatty acids are ground flaxseed, flax oil, hempseed, chia seeds, seaweed, edamame, and walnuts. You can also consider taking an algae-derived omega-3 supplement. (Talk to your healthcare provider about having your omega-3 levels tested to see if your blood levels are adequate.) In addition to omega-3-rich foods, boost your diet with nutritious vegetable fats from nuts, seeds, avocados, and olives to help maintain heart and cardiovascular health.

REMEMBER

Because omega-3 oils are highly sensitive to heat, it's important to use them in warm or room-temperature applications only. Don't sauté or fry anything in flax or walnut oil. Instead, drizzle these oils on foods after they're cooked. An easy way to add flax oil to your diet is by dipping warm bread in it, along with balsamic glaze.

Keeping your iron in check

Both women and men need to be aware of their iron intake in their later years. According to the NIH, these are the iron needs for adults:

>> Men 19 to 50 years old — 8 mg

>> Women 19 to 50 — 18 mg

>> All adults 51 and older — 8 mg

The Food and Nutrition Board suggests that vegetarian and vegan iron needs may be higher than the RDA because non-heme iron isn't absorbed as well as heme iron due to phytates present in plant foods. For this reason, they suggest that vegetarians and vegans could require as much as 1.8 times more iron than those who eat meat. However, it's important to note that they did not factor in the effect of vitamin C, carotenoids, and allium vegetables (onions and garlic) on iron's absorbability. They also didn't weigh in the fact that lower iron stores found in plant-based eaters may actually enhance iron absorption.

Here are some tips for getting iron into your diet:

>> Include a variety of iron-rich plant foods in your weekly menus. Lentils, beans, quinoa, pumpkin seeds, cashews, blackstrap molasses, and tofu are all good sources.

>> Eat foods that contain vitamin C (like tomatoes, oranges, peppers, potatoes, and broccoli) along with iron-rich foods to increase iron absorption.

>> Increase your daily iron intake by using cast-iron cookware.

For more tips on improving absorption and choosing iron-rich foods, check out Chapter 6.

TIP

For a clearer view of your specific iron situation, request a blood workup from your doctor. Of course, we all know that too little iron can lead to anemia. But according to the Institute on Aging, too much iron can damage the pancreas, heart, liver, and even joints, which can lead to arthritis. Talk to your doctor before taking iron supplements.

Improving Cardiovascular Health

Many of the reasons that older people develop cardiovascular or heart disease are avoidable. High blood cholesterol, including high low-density lipoprotein (commonly known as LDL, or "bad" cholesterol), smoking and secondhand smoke exposure, lack of exercise, and unhealthy diet are some of the main culprits, which become more dangerous as humans age.

There's no denying that a diet rich in saturated fats and meats like beef and pork, processed meats, fried foods, and sugary drinks leads to high cholesterol and ultimately heart disease. But some meat eaters believe that choosing poultry and avoiding red meat protects their health. What they may not realize is that the negative impact of red meat on cholesterol may be similar to that of poultry.

A study led by scientists at Children's Hospital Oakland Research Institute in 2019 showed that consuming high levels of red meat or white poultry meat had the same result of higher blood cholesterol levels, as opposed to eating an equal amount of plant proteins. The study, which was published in the *American Journal of Clinical Nutrition*, indicated that plant proteins like beans are healthiest for blood cholesterol.

While the dangers of saturated fat are oft-discussed, the potential negatives of meat eating go beyond that. A 2016 study published in the peer-reviewed journal, *Toxins*, looked at how the body metabolizes animal products. The study showed that *trimethylamine N-oxide* (TMAO), a compound produced by gut bacteria when you eat foods like meat and eggs, may be linked to heart disease and other inflammatory conditions.

A 2022 research article published in *Frontiers* showed that heme iron (the type of iron found in animal flesh) is pro-inflammatory and can lead to inflammatory conditions like heart disease.

On the flip side, many studies have shown that plant foods can be helpful in preventing and treating high cholesterol and hypertension:

>> A study published in the *Journal of the American Heart Association* in 2021 found that eating cholesterol-lowering plant foods (like nuts, soy, oats, barley, okra, eggplant, oranges, apples, berries, and heart-healthy oils) reduced the risk of heart disease in people who were postmenopausal.

This 15-year study found that participants who ate the most of these types of foods were 11 percent less likely to develop any type of cardiovascular disease, 14 percent less likely to develop coronary heart disease, and 17 percent less likely to develop heart failure.

» According to a 2020 study in the *American Journal of Lifestyle Medicine,* "Lifestyle choices, particularly diet, play a significant role in the development and maintenance of hypertension. Research dating back almost a century has demonstrated benefits of plant-based foods on the development and management of hypertension."

The study authors concluded, "The evidence suggests that plant-based diets are a safe and effective way to manage high blood pressure without the side effects of antihypertensive medications. . . . We support the use of a predominantly (or completely) plant-based diet as first-line therapy for the management of hypertensive patients."

» Dean Ornish, MD, received worldwide acclaim in 1990 when he published his classic best-selling book *Dr. Dean Ornish's Program for Reversing Heart Disease.* In it, Ornish details how patients who were prescribed low-fat, vegetarian, or vegan diets, along with exercise and stress-reduction exercises, were able to stop the progression of and reverse their heart disease. Without prescribing cholesterol-lowering drugs (or any other drugs), Ornish was able to show that a plant-based diet can cure heart disease, which is one of the most fatal diseases among older people.

» Caldwell Esselstyn, MD, a retired cardiologist, recommends a stricter, exclusively vegan diet in which total calories from fat are kept under 10 percent of total daily caloric intake. Because strokes are essentially brain "heart attacks," this diet has been used to help people at high risk avoid strokes, the top cause of disability for older adults.

TIP

High consumption of vitamin C is also linked to better heart and cardiovascular health. Eating fresh seasonal fruits and vegetables naturally increases your intake of vitamin C. The best sources of this antioxidant are red bell peppers, parsley, broccoli, cauliflower, strawberries, lemon juice, mustard greens, Brussels sprouts, papaya, kale, grapefruit, kiwifruit, cantaloupe, oranges, cabbage, and tomatoes. These foods also add a healthy dose of fiber to your diet.

The American Heart Association and most medical experts support the idea that a fiber-rich diet decreases the risk of cardiovascular disease. Fiber is only found in plant foods, which means a vegan diet comprising mostly whole-plant foods is naturally chock-full of it.

Managing Menopause

When many people think of menopause, hot flashes are the first thing that comes to mind. What some don't realize, though, is that hot flashes often start during the transitional years before menopause called *perimenopause.* (A person is officially in menopause once menstrual periods have ceased for a year.)

Hot flashes are officially known as *vasomotor symptoms* (VMS), which can also include night sweats and flushes. VMS can be anything from warm flushing to intense heat throughout the head, neck, chest, and upper back. Those fiery feelings are followed by profuse sweating for as long as 5 minutes.

According to a 2019 study published in the *Journal of Mid-Life Health*, 80 percent of those who experience perimenopause or menopause have hot flashes. Hot flashes often begin in a person's 40s and can continue into the 50s and beyond.

Promising research has shown that adding soybeans to a plant-based diet can help reduce hot flashes, thanks to the isoflavones in soy. According to a small 12-week study published in 2021 by the North American Menopause Society in the journal *Menopause*, "In randomized trials, soy products have been shown to reduce the frequency of hot flashes."

Prior to beginning the study, all participants suffered from at least two hot flashes per day. For the study, half the participants were required to eat a low-fat, plant-based vegan diet along with ½ cup of cooked soybeans, which provided 55 to 60 grams of isoflavones per day.

Results of the study suggested that eating a plant-based vegan diet along with soybeans may lead to fewer hot flashes. After embarking on this diet, participants saw a 79 percent reduction in total hot flashes and an 84 percent decrease in moderate-to-severe hot flashes (from 4.9 to 0.8 per day).

Additionally, many in the soybean group reaped the benefits of more energy, better mood, improved sexual health, and weight loss.

The authors of the study noted, "These studies suggest that a plant-based diet and daily soybean consumption may be more helpful than either a diet change or soy supplementation alone."

Lead researcher Neal Barnard, MD, noted that "this is a game changer for women aged 45 and over, most of whom we now know can get prompt relief from the most severe and troubling menopause symptoms without drugs."

One study participant said, "Before you jump to any kind of medication, I would try this route, because it's easy. Anybody can do it."

Here are some simple ways to add soybeans to your diet:

>> Enjoy steamed *edamame* (green soybeans) in the pod. Lightly sprinkle the steamed pods with salt. Then use your teeth to scrape the pods, allowing the beans inside to pop into your mouth. It's a delicious, protein-packed snack.

>> Snack on roasted soybeans.

>> Add ½ cup of boiled soybeans to a grain bowl.

>> Make a delicious vegan BLTA with tempeh bacon, lettuce, tomato, and avocado on toasted bread.

Other studies — like the one published in 2018 in the journal *Maturitas* — have indicated that vegans have fewer hot flashes. The study authors concluded, "Eating a plant-based diet may be helpful for women in menopausal transition who prefer a natural means to manage their symptoms."

Easing Digestion

Older adults are often plagued with chronic constipation. It can be a symptom of various diseases, including irritable bowel syndrome, diabetes, colon cancer, multiple sclerosis, colonic disorders, and Parkinson's disease. Or it may simply be due to lower calorie intake and therefore lower fiber intake.

Plus, certain prescribed medications and supplements like iron and calcium supplements, sleeping pills, antidepressants, painkillers, and antacids can lead to constipation. Combine this with a low-fiber diet and low water intake, and you may find yourself visiting the bathroom less frequently than you'd prefer.

WARNING

Chronic constipation is not only uncomfortable and unhealthy, but can also be dangerous. It can cause pressure inside the veins, which often leads to painful hernias or varicose veins.

The best natural ways to avoid and treat chronic constipation involve your diet, movement, and hydration. Walking, bike riding, swimming, dancing, and weight lifting are all useful for clearing out constipation's effects. And aiming for six to eight 8-ounce glasses of water a day will ensure that you're properly hydrated.

REMEMBER

Getting fiber into your diet helps ease constipation and reduces cholesterol levels. Animal foods have no fiber. However, a vegan diet that includes plenty of whole plant–based foods is naturally packed with it. The RDA for men age 51 and older is 28 grams of fiber a day. Women age 51 and older should get 22 grams a day. To see how easy it is to meet the RDA, take a look at this sample menu:

>> **Breakfast:** Oatmeal with 1 cup raspberries (12 grams)

>> **Lunch:** Lentil soup with 1 cup brown rice (19 grams)

>> **Dinner:** Black bean taco salad in a baked tortilla bowl (11 grams)

That's 42 grams of fiber with this simple menu.

As you can see, you can exceed your daily fiber RDA with little effort. And that's not even including snacks! Consider having three or more servings each of high-fiber whole grains and steamed vegetables every day.

TIP

Some folks develop dental problems as they age. Painful teeth and gum disease can make eating some high-fiber foods like raw vegetables more difficult. You can help break down the fiber by blending plant foods into a smoothie or cooking them. Plus, blending or cooking these high-fiber foods can make them easier to digest. Table 26-1 lists some soft high-fiber plant foods that may be less challenging to eat for folks with dental issues.

TABLE 26-1

Soft High-Fiber Vegan Foods

Food	Serving Size	Amount of Fiber (g)
Split peas, cooked	1 cup	16.3
Lentils, cooked	1 cup	15.6
Black beans, cooked	1 cup	15
Lima beans, cooked	1 cup	13.2
Artichoke, cooked	1 medium	6.84
Peas, cooked	1 cup	8.8
Raspberries	1 cup	8
Pearled barley, cooked	1 cup	5.97
Regular or quick oatmeal, cooked	1 cup	4.32
Broccoli, boiled	1 cup	5.14
Turnip greens, boiled	1 cup	5.04
Brown rice, cooked	1 cup	3.12

Source: U.S. Department of Agriculture's FoodData Central

Planning for Success with Easy Food Choices

Making major dietary changes may seem overwhelming to people who have built up a lifetime of habits. However, eating well as you age can be easy if you keep the following guidance in mind:

>> **Choose a variety of nutrient-dense foods every day.** These foods are high in nutrition but low in calories. Think whole grains, beans, fruits, and vegetables.

>> **Choose whole grain products.** Whole grain products, like whole wheat bread or whole grain pasta, are made with all the edible parts of the seed. The bran, germ, and endosperm are present to contribute fiber, complex carbohydrates, protein, vitamins, and healthy fats.

>> **Include a variety of proteins in your diet every day.** Various kinds of beans, nuts, seeds, whole grains, and soy foods combine over the course of the day to give you all the amino acids you need for complete protein.

>> **Eat smaller, more frequent meals.** People often find that their appetite decreases with age. Eating smaller meals more often throughout the day can help ensure proper nutrient consumption without discomfort.

>> **If chewing or swallowing has become difficult or uncomfortable, make nutrient-dense smoothies with fresh ingredients.** Nondairy milk, nuts, avocado, berries, bananas, and leafy greens can all be blended into tasty, easy-to-digest meals.

7

The Part of Tens

Chapter **27**

Ten Easy Vegan Meals Anyone Can Make

P eople sometimes assume that making a plant-based meal is labor-intensive or difficult. In actuality, it usually requires only a few substitutions or omissions to turn a meat-heavy dish into a vegan one.

You likely already know how to make simple standards like pasta, soup, sandwiches, and salads. In this chapter I share easy swaps you can make to turn familiar meals you already prepare into vegan dishes. (For more tips on "veganizing" recipes, see Chapter 9.)

Cooking Pasta with Ease

For many people, pasta is the ultimate weeknight dinner. After a long day of work, pulling jarred sauce and dried noodles out of the pantry are wonderful shortcuts on the way to a satisfying meal.

WARNING

Check the ingredients on the pasta and sauce before purchasing. Most dried pasta is vegan, but fresh pasta often includes eggs. And while many jarred pasta sauces are vegan, some include dairy-based cheese, meat, or milk.

Cook pasta according to the package directions. While the pasta is boiling, sauté minced garlic and chopped onions with oil in a skillet. Then add one of the following:

>> Brown lentils, cooked

>> Seitan

>> Vegan ground beef

>> Vegan sausage

>> Vegetables like mushrooms or zucchini

Once the ingredients in the skillet are fully cooked, pour in jarred pasta sauce. Then drain the noodles, and add them to the sauce.

Top with a sprinkling of vegan parmesan cheese. Use store-bought or make your own using the Cashew Parmesan recipe in Chapter 14.

TIP

Noodles are also tasty served plain without sauce. Just toss hot noodles with non-dairy butter, granulated garlic, salt, and pepper. Add a side of sautéed mushrooms or steamed broccoli. For another delicious pasta idea, try the recipe for Basil Pesto Pasta with Roasted Chickpeas in Chapter 12.

Enjoying a Variety of Tacos

Who doesn't love tacos? Not only are they delicious, but they're also super easy to personalize! If you wanted, you could make a different type of tacos every day of the week. (Best. Week. Ever.)

For the taco filling, sauté onions and garlic in oil. Then add any of the following:

>> Black beans

>> Brown lentils, cooked

>> Chickpeas

>> Pinto beans

>> Seitan

>> Soy chorizo

>> Vegan ground beef

>> Veggies like mushrooms, peppers, sweet potatoes, and/or cauliflower

Season the filling with cumin, paprika, ancho chili powder, granulated onion, and salt.

Would you prefer to use a taco seasoning packet? Great, do that instead! Most taco seasoning packets call for a pound of meat, so replace the meat with an equal amount of your vegan filling. Add water as needed to distribute the seasonings throughout.

Once it's cooked, add the filling to your preferred tortillas — flour, corn, or hard shells. (As always, just read that ingredient label before buying.)

Then stuff your tacos with any of these toppings:

>> Avocado or guacamole

>> Cabbage

>> Cilantro

>> Green leaf lettuce

>> Nondairy cheese

>> Tomatoes or salsa

>> Vegan sour cream

These basic ingredients also work for burritos, taco salads, or tostadas.

For specific ingredients and instructions, check out the recipe for Black Bean Tacos in Chapter 12.

Preparing Crowd-Pleasing Pizza

Pizza is the great equalizer. It makes almost anyone happy. Luckily, it's a cinch to make a vegan pizza.

For the crust, use any of the following:

>> Shelf-stable premade crust

>> Frozen crust

- » Store-bought refrigerated pizza dough
- » Flatbread
- » Halved baguettes
- » Halved bagels
- » Homemade dough

Cover your crust in jarred pizza sauce or marinara. Then sprinkle on your favorite toppings. Choose from any of the following ingredients:

- » Artichoke hearts
- » Basil
- » Bell peppers
- » Jalapeños
- » Mushrooms
- » Olives
- » Onions
- » Pineapple
- » Sauerkraut
- » Spinach
- » Tomatoes

TIP

There are also a ton of plant-based meat options like vegan pepperoni, sausage, and bacon. For delicious crispy edges, I recommend browning them first with a little bit of oil before adding them to the pizza.

Finish the pizza with a generous sprinkling of shredded vegan mozzarella, or go cheeseless. You may be surprised at how much you enjoy a cheeseless pizza — it allows you to really taste the other toppings.

Bake the pizza in the oven until the nondairy cheese has melted and the bottom of the crust is golden brown.

For an easy start on making pizza at home, flip to the recipe for Pizza Bagels in Chapter 13.

Cleaning out the Fridge with Soup

Soup is the ultimate clean-out-the-refrigerator meal. First, sauté chopped onions, celery, carrots, and garlic in oil. Then add vegetable broth and more chopped veggies of your choice. Finish with your favorite herbs and spices to bring the soup to life.

TIP

If you want soup that's a little more substantive, add rice, noodles, and/or something protein-dense like beans, lentils, seitan, or tofu.

Here are some easy vegan soup ideas:

>> Curried lentil soup

>> Vegan chicken noodle soup (See Chapter 12 for my go to recipe.)

>> Creamy vegan tomato soup

>> Vegan ramen noodles (See Chapter 13 for a recipe that's easy to adjust to your preferences.)

>> Pot sticker soup with store-bought vegetable dumplings

>> Butternut squash soup

>> Miso soup

>> Potato soup

Throwing Simple Sandwiches Together

Sandwiches are a classic effortless lunch — just add mustard, sliced onions, lettuce, and pickles to bread along with vegan deli slices. There are all kinds of vegan deli slices on the market. I'm particularly fond of the options from Tofurky and Field Roast.

Of course, a vegan BLTA is always a winner. Toast bread, slather it with vegan mayo, and add browned seitan bacon, lettuce, sliced tomato, and avocado. Herbivorous Butcher and Upton's Naturals are my favorite makers of vegan bacon.

TIP

If you were a fan of tuna salad sandwiches, use chickpeas instead! Break down drained canned chickpeas in a food processor until they're chunky. Then move them to a bowl and stir in dollops of vegan mayonnaise, a dab of mustard, diced pickles, and chopped celery for vegan tuna salad. Sprinkle in celery seed, dried dill, and a pinch of salt to bump up the flavor.

A toasted bagel sandwich with store-bought or homemade hummus is another option. Finish it with sliced bell peppers and onions, and lettuce. (For more details, check out Chapter 13.) Or kick it old school with a peanut butter and jelly sandwich.

Spicing Things Up with Chili

Chili is easy to veganize. Start by sautéing chopped onions and minced garlic like you usually do. Then instead of ground beef, add any of the following:

» Beans (pinto, black, cannellini, kidney, or great northern)

» Brown lentils, cooked

» Seitan

» Soy chorizo

» Vegan ground beef

Add canned diced fire roasted tomatoes and enough water to make it soupy. Sprinkle in spices like cumin, ancho chili powder, and paprika. For smoky flavor, use smoked paprika. For spicy heat, add a few dashes of hot sauce.

Once it's just the way you like it, ladle the chili into bowls. Then garnish with crushed corn chips, sliced avocado, and/or nondairy sour cream.

If you want more specific directions for vegan chili, see my Ultimate Homemade Chili recipe in Chapter 12.

TIP

Chili is a terrific make-ahead meal, because it tastes even better on day two or three! Repurpose chili by using it to top a baked potato, fries, or tater tots. Slather it on a veggie dog, spoon it into a burrito, or add it to nachos.

Making Colorful Stir-Fries

Stir-fries are simple to make and the perfect way to use whatever vegetables are in the crisper.

Add oil to a skillet and sauté your choice of the following:

>> Bell pepper

>> Bok choy

>> Broccoli

>> Cabbage

>> Carrots

>> Cauliflower

>> Celery

>> Garlic

>> Ginger

>> Kale

>> Mushrooms

>> Onions

>> Sugar snap peas

Once the veggies have softened, add splashes of tamari (or your preferred soy sauce) and rice vinegar. Tamari brings saltiness and *umami* (a rich, savory flavor). Rice vinegar brings tang. If you like, add a small drizzle of toasted sesame oil for nutty flavor, or a few dashes of sriracha for heat.

For a bump of protein, add browned tofu. Top with a handful of cashews and cilantro. Serve over brown rice, cauliflower rice, or rice noodles.

For a complete stir-fry recipe, check out Pineapple Fried Rice in Chapter 12.

Creating Mouthwatering Wraps

Almost anything can go into a wrap! It's a convenient and portable lunch that's ideal when you're on the go.

Start with a warmed tortilla, *lavash* (a thin flatbread), or pita. Then add whatever looks good in the fridge or use one of these ideas:

» **Mediterranean-inspired wrap** with falafel, hummus, romaine lettuce, sliced cucumbers, olives, and cilantro. To make it even more filling, add cooked brown rice. Finish with a drizzle of tahini dressing. (Get the Easy Tahini Dressing recipe in Chapter 14.)

» **California-inspired wrap** with baked tofu, leafy greens, chopped tomatoes, diced onions, and sliced avocado. If you like, add a slathering of vegan mayo inside the tortilla.

» **Vegan chick'n wrap** with store-bought vegan chicken strips, romaine, bell pepper slices, vegan feta cheese, and a drizzle of tahini dressing.

» **Classic deli wrap** with vegan deli meats, vegan cheddar cheese, mixed salad greens, pickles, and chopped red onion. If you like, add a thin layer of vegan mayo, vegan ranch dressing, or mustard.

Fixing Meal-Worthy Salads

Get in your greens with a nourishing salad! Add any of the following ingredients to a bowl:

» Artichoke hearts from a jar

» Bell peppers

» Broccoli

» Carrots

» Cauliflower

» Celery

» Cucumber

» Kale

» Microgreens

» Olives

- >> Romaine
- >> Spinach
- >> Tomatoes

Finish with a drizzle of store-bought or homemade dressing. (Find three delicious dressings to choose from in Chapter 14.)

TIP

Want to make your salad more substantive? Serve it with garlic bread, baked tofu, vegan chick'n strips, or roasted chickpeas. (Grab the Roasted Chickpeas recipe in Chapter 14.)

Feasting on Vibrant Rice Bowls

Rice bowls are a convenient and handy way to repurpose leftovers. They're made with something protein-dense, roasted or raw veggies, and rice. To take the flavor up a notch, finish your bowl with a tasty sauce. (Peanut sauce, tahini sauce, and vegan cashew queso are some of my favorites.)

Rice isn't difficult to make from scratch, or you can buy a box of frozen rice that's already been cooked. You just have to warm it.

Although it's called a rice bowl, feel free to vary the base. Use any of the following:

- >> Barley
- >> Couscous
- >> Grits
- >> Mashed potatoes
- >> Noodles
- >> Polenta
- >> Quinoa
- >> Sheet Pan Potato Hash (Get the recipe in Chapter 11.)
- >> Sweet potatoes, cubed and baked

Then top with your favorite vegan proteins and vegetables. Here are some ideas to get you started:

>> **Burrito bowl** with vegan taco meat, fajita-style vegetables, shredded cabbage, sliced avocado, salsa, and cilantro on a bed of Spanish rice.

>> **Hummus bowl** with store-bought or homemade hummus, chopped cucumbers, cherry tomatoes, olives, spinach, and roasted cauliflower over quinoa.

>> **Black bean bowl** with seasoned black beans, fried plantains, and guacamole on brown rice.

>> **Sushi bowl** with fried or baked tofu, shredded carrots, sliced green onions, chopped cucumber, sliced avocado, microgreens, pickled ginger, and *nori* (dried seaweed) on top of seasoned sushi rice.

Chapter 28

Ten Ways to Create a Satisfying Vegan Lifestyle

In this chapter, I explain how you can turn your veganism into a powerful, productive, and satisfying lifestyle by growing your community, deepening your understanding, and living your values. When you become a curious life-long learner, you realize there's always a new facet of veganism to explore.

Attending a Veg Fest

In the summer months, veg fests are very popular. They include speakers, vendors, and live music. Veg fests can be a helpful resource for discovering more about the vegan lifestyle, as well as a place to meet like-minded people in your community.

Sometimes it can feel isolating to be the odd one out — especially if you live somewhere that veganism is uncommon. So when a bunch of vegans get together, it puts other faces to the movement and reminds you that you're not alone.

While you're there, try delicious plant-based treats from local food trucks and discover restaurants you may not have known about otherwise. It's very handy to sample a variety of dishes in one convenient location. (Bring along a veg-curious friend. Mouthwatering food can be extremely convincing!)

Most veg fests feature interesting and lively cooking demonstrations. See in person how easily a plant-based dish can come together, and get some ideas to try at home. If you have questions about how to prepare new-to-you ingredients, it's a great place to glean information from experts.

To find a veg fest in your area, do a quick Google search, or visit www.happycow.net/events. No veg fests nearby? Consider venturing to a larger city for their fest. It's a good excuse to travel to a new town and explore their vegan scene.

In addition to veg fests, keep an eye out for vegan pop ups, markets, and street fairs. They're not as big of a production as veg fests, but still provide an opportunity to try vegan food in your area and meet other local vegans. Look for notices of these events on the social media pages of your local vegan groups, or on community boards at natural grocery stores and coffee shops.

Making New Vegan Friends — at a Meetup or Online

If you don't already have a bunch of vegan friends, make some! It can be validating to make new friends who share similar sensibilities.

Visit www.meetup.com to find meetups in your area. These get-togethers sometimes happen at local vegan restaurants. Or they're held at nearby parks, where everyone brings a potluck-style dish.

If you're bringing a dish, consider writing down the recipe too. That way if someone has a question about the ingredients, or if they love it and want to make it at home, you'll have it handy.

Some meetups are less food-specific. When I first went vegan, I participated in several vegan hiking meetups. We explored trails all around Southern California. Not only did I make some new pals, but I also discovered a lot of picturesque hikes I wouldn't have known about otherwise.

If you don't see a meetup in your area, consider starting your own.

If in-person gatherings aren't your speed, you can find plenty of places online to meet other vegans. Check out vegan or plant-based groups on Facebook and Reddit. There are city-specific groups on Facebook, where you can hear about new restaurant openings or events happening in your town.

Visiting or Supporting a Sanctuary

Farm animal sanctuaries are safe havens for rescued pigs, chickens, goats, sheep, ducks, and cows. With wide-open spaces, plenty of grass, shady trees, and mud puddles for pig bathing, they're a paradise for animals whose beginnings were bleak.

Visiting a sanctuary is an opportunity to meet animals who were saved from factory farms, abuse, and neglect. While it can be sad to hear their stories and what they've endured, it also warms your heart to know they will live out the remainder of their lives in peace. In their new home, they will be cherished for who they are, not what they can provide. (I'm particularly fond of Farm Sanctuary in Watkins Glen, New York, and Acton, California, where I volunteered as a tour guide, and Iowa Farm Sanctuary in Oxford, Iowa.)

Many animal sanctuaries have open houses during warm-weather months, in addition to special events. These special events often include speakers and local food vendors.

REMEMBER

Be aware that sanctuaries are not the same as petting zoos. Petting zoos are places where animals are used as entertainment in the name of profit. Sanctuaries offer a forever home and lifelong care for their rescued residents.

During open houses, animals who live in sanctuaries have the freedom to decide if they would like to interact with visitors or be touched. When visitors are present, the animal residents can venture deeper into the sanctuary and away from guests if they choose.

TIP

When you go, wear comfortable clothes and shoes you don't mind getting dirty.

If you're interested in volunteering, sanctuaries are often looking for help from people who are willing to muck barns, assist with tours, clean, fix things, do fundraising, and help with animal care. Visit the website of a sanctuary in your area to see what type of assistance they may need.

To find a sanctuary near you, google "farm animal sanctuary" and your state. Or use the search tool from the Global Federation of Animal Sanctuaries (GFAS). On their website, put your location into the relevant field, and write "farm animals" for the type of animals you'd like to visit. Find that tool here: `https://sanctuary federation.org/find-a-sanctuary`.

Don't have a sanctuary nearby? Consider making a donation to one instead. Donations go toward veterinary services, food, and future rescue missions. You can also sponsor specific sanctuary residents on a monthly or yearly basis, which goes toward that animal's food, bedding, and care.

TIP

Most farm animal sanctuaries are committed to protecting animals and keeping them safe for the duration of the animals' lives. However, it's always wise to do your research on any sanctuary you're considering supporting to ensure they're providing the animals with optimum care. One good way to do this is by checking that the sanctuary is accredited by the GFAS. Look for the GFAS seal on the sanctuary's website or visit `sanctuaryfederation.org`.

Watching a Vegan Documentary

Watching a documentary can give you a fuller picture of the whys behind the vegan lifestyle. Whatever your reason for choosing this path, there's a documentary out there that will help illuminate it more fully.

WARNING

Some of these documentaries contain graphic footage that's difficult to watch. I encourage you to look at a trailer before committing.

>> *What the Health* (2017): Examine the link between diet and diseases like cancer, diabetes, stroke, and heart disease.

>> *Forks Over Knives* (2011): See how adopting a whole-food, plant-based diet can help you avoid or reverse chronic diseases.

>> *The Game Changers* (2019): Look at the benefits of plant-based diets for athletes.

>> *Cowspiracy: The Sustainability Secret* (2014): Understand the environmental impacts of animal agriculture and the role it plays in deforestation and water pollution.

>> *Seaspiracy* (2021): Explore the environmental impact of the fishing industry and how the actions of humans affect marine life.

>> *Blackfish* (2013): Examine the ethics of keeping *cetaceans* (marine mammals like whales, dolphins, and porpoises) in captivity.

>> *Dominion* (2018): Take a painful look at the violence within the modern food system.

>> *Slay* (2022): Peek at the underbelly of the fashion industry, and explore the ethical issues behind leather, fur, and wool.

>> *Earthlings* (2005): Take a hard look at the ways animals are used in factory farming and for clothing, entertainment, and scientific research in this graphic film.

Asking Your Library to Carry Vegan Books

Did you know that libraries take requests? It's true! If you've heard of a new cookbook you'd like to try or a helpful book about living a vegan lifestyle, ask your local library to order a copy.

TIP

Simply visit your library's website for a request form. Most of the time when I've asked my library to carry a book, they've said yes. Plus, I was first on the list to read it!

It's a win-win situation.

>> You're able to give the book a test-drive before buying it for your own bookcase. You can see if it will be a book you'll turn to again and again, or if it's just nice to flip through once.

>> After you're done reading it, the book is available as a resource for other folks who are vegan or vegan-curious.

Requesting More Vegan Options at Local Restaurants and Grocery Stores

Is there a restaurant in your town that you'd like to try, but they're short on vegan options? Send them a message online or ask in person if they'll carry some!

Vegans often ignore restaurants that don't have any obvious plant-based options. But that means restaurateurs may assume there isn't any demand for those dishes.

If you go to a non-vegan restaurant with friends and the chef whips up an amazing meal for you, do the following:

1. **Ask them to put that vegan dish on the menu for others to enjoy.**
2. **Post about it on your social media pages and tag the restaurant.**
3. **Let others in your life know about the fabulous dinner you enjoyed.**

Having an increased interest in vegan dishes makes a good argument for the restaurant to grow that portion of their menu.

When you visit a restaurant that has great vegan options, suggest that they label the vegan or veganizable items on their menu. It makes ordering much easier, and it alerts other plant-based eaters to the vegan options. (Now that many menus are online, it's not that difficult to add a small symbol next to plant-based dishes.)

Several years ago, I became friendly with the manager of a favorite Indian restaurant. The restaurant had several vegan options available, and I asked if he'd be willing to add asterisks on the menu to denote vegan items.

He took me up on it! When the new menu came out, I was surprised that there were so many more options than I realized were available.

It worked out well for me and for the restaurant. I had a larger variety of choices, and that meant I visited more often. I'm sure other area vegans did the same, which is good for business.

TIP

Similarly, if you hear about a new nondairy cheese or plant-based meat, but it's not available in your area, reach out to the purchasing manager at your local grocery store. You can talk to them directly at the store, use their website contact page, or message them on their social media channels.

Oftentimes stores are able to order new items if they know they have customers who want to buy them. It will depend on the availability of shelf space and their ability to source the item. It's worth a shot!

Taking a Vegan Cooking Class

When you're trying a new way of eating, it can be helpful to have someone knowledgeable as a guide. The next time you get a flyer from your local community college in the mail, see if they're offering any vegan cooking classes. If they are, sign up!

TIP

Other places to look for classes include culinary schools, kitchen stores, or pop-up events by local chefs and health counselors. Even restaurants sometimes offer them.

When I went vegan back in 2007, a favorite upscale restaurant held vegan cooking classes once a month. It was a pretty fancy place, and I adored their food. But it wasn't somewhere I could afford to dine all the time.

So it felt like quite the coup to be able to go into their kitchen and watch the head chef and owner work his magic. After he finished his demonstration, all the students got to eat what he'd made. Then we were given printouts of the recipes to take home.

If you can't find any local classes, lots of people offer online courses. Some of them are live, and you can cook along with the instructor. Others are filmed, and you can go at your own pace.

You can also find many vegan cooking videos on YouTube and TikTok. They can be terrific free resources for finding vegan recipes and mastering culinary techniques.

Trying a New Vegan Recipe or Food Every Week

It can be easy to stick to the same foods meal after meal. But to really keep your vegan diet interesting, I encourage you to try a new recipe or food every week.

When you go to the grocery store, see if there's a fruit, vegetable, grain, or bean you've never tried before. Put that watercress, *rambutan* (spiny red fruit with white flesh similar to a lychee), *purslane* (succulent plant known for its omega-3s), or package of calypso beans into your cart. Then when you get home, do a search online to see how to use it. I've found some of my favorite foods that way!

If you see something unfamiliar at the farmers market, ask the person working the stand about it. They can tell you what it is and how it's grown, and suggest different ways to prepare it. Farmers are often happy to tell you about the food they grow. Plus, you know it's going to be at its best, because it was picked fresh.

Every week, check out a new vegan cookbook at the library, or pick a book from your collection. Flip through it until you've found a recipe that calls your name. Then get all the ingredients together and have a feast.

TIP

If the cookbook is one you own, I encourage you to make notes in the margins. Mark down what you loved, what you disliked, how your family felt about it, or what you'd do differently next time. It's extremely helpful for future dinners.

To take the fun up another level, get some friends involved! Have a regular cooking party at which you all prepare different dishes from a specific cookbook or blog. You can pick a different cookbook or website every month. It's a terrific way to explore new dishes without doing all the work yourself.

Seeking Vegan Options When You Travel

One of the best parts about being vegan is trying new-to-you plant-based restaurants in other cities. I've based whole vacations around the vegan restaurants I wanted to try.

TIP

Before you go on your next adventure, google vegan restaurants in that area, read blog posts about the city's options, look at relevant hashtags on Instagram, and check out online resources like HappyCow or Yelp for vegan or vegan-friendly listings.

See if any restaurants make plant-based versions of local specialties. It can really up the fun quotient.

Consider feasting on:

>> Soy chorizo tacos in Austin, Texas

>> Seitan cheesesteaks in Philadelphia, Pennsylvania

>> Vegan meat pies in Sydney, Australia

>> Impossible Juicy Lucy burgers in Minneapolis, Minnesota

>> Vegan poutine (fries covered with gravy and nondairy cheese curds) in Vancouver, Canada

>> Chickpea tenderloins in Des Moines, Iowa

>> Banana blossom fish and chips in London, England

>> Plant-based deep-dish pizza in Chicago, Illinois

Taking Care of Yourself

Going vegan can be challenging sometimes. It can feel awkward going against the grain. You can't be vegan for 10 or 20 years until you've been vegan for one or two days. That first year you have to figure out what to eat. Plus, you have to navigate any sticky social situations that arise when you choose a different path from the norm.

Here's the good news: It gets easier. With time you find your voice. You get more comfortable speaking up for yourself and asking for what you need. Your vegan lifestyle becomes natural and seamless.

Create an attitude of enthusiasm and curiosity. Be open to trying new things. Make new traditions. That's what makes veganism sustainable and fun. Be gentle on yourself, and remember that simply doing your best as a vegan can make a big impact on your life, the animals' lives, and on the planet.

Index

About the Author

Cadry Nelson is the founder, writer, and recipe creator at Cadry's Kitchen (https://cadryskitchen.com), where she shares vegan comfort food classics that come together in about 30 minutes. After going vegan in 2007, Cadry knew she wanted to help others who are interested in transitioning to a plant-based diet. She'd grown up eating the standard American diet and understood that changing your habits can feel intimidating. So Cadry created easy, user-friendly recipes that would satisfy any craving, while using plant-based ingredients. Since starting her website in 2009, she's developed hundreds of recipes, taken countless photos, and helped readers all over the globe to prepare vegan dishes in their own kitchens.

Cadry's work has been featured on NBC News, Mashable, Yahoo, Buzzfeed, Parade, HuffPost, VegNews, and Vegan Food and Living. She has spoken at veg fests and blogging conferences, as well as doing public cooking demonstrations. Cadry has collaborated with a variety of brands to develop recipes using their products, as well as showcase their vegan goods. She has also worked with tourism boards and hotels to promote vegan options in their cities and restaurants. She delights in showing that tasty vegan fare can be found anywhere — even in the most unlikely of places.

Cadry earned a degree in theater from the University of Iowa and worked as a professional actor in Los Angeles, California, for more than a decade. She loves bringing that performance background to her cooking videos and social media posts. Her other passions include traveling, having amazing vegan meals in restaurants, visiting unique grocery stores, making independent films, and spending quality time with her husband and their cats.

Dedication

This book is dedicated to my husband, David, whose love and support makes every day sweeter. Thank you for reading every chapter, tasting every recipe, bringing me coffee, and knowing when a Trader Joe's run was in order.

Author's Acknowledgments

I am forever grateful to the many readers of Cadry's Kitchen, who have brought my recipes to life in their homes, and let me be a small part of their everyday moments.

Heartfelt thanks to my parents, Jim and Sharon Nelson, for always believing in me. Thank you to Michelle Wetmore for your enthusiasm, support, advice, and lifelong friendship. Thanks to my family and friends, who have been my cheerleaders every step of the way, including David Busch, Jim and Sonja Nelson, Brian and Teri Nelson, Susie Patterson, Darcy and Tim Wheeldon, Ashley Peterson-DeLuca, Adam DeLuca, and Jenn Sebestyen. Special shout-out to my cats, Avon and Cally, who offered copious amounts of cuddles while I wrote.

Many thanks to everyone at Wiley Publishing who made this book possible, including Tracy Boggier (senior acquisitions editor), Donna Wright (project editor), Kelly Brillhart (copy editor), Nichole Dandrea-Russert, MS, RDN (technical editor and author of *The Vegan Athlete's Nutrition Handbook*), and Rachel Nix, RD (recipe tester and nutritional analysis).

Publisher's Acknowledgments

Acquisitions Editor: Tracy Boggier

Project Editor: Donna Wright

Copy Editor: Kelly Brillhart

Technical Editor:
  Nichole Dandrea-Russert, MS, RDN

Recipe Tester: Rachel Nix, RD

Nutritional Analysis: Rachel Nix, RD

Proofreader: Debbye Butler

Production Editor: Tamilmani Varadharaj

Cover Image: © Cadry Nelson/cadryskitchen.com